Handbook of Sports Medicine and Science
Sports Nutrition

EDITED BY
Ronald J. Maughan

University Medical School
Aberdeen, UK

Louise M. Burke

Department of Sports Nutrition
Australian Institute of Sport
Bruce ACT 2617
Australia

Blackwell
Science

© 2002 by Blackwell Science Ltd
a Blackwell Publishing company
Blackwell Science, Inc., 350 Main Street, Malden, Massachusetts 02148-5018, USA
Blackwell Science Ltd, Osney Mead, Oxford OX2 0EL, UK
Blackwell Science Asia Pty Ltd, 550 Swanston Street, Carlton, Victoria 3053, Australia
Blackwell Wissenschafts Verlag, Kurfürstendamm 57, 10707 Berlin, Germany

First published 2002

Library of Congress Cataloging-in-Publication Data
Sports nutrition / edited by Ronald J. Maughan, Louise Burke.
        p. cm. — (Handbook of sports medicine and science)
Includes index.
   ISBN 0-632-05814-5
   1. Athletes—Nutrition.   I. Maughan, Ron J., 1951–   II. Burke, Louise.
III. Series.
   TX361.A8 S663 2002
   613.2′024′796—dc21

                                        2002007304

ISBN 0-632-05814-5

A catalogue record for this title is available from the British Library

Set in 8.75/12pt Stone by Graphicraft Limited, Hong Kong
Printed and bound in Great Britain by
MPG Books Ltd, Bodmin, Cornwall

Commissioning Editor: Andrew Robinson
Production Editor: Julie Elliott
Production Controller: Kate Charman

For further information on Blackwell Science, visit our website:
www.blackwell-science.com

Contents

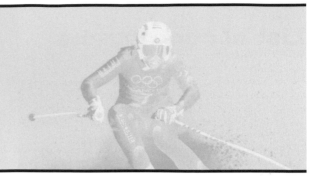

List of contributors

The following are contributors to the Expert comment and Case Studies found throughout the book.

Louise M. Burke PhD, *Department of Sports Nutrition, Australian Institute of Sport, Bruce, ACT 2617, Austalia*

Priscilla M. Clarkson PhD, *Department of Exercise Science, University of Massachusetts, Amherst, Massachusetts 01003, USA*

Gregory R. Cox, MSc (Nut), *Department of Sports Nutrition, Australian Institute of Sport, PO Box 176, Belconnen, ACT 2616 Australia*

Mikael Fogelholm ScD, *The UKK Institute for Health Promotion Research, PO Box 30, FIN-33501 Tampere, Finland*

Mike Gleeson PhD, *School of Sport and Exercise Sciences, University of Birmingham, Birmingham B15 2TT, UK*

John A. Hawley PhD, *Department of Human Biology and Movement Science, Faculty of Biomedical and Health Science, RMIT University, PO Box 71, Bundoora, Victoria 3083, Australia*

Linda Houtkooper PhD, *Department of Nutritional Sciences, Special Assistant—Cooperative Extension Director, University of Arizona, Tucson, Arizona 86721*

Peter W.R. Lemon PhD, *3M Centre, University of Western Ontario, London, Ontario N6A 3K7, Canada*

Henry C. Lukaski PhD, *USDA ARS Grand Forks Human Nutrition Center, PO Box 9034, Grand Forks, ND 58202-9034, USA*

Melinda M. Manore PhD, *Nutrition and Food Management Department, Oregon State University, 108 Milam Hall, Corvallis, Oregon, 97331-5109, USA*

Ronald J. Maughan PhD, *Department of Biomedical Sciences, University Medical School, Foresterhill, Aberdeen AB25 2ZD, UK*

Robert Murray PhD, *Exercise Physiology Laboratory, Quaker Oats Company, 617 West Main Street, Barrington, Illinois 60010, USA*

Helen O'Connor PhD, *Department of Exercise and Sport Science, University of Sydney, Lidcombe, NSW 2141, Australia*

Bente Klarlund Pedersen MD, *Department of Infectious Diseases M, Rigshospitalet, Tagensvej 20, Copenhagen N, Denmark*

Karin Piehl-Aulin MD, *Section for Sports Medicine, LIVI, Box 1992, S-791-19 Falun, Sweden*

Susan M. Shirreffs PhD, *Department of Biomedical Sciences, University Medical School, Foresterhill, Aberdeen AB25 2ZD, UK*

Patricia Thompson MSc(Nut), *3 York Castle Avenue, Kingston 6, Jamaica W.I.*

Anton J.M. Wagenmakers PhD, *Department of Human Biology, Maastricht University, PO Box 616, 6200 MD Maastricht, The Netherlands*

Clyde Williams PhD, *Department of PE and Sports Science, Loughborough University, Loughborough, Leicestershire LE11 3TU, UK*

Forewords by the IOC

The scientific area of Sports Nutrition has experienced a phenomenal expansion of knowledge during recent years. Even 30 years ago, the athletes and the associated health care professionals who worked with the athletes lacked very basic information on the possible relationships among food intake, nutritional status, conditioning programmes, and competitive performance.

During the past three decades of laboratory and field research, a broad foundation of science has been laid in scientific literature. An area of science called Sports Nutrition has now been established and it has served as the basis for careful planning of the dietary patterns and food ingestion for athletes during periods of training and as directly related to competition.

I would like to thank the IOC Medical Commission and its Sub-commission on Publications in the Sport Sciences for this valuable contribution to the literature in sports medicine and the sport sciences.

Dr Jacques Rogge
IOC President

To supplement and complement the earlier volumes in the Handbook series that have dealt with either individual or team sports, this Handbook on Sports Nutrition deals with the general considerations of the energy demands of physical exercise and sport and the associated demands for appropriate nutrient intake.

All of the different aspects of nutrition related to sports have been taken into consideration, including age, sex, competition, and training. Each area is clearly explained and easily accessible for anyone dealing with athletes.

This Handbook will certainly be of great interest to nutritionists, sports medicine physicians, athletic trainers, and knowledgeable athletes alike. It will serve as the most practical reference available concerning nutrition applied to exercise and sport for many years to come.

I would like to congratulate Ronald Maughan and Louise Burke, for having taken such a unique approach with the formulation of this volume in the series, "Handbooks of Sports Medicine and Science".

Prince Alexandre de Merode
IOC Medical Commission Chairman

Preface

In the modern world of sport, performing at your best requires commitment at many levels. It is no longer enough to rely on natural talent, hard training, superior equipment or a will to win—in fact, among the top competitors in any sport these factors are often equalized. Under these conditions, sound nutritional practices can make the difference between winning and losing, or between doing a personal best and just finishing the event. Whether the stakes are fame and millions of dollars, or the satisfaction of achieving a sporting goal, there are clear rewards for eating well. This book is designed to provide an up-to-date summary of the science and practice of sports nutrition.

The importance of sports nutrition is reflected at all levels of sport. The International Olympic Committee has conducted extensive reviews of the available scientific knowledge on nutrition for athletes at its 1991 Consensus Conference, and in its 51-chapter textbook *Nutrition in Sport*, Volume VII of the Encyclopaedia of Sports Medicine. Other international governing bodies of sport have produced position stands on this topic. At the practical level, most professional teams and serious athletes use the services of a sports dietitian or sports nutritionist to advise them on how to eat to perform at an optimal level. Many other sports medicine professionals, sports scientists, coaches, and trainers are involved in this education process or in the implementation of sound sports nutrition strategies. Athletes and their families must have a good understanding of the practice of sports nutrition as well as the principles that support it.

This book is divided into three sections. The first deals with issues relating to training, where the goal is to prepare the athlete to reach the starting line in the best possible form. Everyday eating patterns must supply the athlete with the fuel and nutrients needed to optimize their performance during training sessions and to recover quickly afterwards. Increasing evidence now suggests that nutrient intake in the period after training can influence the responses taking place in the muscles and other tissues, allowing more effective adaptation to the training session. The athlete must also eat to stay in good health and in good shape. Special strategies of food and fluid intake before, during, and after a workout may help to reduce fatigue and enhance performance. These will often be important in the competition setting, but must be practised and fine-tuned during training so that successful strategies can be identified.

Section 2 on competition eating deals with the nutritional challenges that cause fatigue or limit performance during sport and exercise. Many of these relate to the fuel and hydration status of the athlete. Strategies that reduce the disturbance to fluid and fuel status caused by exercise can reduce or delay the onset of fatigue, thus enhancing performance, and these strategies can be undertaken before, during, or after exercise.

Finally, Section 3 deals with the practical side of sports nutrition, looking at the ways that scientific knowledge can be translated into eating strategies and menu choices. This includes some of the hot topics in sport—such as changing physique or using supplements to optimize performance. The individual needs of specific populations or for special environments are also be covered.

This book provides a accompaniment to the other IOC textbooks and handbooks on sports medicine, and we hope that it will provide a useful addition to resources used by athletes and coaches to prepare themselves to perform at the highest level.

Ron Maughan and Louise Burke, 2002

PART 1
NUTRITION NEEDS FOR TRAINING

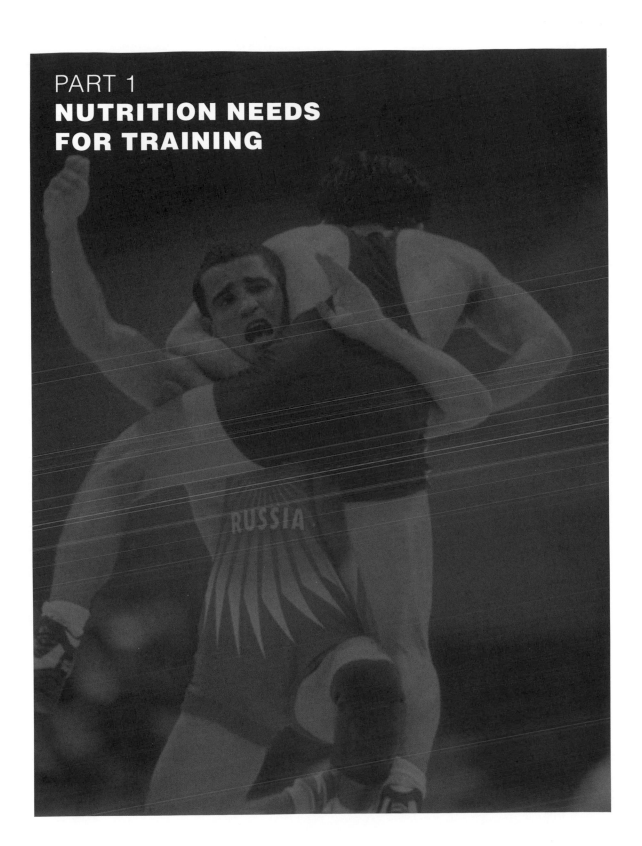

Chapter 1
Exercise and energy demands

Introduction

Many of the world's nutrition problems relate to a failure to match energy intake to energy requirements. In many countries, chronic undernutrition is a leading cause of mortality, especially in infants and children. In most industrialized countries, however, excess dietary energy is the major problem, with obesity and its sequelae being a major cause of morbidity and mortality. Most adults succeed in maintaining their body weight within fairly narrow limits, indicating that the match between energy intake and energy expenditure is quite close. These control mechanisms are not perfect, however, and it has been estimated that the body fat content of the average male doubles between the ages of 20 and 50 years, and that of women typically increases by 50%.

Training and competing in sport involve a range of activities of varying energy demands. Athletes face a spectrum of challenges in meeting their individual energy demands—ranging from difficulties in achieving sufficiently high energy intakes to meet very high energy needs, to the need to restrict energy intake to achieve and maintain a low weight (body mass) and body fat level. This chapter will overview the factors that determine the energy needs of athletes and recreationally active people, and will comment on the energy intakes reported by athletes in a variety of sports.

Determination of energy needs

The food that we eat provides the fuels and building materials for life, supplying both the structural elements of the body and the means of sustaining the body's energy-requiring processes. Energy is needed for all biosynthetic pathways and for maintaining the internal environment of the body. After the body's basal needs have been met, additional energy is needed to fuel muscular activity, whether this is carried out for occupational, recreational, or sporting purposes.

The individual components considered to make up total energy requirements of an individual are summarized in Fig. 1.1, and include:
• Basal or resting metabolic rate (the energy required to maintain body systems). This should be measured in a thermoneutral environment.
• Thermic effect of food (the increase in energy expenditure following the intake of food that is associated with the digestion, absorption, and metabolism of food and nutrients).
• The thermic effect of activity, including the energy cost of spontaneous movements as well as planned muscular activities such as exercise.
• The cost of growth.

The primary factors that determine the energy requirement of athletes in training are body size and the training load. The importance of body mass is often underestimated, but the active tissue mass influences the basal metabolic cost of living as well as the energy cost of exercise. Total energy

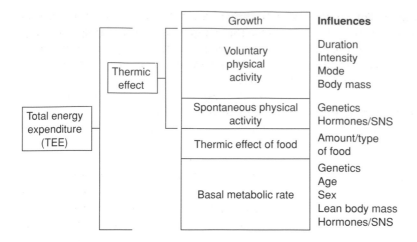

Fig. 1.1 The components of energy expenditure.

expenditure can be expected to vary between athletes who range in size from the female gymnast or marathon runner at less than 40 kg to the heavyweight weightlifter at 120 kg and the sumo wrestler in excess of 200 kg. The total training load will increase energy requirements above those of normal daily living and in some individuals may be as high as 50% of total daily energy expenditure. The three important components of any training program—intensity, duration, and frequency—will all influence total energy expenditure.

Energy costs of exercise

In the simple locomotor sports that involve walking, running, or cycling, the energy cost of activity is readily determined and can be shown to be a function of speed. Whether body mass is supported by the muscles as in running, or the athlete is seated as in rowing or cycling, or where it must be moved against gravity as in cycling uphill, then this too is an important factor in determining the energy cost. For walking, running, and cycling at low speeds, there is a linear relationship between velocity and energy cost, if the energy cost is expressed relative to body weight. At higher speeds, the relationship becomes curvilinear and the energy cost increases disproportionately. In cycling a large part of this is due to the need to overcome air resistance, which increases as the square of velocity. The effect of air resistance becomes significant at the speeds involved in cycling, and explains the attention paid by elite

cyclists to methods of reducing it. Bicycle design, cycling position, and clothing all affect the aerodynamics and hence the energy cost.

At the speeds involved in walking and running through still air, air resistance is not a significant factor, but the relationship is nonetheless curvilinear. The reason for this seems to be a reduced mechanical efficiency as velocity increases. At very low speeds, the energy cost of walking is less than that of jogging, because of the smaller vertical displacements of the centre of mass; as velocity increases, however, the cost of walking increases faster than that of running, and at speeds in excess of about 6–7 km·h^{-1}, running is less energetically demanding than jogging. As a rough approximation, the energy cost of walking or jogging is about 1 kilocalorie per kilogram of body mass per kilometer of distance covered. There are, however, large differences between individuals in the energy cost of even simple activities such as running, and these differences in the efficiency of movement may translate into substantial differences in energy demand.

It is often recommended that 20–30 min of moderate intensity exercise three times per week is sufficient exercise to confer some protection against cardiovascular disease: if this exercise is in the form of jogging, the energy expenditure will be about 4 MJ (1000 kcal) per week for the average 70-kg individual. The energy cost of running a marathon is equivalent to only about 12 MJ (3000 kcal). However, even a small daily contribution from exercise to total daily energy expenditure will have a cumulative effect on a long-term basis. For obese individuals, whose exercise capacity is low, the role of physical activity in raising energy expenditure is necessarily limited, but this effect is offset to some degree by the increased energy cost of weight-bearing activity.

There have been several attempts to identify the factors that might account for the differences in running economy which exist among runners. When elite and non-elite runners are compared, there is generally a slightly shorter stride length and correspondingly higher stride frequency in the elite runners when running at the same speed. Some studies have shown that the extent of vertical oscillation of the centre of gravity does not vary between runners of different levels of ability, but other studies have found differences. It seems unlikely that any single variable can account for differences in running economy, but rather that many different factors each make a small contribution to the observed differences that exist between individuals.

In most sports, the pattern of energy is variable, and is therefore even more difficult to quantify: in field games such as soccer, play consists of sprints, periods of jogging at submaximal speed, walking, and resting. The overall energy cost depends on many factors, including the total distance covered. It must also always be remembered that the fitter the individual, the higher the overall rate of energy expenditure. Estimates made from match analysis suggest that most top-class soccer players cover a total of about 8–12 km during a game. The distance may vary between the two halves, and also depends on the level of play and the position of the individual in the team. The daily energy expenditure during typical training of English professional players has been estimated to be approximately 6.1 MJ (1500 kcal). The only technique that might be expected to give a reliable estimate of energy expenditure in a situation such as this is the doubly labeled water method, but this has not yet been applied to the wide range of team sports.

Tables of the energy cost of a wide range of different sports activities are available, but these have to be considered as crude approximations at best. The body mass and fitness level of the performer will have major influences on the energy cost of training, and even when these factors are similar, there

may be differences in the mechanical efficiency, as well as in the energy expenditure during other daily activities. Because of this, applying mean values may not be helpful when providing advice for an individual.

Evidence suggests that the metabolic rate may remain elevated for at least 12 and possibly up to 24 h after very prolonged intense exercise. The athlete training at near to the maximum sustainable level, who already has a very high energy demand, will find this increased further by the elevation of postexercise metabolic rate, and this will increase the difficulties that many of these athletes have in meeting their energy demand. It seems unlikely, however, that metabolic rate remains elevated for long periods after more moderate exercise. The recreational exerciser, for whom the primary stimulus to exercise is often control of body weight or reduction of body fat content, will not therefore benefit to any measurable extent from this effect.

Energy costs of growth or changing body mass

The requirement for growth is an important factor in the energy needs of young athletes who have not reached full maturity. In these cases, energy intake must exceed expenditure if growth is to take place. Some athletes, mostly in events where a high power output is an important part of successful performance, will also benefit from an increased body mass, and an increase in muscle mass rather than in fat mass is usually desired. In some events, such as the heaviest weight categories in weightlifting and in the combat sports, and in the throwing events in track and field, a high absolute mass may be important, and a high body fat content is often seen in the most successful competitors. If the body mass is to increase, there must be an excess of energy intake over expenditure. The reverse situation, a need to reduce body mass and especially to reduce the body fat content, is also frequently encountered. There are particular problems in reducing the energy take to a level that will result in a loss of body mass without compromising the ability to sustain the training load. In seasonal sports such as soccer or rugby, a substantial gain in body fat is not unusual in the off season, and the preseason training for these athletes often involves a combination of sudden increases in the training load in combination with a restriction of energy intake.

Dietary strategies which assist athletes to manipulate their body mass and body composition are discussed in more detail in Chapters 11 and 13.

Determining individual requirements for energy

As with the general population, there is likely to be a large variability in energy requirements between athletes, even when body mass and training loads are similar. The reasons for this remain obscure. However, as shown in Fig. 1.1, the determinants of the components of energy expenditure are complex and multifactorial.

Each athlete must identify their own energy requirement and their own ideal body mass and body fat content. An adequate energy intake is achieved when body weight and body fat content are maintained at a level that is appropriate for the sport and healthy for the athlete. In a small number of sports situations, there appears to be a conflict between the demands of performance at elite level and a body composition level that is optimal for health. Examples of such sports are primarily those where performance is based on subjective aesthetic assessment, including women's gymnastics and ice dancing, but also include long-distance running. Additional needs for growth and development must be added to the cost of daily activity where young athletes are involved, and an increase in body mass, and in body fat content, is a normal part of the maturation process.

The energy requirements of an individual can be determined by a number of methods, each of which has some advantages and disadvantages. The most common laboratory-based method is indirect calorimetry, in which energy expenditure is calculated from the rates of oxygen consumption and production of carbon dioxide. Of course this requires equipment such as a Douglas bag, ventilation hood, or metabolic chamber in which expired air samples can be accurately collected and analysed. Disadvantages of this technique include expense and the

need for specialized equipment and trained personnel. Most importantly, the technique usually interferes with the performance of normal daily living and exercise activities, meaning that it measures an artificial situation of daily energy expenditure. On the other hand, it can be used to measure the individual components of energy expenditure —for example resting metabolic rate, the thermic response to a meal, and the energy cost of various exercise activities.

More recently, the doubly labeled water (DLW) technique has been developed and validated to estimate energy expenditure. In this technique, the subject ingests a sample of water that has been labeled with stable (non-radioactive) isotopes of both hydrogen and oxygen ($^2H_2^{18}O$). Energy expenditure can be calculated via the periodic monitoring of the concentration of these isotopes in body fluids to compare the different rates of disappearance of these isotopes (see Expert Comment 1). This technique has no effect on the daily activities of the subject and measures the total energy expenditure, so it is particularly useful for monitoring energy expenditure in the field over a period of days or weeks. Nevertheless, the cost and availability of the DLW sample and analyses restrict the use of this method to the realms of research. Indirect calorimetry and DLW estimates are rarely used in the management of individual athletes, except perhaps where they are used to investigate the case of an athlete who has an apparent disturbance of energy balance.

The most accessible and practical way to assess the energy requirements of the athlete is to use prediction equations based on assessments of resting metabolic rate and the energy cost of daily activities. Several equations are available to predict resting metabolic rate from factors such as age, height, weight, or lean body mass. Once resting metabolic rate is estimated, it must then be multiplied by various activity factors to determine the total daily energy expenditure. At the simplest level, an overall activity factor is applied to the whole day to represent the athlete's typical exercise level. At the most complex level, an athlete might complete an intricate activity diary, with the energy cost of each activity undertaken over the day being separately added to calculate the final prediction of total energy expenditure. In most cases the factorial information used to predict the cost of activities is generically derived. However in some research projects or cases of individual therapy, measurements may be made of the exact energy cost of an individual's exercise activities—for example, the cost of their typical training and competition activities. While this protocol can provide a general estimation of an athlete's energy requirements, the possibility for substantial error should be taken into account.

Even if athletes do not have access to facilities for estimation of their energy requirements, they should be able to identify when they are in energy balance by monitoring long-term changes in body mass as part of their training diary. The athlete should be weighed at the same time of day, and under the same conditions—many athletes use their early morning weight, taken just after waking and going to the toilet but before breakfast, as their true body weight. Small fluctuations from day to day should be ignored, and hydration status should also be taken into account as a cause of variations in body weight. However, trends in weight change over a week or more, whether upwards or downwards, indicate an imbalance between energy intake and expenditure. Assessment of body composition, and more specifically of body fat content, requires more sophisticated procedures (see Chapter 11).

Energy intake of athletes

If body weight and performance levels are to be maintained during periods of intense training, the high rate of energy expenditure must be matched by an equally high energy intake. Available data for most athletes suggest that they are in energy balance within the limits of the techniques used for measuring intake and expenditure. This is to be expected, as a chronic deficit in energy intake would lead to a progressive loss of body mass. Because they often fall at or beyond the extremes of the normal range, the dietary habits of athletes in different sports have been extensively studied.

Extreme endurance activities that involve very high levels of energy expenditure on a daily basis are now rarely encountered in occupational tasks. The average daily metabolic rate of lumberjacks was estimated in the 1930s to be about 4 times the basal metabolic rate, and similar values have been reported elsewhere, suggesting that this may be close to the upper limit of physical exercise that can be sustained on a long-term basis. In the short term, sporting activities can involve much higher levels of energy output: the world record for distance run in 24 h is 286 km, which requires an energy expenditure of about 80 MJ (20 000 kcal). Such an effort, however, results in considerable depletion of the body's energy reserves, and must be followed by a period of recovery.

Very high levels of daily energy expenditure are more often a feature of training than of competition, but there are some competitive events that require high levels of activity to be sustained for many consecutive days. One of the most obvious examples is the multistage cycle tour, of which the most famous is the Tour de France. Measurements on some of the competitors have shown that the successful riders manage to maintain body weight in spite of a mean daily energy expenditure of 32 MJ (8000 kcal) sustained over a 3-week period. Those cyclists who are unable to meet the daily energy requirement are unable to complete the race. In multiday running events, it appears that intake and expenditure may be less well balanced, although individual case histories of successful runners undertaking non-stop races have reported intakes of 25–50 MJ (6000–12 500 kcal) per 24-h period over periods of 5–9 days. There is a tendency in these races for performance to deteriorate over time, and this may be in part due to the growing energy deficit.

Of course, most athletes spend more time in the training phase then they do in competition, and in many cases, the energy requirements of the one or more sessions of daily training are greater than the energy cost of the event. The results of recent dietary surveys of groups of athletes training for different sports are summarized in Figs 1.2 and 1.3 (female athletes), and Figs 1.4 and 1.5 (male athletes). These are divided into sports involving a strong endurance base and lengthy training sessions (e.g. distance running, cycling, triathlon, rowing, and swimming) as well as sports with a greater emphasis on skill, speed, and power (e.g. team sports, gymnastics, track and field athletics, lifting sports). It is difficult to make direct comparisons of

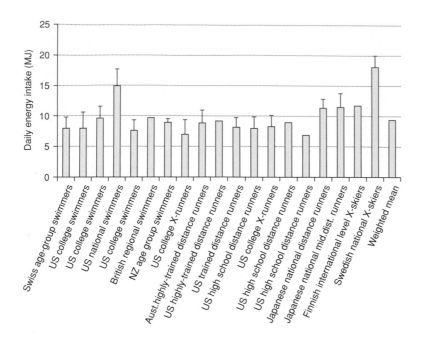

Fig. 1.2 Daily energy intakes reported by groups of female endurance athletes from dietary surveys published 1990–2000.

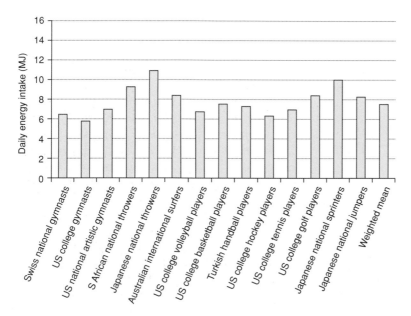

Fig. 1.3 Daily energy intakes reported by groups of female non-endurance athletes from dietary surveys published 1990–2000.

the results of different studies since they are usually conducted on athletes of different levels of ability from different countries, as well as being influenced by the technique used to collect the dietary survey results. Nonetheless, it is interesting to see how the components of daily energy expenditure (Fig. 1.1) predict the typical energy intakes reported in different types of sport. For example, higher energy intakes are typically reported by endurance athletes than non-endurance athletes due to the substantial energy demands of prolonged sessions of moderate-to high-intensity training. On the other hand, athletes with large body mass, particularly due to high levels of lean body mass or muscle mass

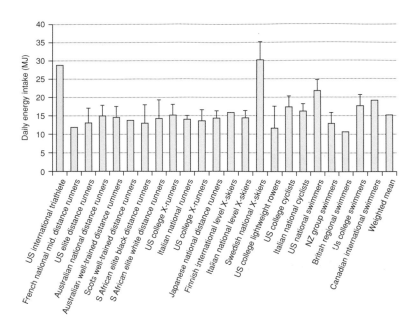

Fig. 1.4 Daily energy intakes reported by groups of male endurance athletes from dietary surveys published 1990–2000.

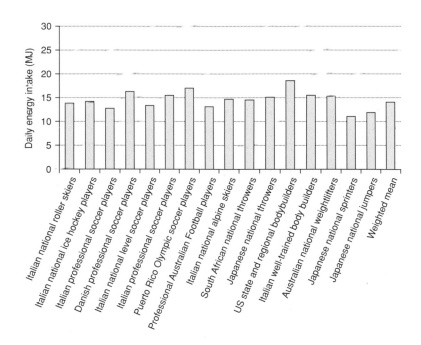

Fig. 1.5 Daily energy intakes reported by groups of male non-endurance athletes from dietary surveys published 1990–2000.

(e.g. body builders and throwers) reported higher energy intakes than athletes of small stature (e.g. gymnasts).

It should be remembered that dietary surveys cannot present the *actual* and *usual* energy intakes of athletes. Rather they present the results of what athletes *report* eating during a *particular* period of time. Experts in dietary survey methodology are keenly aware that such studies rely on the athlete accurately reporting what they consumed, and on the study period being a true representation of their usual eating patterns. Errors occur because athletes eat differently during the period of the dietary survey, or because they fail to be accurate and truthful about everything they eat and drink. In general, dietary surveys underestimate the true intakes of most people, because subjects undereat or under-report their usual intake while they are being studied.

The female athlete

There has been much interest recently in the eating patterns of female athletes. Across the board, female athletes tend to report a lower energy intake than male athletes involved in the same sporting activities, even when differences in body mass and lean body mass are taken into account. For example, when the reported energy intakes of the groups of athletes presented in Figs 1.2–1.5 are presented per kilogram of body mass, the typical female athlete reported a daily energy intake of 172 kJ·kg^{-1} for endurance sports and 125 kJ·kg^{-1} for non-endurance sports. By contrast, male athletes typically reported daily energy intakes of 227 kJ·kg^{-1} (endurance) and 183 kJ·kg^{-1} (non-endurance). Even allowing for differences in the range of athletes studied. The modern female athlete trains at a similar volume and intensity to that of her male counterpart. None the less, some studies have found that female athletes report energy intakes that seem barely able to cover the energy cost of their training, let alone basal metabolic needs, or intakes that are similar to the reported energy consumption of sedentary controls. These reports are more understandable in the case of "aesthetic sports" where a low body fat level must be achieved primarily by energy restriction rather than energy expenditure. However, it is also prevalent in the case of female endurance athletes such as distance runners where low energy intakes are an anomaly in view of the considerable training requirement.

There is no obvious physiological explanation for this finding. There are, of course, many possible sources of methodological errors in the calculation of energy intake and expenditure, but it seems odd that these should apply specifically to female athletes in sports where low body mass is important. It is tempting to try to explain low energy intakes in terms of metabolic adaptations leading to a lower resting metabolic rate or a reduced energy cost of activity in these athletes. This is a common excuse or frustration claimed by the many female athletes who feel that they can't lose weight/body fat despite "hardly eating anything". In fact, if metabolic "efficiency" does occur, it is found in individuals and isolated situations rather than the widespread situations in which it is claimed. Several studies have convincingly shown that there are no aberrations in the energy requirements of groups of female athletes. The use of the doubly labeled water method for the assessment of energy expenditure has been particularly useful in addressing this issue (see Expert Comment 1). Studies using this technique to investigate energy balance in female athletes have shown that energy expenditure is generally greater than reported energy intake, even though body weight is maintained, suggesting an under-reporting of energy intake.

If under-reporting is the major contributor to energy discrepancies, the true energy intakes of female athletes will be higher than estimated from the present overview of dietary surveys. However, it is also likely that some level of energy restriction occurs either chronically or periodically in these athletes compared to true energy requirements, due to activities related to body fat loss. This pattern will vary between individual female athletes or over time in the same athletes. There is considerable evidence that restrained eating practices or low energy availability may be involved in the development of the menstrual dysfunction that is common among female distance runners, gymnasts, and other athletes who are preoccupied by weight and body fat issues. This issue is discussed in greater detail in Chapter 11.

Practical considerations for achieving energy intake

Most people manage to balance energy intake and energy needs over the long term, but situations of extreme energy requirement are harder to manage. Athletes in endurance sports often find it difficult to achieve the very high energy intakes necessary to sustain hard training on a daily basis, and may need advice on dietary strategies to achieve this. This becomes particularly important for the athlete who has to work or study in addition to training, and whose opportunities for eating are therefore limited. The athlete who trains two or even three times per day also has particular problems. Most athletes do not like to eat for some hours before training, and the appetite is likely to be suppressed for some hours after a hard session. By contrast, other athletes need to restrict energy intake to reduce or maintain body weight and body fat levels. This can be difficult to achieve in the face of hunger, customary eating patterns, or the eating habits of peers. These athletes may also need to address their requirements for other nutrients within a reduced energy allowance.

Practical considerations for manipulating energy intake to achieve high or low energy goals are demonstrated in the case histories provided in this chapter. These issues are also explored in greater detail in Chapter 11, in the context of changing physique to increase muscle mass or reduce body fat levels. Practical guidelines for achieving energy restriction and a high energy intake are discussed in Chapter 13.

Reading list

Burke, L.M. (2001) Meeting energy needs. *Canadian Journal of Applied Sports Science* **26**, s202–s219.

Burke, L.M., Cox, G.R., Cummings, N.K. & Desbrow, B. (2001) Guidelines for daily CHO intake: do athletes achieve them? *Sports Medicine* **31**, 267–299.

Ebine, N., Feng, J.-Y., Homma, M., Saitoh, S. & Jones, P.J.H. (2000) Total energy expenditure of elite synchronized swimmers measured by the doubly labelled water method. *European Journal of Applied Physiology* **83**, 1–6.

Edwards, J.E., Linderman, A.K., Mikesky, A.E. & Stager, J.M. (1993) Energy balance in highly trained female endurance runners. *Medicine and Science in Sports and Exercise* **25**, 1398–1404.

Haggarty, P., McGaw, B.A., Maughan, R.J. & Fenn, C. (1988) Energy expenditure of elite female athletes measured by the doubly labelled water method. *Proceedings of the Nutrition Society* **47**, 35A.

Jones, P.J. & Leitch, C.A. (1993) Validation of doubly labelled water for measurement of caloric expenditure in collegiate swimmers. *Journal of Applied Physiology* **74**, 2909–2914.

Jonnalagadda, S.S., Benardot, D. & Dill, M.N. (2000) Assessment of under-reporting of energy intake by elite female gymnasts. *International Journal of Sports Nutrition and Exercise Metabolism* **10**, 315–325.

Manore, M.M. (2000) The overweight athlete. In: *Nutrition in Sport* (ed. R. J. Maughan), pp. 469–483. Blackwell Science, Oxford.

Manore, M. & Thompson, J. (2000) Energy requirements of the athlete: assessment and evidence of energy efficiency. In: *Clinical Sports Nutrition* (eds L. Burke & V. Deakin), 2nd edn, pp. 124–145. McGraw-Hill, Sydney, Australia.

Schoeller, D.A. & van Santen, E. (1982) Measurement of energy expenditure in humans by the doubly labelled water method. *Journal of Applied Physiology* **53**, 955–959.

Schoeller, D.A., Bandini, L.G. & Dietz, W.H. (1990) Inaccuracies in self-reported intake identified by comparison with the doubly labelled water method. *Canadian Journal of Physiology and Pharmacology* **68**, 941–949.

Schulz, L.O., Alger, S., Harper, I., Wilmore, J.H. & Ravussin, E. (1992) Energy expenditure of elite female runners measured by respiratory chamber and doubly labelled water. *Journal of Applied Physiology* **72**, 23–28.

Westerterp, K.R., Saris, W.H.M., van Es, M. & ten Hoor, F. (1986) Use of the doubly labelled water technique in humans during heavy sustained exercise. *Journal of Applied Physiology* **61**, 2162–2167.

EXPERT COMMENT 1 Energy intakes of athletes: discrepancy between reported and measured values. Henry C. Lukaski

Determination of dietary intake in free-living persons usually relies on some form of self-reporting. The self-reports include an interview with a dietitian to recall the food consumed during the previous 24-h period, multiple-day recording of each food item and the amount consumed, and semiquantitative food (e.g. food groups such as dairy, meat, etc.) questionnaires that are reviewed during a dietetic interview. These methods yield data that are used to estimate the nutrient and energy intakes, and hence needs, of various groups of individuals, including athletes. Measurements of body weight and body composition are coupled with the self-reported energy intakes to assess energy balance.

A more objective method is the use of doubly labeled water (DLW) to determine total energy expenditure and, by inference, intake. This approach measures the fractional rates of excretion of an orally administered dose of the stable isotopes of hydrogen (deuterium, $D = {}^2H$) and oxygen (^{18}O) in body fluids (e.g. saliva), during time periods ranging from 3 to 21 days. The rate of loss of deuterium is proportional to water flux and the rate of elimination of ^{18}O is proportional to the sum of water and carbon dioxide losses. The difference between the two elimination rates is proportional to carbon dioxide production and, thus, to total energy expenditure, determined either as an average daily energy expenditure or as total expenditure over a specified number of days. This method yields highly accurate (1%) and precise (3%) estimates of total energy expenditure in free-living individuals, including infants, children, and adults over periods of up to 10–14 days.

Comparisons of self-reported energy intakes and total energy expenditure using the doubly labeled water method consistently show discrepancies in individuals regardless of the level of daily energy expenditure. Among adolescents, boys and girls with measured daily energy outputs of 13.8 MJ (3300 kcal) and 10.7 MJ (2557 kcal) under-reported energy intake by 18 and 22%, respectively. Similarly, male soldiers participating in strenuous field maneuvers and training under stressful environmental conditions (cold and high altitude or heat and high humidity) regularly underestimated total energy intake by 5–15% in self-reports of food intake at levels ranging from 14.2 MJ·day^{-1} (3400 kcal·day^{-1}) to 32.4 MJ·day^{-1} (7720 kcal·day^{-1}).

Limited studies of athletes participating in various sports have also found similar discrepancies between reported and measured energy intakes. Male cyclists who completed the Tour de France, consistently under-reported energy intake compared to energy expenditure estimated with doubly labeled water. Furthermore, the underestimate increased progressively throughout the 23-day competition from 13% to 22% then 36% during days 1–7, 8–15 and 16–23, respectively. Among elite female runners with daily energy intakes ranging from 11.8 MJ (2826 kcal) to 14.6 MJ (3492 kcal) over a period of 21 days, self-reports of food intake were 10–34% lower than determinations of total energy expenditure determined with doubly labeled water. Similarly, international female synchronized swimmers under-reported by 23% their daily energy intake from food records (8.9 MJ or 2128 kcal) compared to estimates derived from the doubly labeled water method (11.5 MJ or 2738 kcal). In another study, 61% of elite female gymnasts substantially under-reported energy intake. Interestingly, among athletes who obtain food under supervised conditions (e.g. training centers), there is a negligible discrepancy (~ 1%) in total energy intake from reported food intake and the doubly labeled water method.

There are some fundamental points to be derived from these studies. The key finding is that self-reported food and energy intake almost always underestimates actual intake. The magnitude of this discrepancy is substantial; it may vary from 2.4 MJ (575 kcal) in adolescents to 7.5 MJ (1800 kcal) on a daily basis during sustained, heavy exercise over a period exceeding 21 days. There is also considerable between-athlete variability in the observed differences between reported energy intake and objectively determined energy expenditure; it ranges from 1–2% to more than 20%. In general, this variability has been attributed to a failure to record total food consumption or to undereat during the period of recording. In general, people who are overweight tend to be more at risk of underestimating food and energy intakes, or likely to underestimate to a greater extent. Female athletes may underestimate food intake more than male athletes; similarly, athletes who are concerned with maintenance of a lower body weight or dissatisfied with their present body weight and composition may be more likely to under report. Coaches should be aware of this behavior and of the limitations of the self-report method to estimate the energy needs of an athlete. Furthermore, attempts to evaluate self-reports of food and energy intake should include independent measures of validity to identify more accurately nutritional problems experienced by individual athletes.

CASE STUDY 1 Athlete with low energy needs: ballet dancer. Helen O'Connor

Athlete

Alexandria was a 14-year-old classical ballet dancer studying for her Royal Academy of Dancing Intermediate Ballet Examination. She was 167 cm and 66 kg (90th percentile)*. She attended a 1.5-h classical ballet class four times per week and completed one class of repertoire, contemporary, and jazz ballet each Saturday. Alexandria had recently moved from her local suburban dancing school to one that provided a highly regarded but rigorous dance training program.

Reason for consultancy

Alexandria's ballet teachers were concerned about her increasing weight, which was 6 kg higher than when she first started at their school 9 months previously. In addition to the weight concern, Alexandria had recently become moody, tired, and less motivated.

Existing dietary patterns

Alexandria had been dieting in an attempt to reduce weight with little success since her menstrual cycle began 18 months previously. She tried almost every diet given to her by other ballet students, but any weight loss achieved seemed to rapidly reappear. The experience of "nothing seeming to work" left Alexandria convinced that her metabolism was slow and that she would never be able to lose weight. A sample of her precounseling eating plans is outlined below.

Professional assessment

Mean daily intake from this self-reported eating plan was assessed to be ~ 7050 kJ (1680 kcal); 198 g carbohydrate (3 g·kg body mass^{-1}); 53 g protein; 79 g fat (42% of energy). This diet failed to meet the recommended dietary intake (RDI) for calcium (reported intake 637 mg·day^{-1} vs. goal of 1000 mg) and iron (7.9 mg·day^{-1} vs. goal of 12–15 mg). Alexandria was initially anxious to discuss her "craving" for chocolate. However, over time she realized that she needed help to control her often excessive intake of chocolate at the expense of other foods. Although not overweight by health standards, Alexandria needed

*Data from the National Center for Health Statistics (NCHS) Hyattsville, Maryland. (Hamill, P.V.D., Drizd, T.A., Johnson, C.L., Reed, R.B., Roche, A.F. & Moore, W.M. (1979) Physical growth: National Center for Health Statistics percentiles. *American Journal of Clinical Nutrition* **32**, 607–629.)

to be at the lower end of the healthy range to be successful at ballet.

Intervention

The following suggestions were made to improve calcium, iron, and general nutrient intake, control cravings, and facilitate weight loss.

1 Consume a balanced breakfast each day, which is high in fiber and includes low glycemic index carbohydrate and protein to boost satiety. Examples include a bowl of wholegrain cereal or oats with calcium-fortified milk, fresh citrus fruit to enhance iron absorption, and water or a small citrus juice or milk instead of tea (to avoid inhibition of iron absorption).

2 Include nutritious, nutrient-dense snacks between meals: examples include fresh fruit, reduced-fat yoghurt, reduced-fat milk, or a slice of wholegrain bread or toast.

3 Include protein-rich foods at lunch (e.g. lean meat, poultry, seafood or reduced-fat cheese) to boost iron and/or calcium intake. Team this with plenty of vegetables or salad to increase the feeling of fullness, and add a small serving of carbohydrate (e.g. grain bread, pasta, rice, potato, etc.) to maintain blood glucose and glycogen stores. For example, try a wholegrain roll filled with salad and lean chicken.

4 Use the same principle with the evening meal, with particular focus on adding a carbohydrate serving. For example, try a lean meat or chicken stir-fry with vegetables, served with rice or pasta.

5 Use a food diary to monitor food intake, cravings, and feelings. Allow chocolate or another treat once or twice a week to help prevent binge eating.

6 Obtain a body composition assessment to properly assess and monitor changes in body fat levels.

7 Also consider the possibility of low-impact aerobic training (e.g. walking, cycling, swimming, or deep-water running) to help weight loss via increasing energy expenditure.

Outcome

Alexandria managed to implement the dietary strategies suggested. This decreased her average energy intake slightly to 5640 kJ (1340 kcal) and increased calcium intake to 800 mg and iron to 14 mg per day. Alexandria's weight initially stabilized and then gradually began to fall. Body composition measures provided additional information and motivation about losses of body fat. An important benefit of these changes was the improvement in her mood and concentration levels. As a result of her dietary program she finally began to enjoy class and life again.

Breakfast	Lunch	Dinner	Snacks
Nothing or one slice wholemeal toast with jam (no butter)	Green salad	Steamed chicken or fish with steamed vegetables	Diet cola and if feeling really low before class a chocolate bar or two
1 cup tea	One apple	1 cup tea	
	Diet cola		

CASE STUDY 2 Athlete with high energy needs: vegetarian distance runner. Gregory R. Cox

Athlete

Damien was a 24-year-old male training for his first marathon. He weighed 68 kg and his previous training history included 30–40 km per week or running, three gym sessions per week and touch football twice a week. Twelve weeks before the marathon, Damien joined a running group, and effectively doubled his weekly training distance to around 85 km.

Reason for consultancy

Damien had lost 3 kg in body mass over his first 6 weeks of increased running training, was suffering excessive fatigue, and was unable to recover between training sessions. He struggled to maintain pace during the long group runs and dropped his gym workouts due to lack of energy.

Existing dietary patterns

Damien followed a vegetarian eating plan based on organic wholesome grains, nuts, and legumes. He used vegetable oil liberally in cooking and avocado on sandwiches and in salads. However, he avoided many sugary foods and drank only water and freshly squeezed fruit juices. Although he had tried to increase his food intake to combat the weight loss, this attempt left him feeling too full after meals. During training and touch football games he consumed water only. A sample of his precounseling eating plans is outlined below.

Professional assessment

Mean daily intake from this self-reported eating plan was assessed to be ~ 10 700 kJ (2550 kcal); 315 g carbohydrate (4.6 g·kg body mass^{-1}); 86 g protein; 106 g fat (37% of energy). This diet failed to meet his RDI for calcium (reported intake estimated at 520 mg·day^{-1} vs. goal of 1000 mg) and was excessive in fiber content (73 g·day^{-1}). Damien was motivated to make dietary modifications.

Intervention

The following suggestions were made to reduce his daily fiber intake, increase his daily energy and carbohydrate intake, and meet the RDI for calcium.

1 Replace high-bran breakfast biscuit with regular variety and remove added unprocessed bran. Add a dessertspoonful of honey to breakfast cereal, and have toast with banana and honey to finish breakfast. Realize the importance of consuming carbohydrate while exercising; consume sports drink during training sessions and touch football.

2 Include a banana smoothie made with low-fat soy milk, banana, honey, and low-fat fruit yoghurt after a long training session or as a snack between meals.

3 Reduce serving size of low-energy salad items at the evening meal, in order to include a carbohydrate-rich dessert such as soy custard and tinned fruit.

4 Replace current full-fat, non-fortified soy milk with a calcium-fortified low-fat soy milk alternative.

Outcome

Damien managed to implement suggested dietary modifications successfully. As a result his weight stabilized and his performance during long training sessions improved, along with his recovery from these sessions. New reported dietary patterns showed an increase in energy intake (14 020 kJ·day^{-1} or 3380 kcal·day^{-1}), carbohydrate intake (550 g·day^{-1}; 8 g·kg body mass^{-1}) and calcium (1450 mg·day^{-1}). Despite the increase in total daily energy, fiber intake was reduced by 20 g·day^{-1} and energy derived from fat decreased to 20%. Damien successfully completed his first marathon in a time of 2 h 50 min and was ready to tackle his next challenge.

Breakfast	Lunch	Dinner	Snacks
Six high-bran breakfast biscuits with full-fat soy milk, sliced banana, and unprocessed bran Glass of juice	Wholemeal lavash bread with hummus, avocado, and salad Two pieces of fruit and large handful of almonds	Dahl with brown rice and large side salad	Bowl of dried fruit, nut, and seed mix Warm mug of carob drink made with soy milk

Chapter 2
Fuels used in exercise: carbohydrate and fat

Introduction

All exercise imposes an increased energy demand on the muscles. If the muscles are unable to meet that demand, the exercise task cannot be performed. When the exercise intensity is high or the duration is prolonged, there may be difficulty in supplying energy at the required rate, and fatigue ensues. For simple activities such as running or swimming, the rate at which energy is required is a function of speed, and the time for which a given speed can be maintained before the fatigue process intervenes is inversely related to speed. In most sports situations, however, the exercise intensity, and hence the energy demand, is not constant. For example, games such as soccer or tennis involve brief periods of high-intensity effort interspersed with variable periods of rest or low-intensity exercise. Even in sports such as running or cycling, the energy demand will vary with changes in pace or in other factors such as wind resistance or the topography of the course. Muscles have adapted, and can be trained, to meet the varying demands as far as possible. Given the wide range of the requirements placed on muscle it is not surprising that several different strategies are employed to meet these demands.

Fuels available to the muscle

Energy is required by muscle cells to perform work and can only be used in the form of adenosine triphosphate (ATP). All the energy-requiring processes in muscle are powered by the energy released when ATP is converted to adenosine diphosphate (ADP) with the release of an inorganic phosphate group (PO_4^2, P_i); this applies as much to the pumping processes that maintain the ionic gradients across muscle membranes as to the contractile mechanisms that make the muscle "move".

Only a small amount of ATP is present within the muscle cells, amounting to about 5 mmol·kg^{-1}. This is about 3.4 g, so with about 20 kg of skeletal muscle in the average healthy young man, this is about 70 g of ATP in total. Most activities, however, use only a fraction of the total muscle mass, so much less than this is available. The ATP content of the muscle is never allowed to fall by more than about a third, but even if it fell to zero the amount of energy available is very small and would only sustain about one second of exercise at maximum intensity. Because the content is so small and must be maintained, the ATP present in the muscle cannot be considered to be an energy store. Storage of ATP sufficient to support exercise of more than a few seconds' duration would impose an impossible weight burden. The muscle does have a second source of readily available energy in the form of creatine phosphate (CP), which is present within the muscle cell at a concentration about 3–4 times

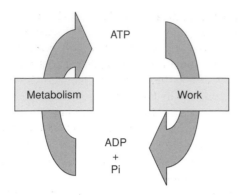

ATP

Metabolism

Work

ADP
+
Pi

Fig. 2.1 The hydrolysis of adenosine triphosphate (ATP) to adenosine diphosphate (ADP) provides energy for almost all energy-consuming processes in the body. Regeneration of ATP by transfer of a phosphate group from creatine phosphate (CP) allows rapid resynthesis of ATP, but the other metabolic pathways have the advantage of allowing more sustained exercise to be performed.

that of ATP (Fig. 2.1). Although the muscle content of ATP is closely regulated, that of CP can fall to almost zero after a few seconds of maximum exercise. The resynthesis of ATP from ADP by transfer of a phosphate group from CP is catalysed by the enzyme creatine kinase in a reaction that is extremely rapid. These mechanisms can supply energy at a very high rate and can thus support a high power output, but their capacity is limited and they cannot sustain this level for long (Table 2.1). For more prolonged exercise, an alternative fuel must be used.

Glycogen, consisting of very large branched polymers of glucose, is stored within the muscle cells, and glycogenolysis can supply relatively large amounts of energy to the muscles. Unlike the CP content of muscle which is small and, at least in the resting state, rather constant, the amount of energy

Table 2.1 Maximum rates of ATP resynthesis (μmol·min^{-1} gram muscle^{-1}).

Creatine phosphate hydrolysis	440
Lactate formation	180
Carbohydrate oxidation	40
Fat oxidation	20

Table 2.2 Integration of the different energy sources available to muscle allows the best combination of power and endurance. The capacity of oxidative metabolism is essentially unlimited as the system can be continually refueled even during exercise.

	Capacity (J·kg^{-1})	Power (W·kg^{-1})
ATP/CP hydrolysis	400	800
Lactate formation	1000	325
Oxidative metabolism		200

available from the glycogen store is large and highly variable. Human skeletal muscle normally contains about 14–18 g·kg^{-1} of glycogen (80–100 mmol glucosyl units per kg wet weight of muscle), but the range can be much wider than this. If glycogenolysis proceeds only as far as lactate, the muscles can produce 4 mol of ATP for each mol of glucosyl units consumed. This series of reactions, which constitutes anaerobic glycogenolysis, is rapid although the maximum rate of ATP production that can be achieved is less than can be supplied from CP. As the name indicates, it proceeds without the involvement of molecular oxygen. When rates of glycogenolysis are high, much of the lactate formed will leave the muscle and appear in the blood. If glycogenolysis is allowed to go to completion with the oxidation of the pyruvate through the tricarboxlic acid cycle (TCA cycle) to carbon dioxide and water rather than to lactate, the amount of ATP formed is much greater, being 39 mol per mol glucosyl units. Although the amount of energy that can be liberated from the glycogen stores is thus increased, the rate at which it is available is much less (Table 2.2).

An alternative source of carbohydrate fuel available to the muscles is blood glucose, which is derived from the liver. The total amount of glycogen stored in the liver varies greatly: in the postabsorptive state, a range from 14 to 80 g·kg^{-1} has been reported. Assuming a liver weight of 1.8 kg, the mean value from these studies for the total liver glycogen content is about 80 g, which is much less than the amount of glycogen stored in the muscles (about 300–400 g). Although short-term fasting has little effect on the muscle glycogen content if no exercise is performed, a 12-h fast can cause the liver glycogen to fall by more than half. This reflects the important role of the liver in maintaining the blood glucose concentration and thus ensuring a constant supply of glucose to vital tissues, especially the brain. To do this, liver relies on the enzyme glucose 6-phosphate dehydrogenase, which releases free glucose that is then able to leave the cells. This enzyme is not present in muscle, so the sugar phosphates that are formed when glycogen is broken down are trapped within the cells. If glucose rather than glycogen is the starting point, one ATP molecule is needed to convert the glucose to glucose 6-phosphate, so the net gain in energy to the cell is three molecules of ATP for each molecule of glucose broken down rather than the four when glycogen is the starting point. This, together with the limitation on the rate at which glucose can enter the muscle cells, makes glycogen a more suitable fuel when the energy demands are high.

Manipulation of diet and exercise patterns can cause the glycogen content of both liver and muscle to vary widely. In addition to its store of glycogen, the liver can release glucose produced by the process of gluconeogenesis in which glucose is synthesized from other substrates, including lactate and amino acids as well as glycerol derived from triglycerides. Although the process is relatively expensive in energy terms—12 molecules of ATP are required for each molecule of glucose produced—gluconeogenesis can account for more than half of the glucose released by the liver in some situations, and may be particularly important in prolonged exercise when the liver glycogen store is depleted. The supply of gluconeogenic precursors is generally increased during exercise and in starvation, both situations where there may be a need for extra carbohydrate to be made available.

Not all of the lactate produced by active muscle fibers will be used by the liver for gluconeogenesis. Although muscle is often a net producer of lactate, it also has a high capacity for the oxidation of lactate. Heart muscle cells are exceptionally good at using lactate as a fuel for energy supply, but skeletal muscle, especially the Type I muscle fibers, can also do this. In many exercise situations, lactate produced by one muscle, which is working at a high percentage of its capacity, will be taken up and oxidized by another muscle. This may also happen

within the same muscle: lactate released by one muscle fiber may be taken up and used as a fuel for oxidation by another fiber within the same muscle without ever reaching the bloodstream. This depends on the biochemical characteristics of the muscle fibers, which determine the relative capacities for lactate production and oxidation, and on the fiber recruitment patterns. The significance of muscle fiber composition for exercise performance and substrate utilization is described in more detail in Expert Comment 1.

Muscle also has the capacity to obtain energy from the oxidation of fat in the form of free fatty acids derived from triglyceride: each triglyceride molecule can be broken down to release three molecules of fatty acids and one of glycerol. The body stores large amounts of triglycerides within the adipose tissue and, to a much smaller extent, within the muscle cells themselves. Again, the extent of these stores varies greatly between individuals, although, unlike the body's carbohydrate stores, they are not susceptible to large changes in the short term. Free fatty acids released from the adipose tissue are transported to the muscle in the plasma where they are bound to albumin. Within the muscle cells, the fatty acids are oxidized to carbon dioxide and water. The rate at which energy can be produced by fat oxidation is, however, much less than can be achieved by oxidation of carbohydrate, and the amount of energy released per unit of oxygen consumed is less for fat (19.7 kJ·l O_2^{-1}) than for carbohydrate (21.4 kJ·l O_2^{-1}). Translated into marathon running terms, this difference may be highly significant. The 70-kg runner who completes the race in about $2^1/_2$ h requires a power output of about 80 kJ·min^{-1} throughout the race. If carbohydrate (CHO) oxidation met the entire energy requirement, the oxygen consumption would be about 3.74 l·min^{-1} whereas an oxygen consumption of about 4.06 l·min^{-1} would be necessary if fat oxidation provided all the energy. Assuming a maximum oxygen uptake of 5 l·min^{-1}, CHO oxidation requires that the runner uses 75% of his maximum, compared with 81% if fat was the sole fuel. The main advantage of fat as a fuel is that it is an extremely efficient storage form, releasing approximately 37 kJ·g^{-1} compared with 16 kJ·g^{-1} for carbohydrate. Each gram of CHO stored also retains

Table 2.3 Energy stores in the average man. This assumes a body weight of 70 kg and a fat content of 15% of body weight. The figure for blood glucose includes the glucose content of the extracellular fluid. Not all of this, and not more than a very small part of the total protein, is available for use during exercise.

	Weight (g)	Energy (kJ)
Liver glycogen	80	1280
Muscle glycogen	350	5600
Blood glucose	10	160
Protein	12 000	204 000
Fat	10 500	388 500

some additional water because of the osmotic effect it exerts, further decreasing the efficiency or "compactness" of CHO as an energy store. The energy cost of running a marathon is about 12 000 kJ; if this could be achieved by the oxidation of fat alone, the total amount of fat required would be about 320 g, whereas 750 g of CHO and additional associated water (perhaps as much as 2 kg) would be required if CHO oxidation were the sole source of energy. Apart from considerations of the weight to be carried, this amount of CHO exceeds the total amount normally stored in the liver and muscles. The total storage capacity for fat is extremely large, and for most practical purposes the amount of energy stored in the form of fat is far in excess of that required for any exercise task (Table 2.3).

All of these fuels are used by muscle to produce energy during exercise, but the proportions in which they contribute to the total energy requirement will depend on a number of different factors including the intensity and duration of the exercise, nutritional status, and the physiological and biochemical characteristics of the individual.

Physiological factors affecting exercise metabolism

The capacity to perform exercise and the metabolic response to exercise both vary greatly between individuals. Many factors contribute to these differences, which are particularly apparent in highly trained elite athletes. The key to successful sprinting is the ability to generate a high power output, and elite sprinters are characterized by a large muscle mass and a highly developed capacity for anaerobic energy production. The muscles of endurance athletes are not large, but have a high capacity for aerobic metabolism. These athletes also have a cardiovascular system that is extremely effective at delivering oxygen to the muscles. Measurement of the maximum oxygen uptake ($\dot{V}_{O_{2max}}$) shows that sprinters commonly achieve values that are little greater than those of untrained individuals, whereas the $\dot{V}_{O_{2max}}$ of endurance athletes may be twice as great. The physiological and biochemical response to an exercise task is largely determined by the fraction of the individual's $\dot{V}_{O_{2max}}$ that the task represents. Running at a speed that requires 100% of $\dot{V}_{O_{2max}}$ for the sedentary individual may require less than 50% of $\dot{V}_{O_{2max}}$ for the distance runner. Where technique is important, as for example in swimming or cross-country skiing, the differences between the elite competitor and the novice are even more marked. Whereas fatigue will occur within a few minutes of the onset of exercise at 100% of $\dot{V}_{O_{2max}}$, exercise at 50% of $\dot{V}_{O_{2max}}$ represents a fairly comfortable level of effort that can be continued for many hours.

The metabolic response to exercise is also influenced by the biochemical characteristics of the muscles performing the work. Although muscle is often considered to be a homogeneous tissue, skeletal muscle fibers may have very different biochemical and contractile properties. Type I muscle fibers are often referred to as slow-twitch or oxidative fibers, whereas Type II fibers are also classified as fast-twitch or glycolytic fibers (see Expert Comment 1). Although the classifications based on the speed of muscle shortening (twitch times) or on the enzyme activities may appear more useful, they may be misleading. Type II fibers all have a relatively high glycolytic capacity, but some, the Type IIa fibers, also have a high oxidative capacity, which may be even greater than that of the Type I fibers. The Type II fibers, which were formerly referred to as Type IIb fibers have a low oxidative capacity and a high glycolytic capacity. Type I fibers are well supplied with blood due to the large number of capillaries around each fiber, and have a high capacity to oxidize a range of substrates, including glycogen, blood glucose, lactate, and fat.

The individual muscle fibers are organized into motor units. All the fibers in a motor unit belong to the same fiber type, and the same nerve serves all fibers in the unit so that all are activated simultaneously. The recruitment pattern of the muscle fibers is determined by the effort required, and is organized such that the motor units consisting of Type I fibers are the first to be recruited. Only sufficient motor units to accomplish the required task are activated. In low-intensity exercise, this can be achieved by the activation of some of the Type I fibers with no involvement of Type II fibers, but if high forces are required, then the Type II fibers are recruited to help (see Expert Comment 1).

Thus the patterns of substrate metabolism that are observed during exercise can be largely explained in terms of the biochemical characteristics of the muscle fibers and their recruitment patterns. The biochemical characteristics of the muscle fibers can be modified by the patterns of use or disuse imposed upon them, but the speeds of contraction are relatively fixed. Endurance training has the effect of increasing the capacity of all of the muscle fiber types for oxidative metabolism, and may lead to the Type II fibers of the well-trained individual having a higher oxidative capacity than that of the Type I fibers of the sedentary individual.

Substrate utilization in high-intensity exercise

In the transition from rest to maximum exercise, the rate of energy turnover in the exercising muscles can increase by as much as 1000-fold. The supply of oxygen to the working muscles increases only rather slowly at the onset of exercise, and takes at least 1–2 min to reach its peak value. The maximum rate at which the aerobic system can supply energy exercise is also rather low relative to the rates of energy demand in high-intensity exercise (Table 2.2). The duration of maximal-intensity activity is severely limited, however, as fatigue occurs rapidly. Studies on animal muscle in which the resynthesis of ATP is prevented have shown that the amount of work that can be performed is very small—only

about three normal twitch contractions are possible under these conditions. However, the maximum activity of the enzyme creatine kinase, which transfers a phosphate group from creatine phosphate (CP) to ADP resulting in the resynthesis of ATP, is higher than that of ATPase which catalyses the breakdown of ATP to ADP. This ensures that the ATP content of the muscle is kept high as long as there is adequate CP available. Only when the CP content has fallen to less than half the resting value will a fall in the ATP level be apparent. When only a few muscle contractions are involved and the duration of the exercise is no more than 1–2 s, all of the energy required will be provided from these sources. In the postexercise period, the muscle CP and ATP content will return to normal within a few minutes, with the energy for their resynthesis being derived from oxidative metabolism.

When the duration of the exercise is increased to a few (5–10) seconds, significant falls in the muscle ATP and CP content are observed. Although it was thought at one time that no lactate would be produced in exercise lasting less than 10 s, sprinting over a distance of 40 m (in about 5 s) has been shown to cause a large increase in the lactate content of the quadriceps muscles. There was no change in the muscle ATP content in that study, even when the distance run at full speed was extended to 100 m. Muscle CP content fell significantly after 40 m of sprinting, but did not fall further when the distance was extended, indicating that CP breakdown did not contribute to energy provision at this stage. In a maximal cycling task of 30 s duration, CP breakdown and lactate formation by glycolysis contribute about equally to the total energy requirement during the first 6 s of exercise. Only about 35% of the muscle CP content is used in the first 6 s of exercise, and a further substantial contribution is made over the next 24 s during which time the power output falls progressively. The muscle ATP content remains essentially unchanged after 6 s, but falls by almost half at the end of the 30-s period. Large amounts of muscle glycogen are used, with reductions of about 16% of the resting value after 6 s and 30% after 30 s. These findings suggest that major demands on the muscle glycogen store will be made in training sessions consisting of multiple short sprints.

The rate of energy provision by glycogenolysis is not normally limited by the availability of glycogen within the muscle. Even in maximum exercise, large amounts of glycogen remain within the muscle at the point of fatigue. If repeated sprints are performed, however, the glycogen content of the muscles will be reduced. In particular, the Type IIx muscle fibers, which have a high capacity for glycogenolysis, may lose most of their glycogen. If this happens, sprinting ability will be seriously impaired. It is important therefore to ensure that the muscle has an adequate glycogen store before exercise begins. Where high-intensity training or competitions occur on successive days, replacement of these stores by consumption of a diet rich in carbohydrate is essential to ensure optimum performance. The need for a high CHO intake is well recognized among endurance athletes, but sprinters and games players often do not appreciate that the muscle glycogen stores may be substantially depleted in training as well as in competition and must be replaced.

It has long been known that the maximum speed which can be achieved by elite sprinters begins to decline towards the end of a 100-m race, and in maximal cycle ergometer tests the peak power output is observed within 1–3 s of the onset of exercise. The reasons for this now become apparent. In the initial acceleration phase, most of the energy is derived from CP breakdown, and after only a few seconds the CP content of the muscle has fallen to the point where the rate of resynthesis of ATP by this mechanism cannot be sustained. Almost immediately during the exercise, the rate of glycolysis is dramatically increased but the maximum rate of energy production is still less than can be achieved by transfer of phosphate groups from CP (Tables 2.1 & 2.2).

In most field games such as soccer, the pattern of activity consists of sprints lasting no more than a few seconds (typically 1–2 s) followed by recovery. During these high-intensity bursts, most of the energy will be supplied by CP, with glycolysis contributing more as the distance increases or if there has not been complete recovery from the previous sprint. The resynthesis of CP after exercise has been reported to be complete within a few minutes after work, but more recently it was shown that the CP

Table 2.4 Contributions of anaerobic and aerobic energy metabolism in maximal work of different durations.

Time	% Anaerobic	% Aerobic
10 s	90	10
60 s	70	30
5 min	30	70
30 min	5	95
60 min	2	98
120 min	1	99

content of muscle did not return to the pre-exercise level even 60 min after high-intensity exercise where exhaustion was reached after about 3 min. If a second sprint is performed before CP levels have been restored, the speed and duration may be reduced. Restoration of CP levels during recovery will not be delayed if low-intensity exercise is performed, even though this increases the total energy demand on the muscles.

As the exercise becomes more prolonged, the contribution of glycolysis to energy production is increased, leading to the accumulation of the end-product lactate in the muscle and blood. In exercise lasting from about 10 s to about 2–3 min anaerobic glycolysis will be the main source of energy. In longer events, oxidative metabolism gradually becomes more important (Table 2.4). When the exercise duration exceeds about 2–3 min, aerobic processes supply more than half the total energy requirement. In the shorter events, most of the fuel used will be in the form of muscle glycogen, but glucose derived from the blood becomes more important as the duration increases.

At the pH that exists within muscle, the lactic acid that is formed by glycolysis is almost totally dissociated to form the negatively charged lactate anion and a proton (a positively charged hydrogen ion, H^+). Some of these protons are buffered within the muscle, and some leave the muscle, but if the exercise is sufficiently intense and prolonged the accumulation of protons will cause the intramuscular pH to fall. This may reduce the rate of energy production by glycolysis as a result of inhibition of phosphofructokinase (PFK), one of the key enzymes, although other changes in the muscle have the effect of stimulating PFK activity. It may also inter-

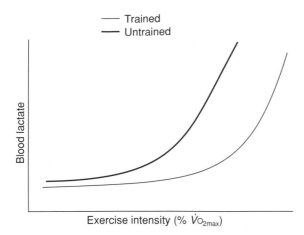

Fig. 2.2 Effects of endurance training on the blood lactate response to exercise. Note that this is a smooth curve, and there are no distinct "threshold" points.

fere more directly with the contractile process within the muscle. Whatever the mechanism involved, the end result is a subjective sensation of fatigue and an inability to continue exercising.

One of the most striking effects of endurance training is to increase the rate at which work can be performed before significant accumulation of lactate and protons occurs within the muscle and blood. A running speed which, in the untrained state, results in a high rate of anaerobic glycolysis with its associated lactate production, fall in muscle pH, and fatigue, can be accomplished with little or no anaerobic glycolysis in the trained state (Fig. 2.2).

Substrate utilization in prolonged exercise

During prolonged exercise at constant intensity, the muscle relies almost entirely on oxidative metabolism for energy production. The exception to this is the first few minutes of exercise when anaerobic metabolism will make a contribution to energy production until a more or less steady state of oxygen consumption is attained. In the competitive situation, of course, the exercise intensity is rarely constant, and anaerobic metabolism may be required during prolonged races where there are tactical

bursts during the event, where uphill stretches are encountered, and during a sprint finish. In many games, the total exercise duration is about 90 min; the oxygen uptake will normally be elevated throughout this period, but the immediate energy requirements of the many short bursts of activity will be met by anaerobic metabolism. Oxidative metabolism will provide energy for the resynthesis of ATP and CP and the removal of lactate during recovery periods.

The major fuels contributing to oxidative metabolism during prolonged exercise are fat and carbohydrate. It is often assumed that protein breakdown does not contribute to energy production during exercise, but, although there is disagreement as to the extent to which this occurs, some protein is oxidized during prolonged exercise (see Chapter 3). The use of protein as a fuel will be increased when other substrates, especially carbohydrate, are not available, but under normal conditions, protein oxidation probably accounts for not more than about 5% of the total energy requirement in exercise lasting up to 2–3 h. Although the body's protein content can be used as a source of substrate for oxidation, there is no significant store of protein. The loss of structural and functional proteins can only be tolerated to a limited extent without some impairment of health and performance.

The relative contributions of fat and CHO are determined largely by the intensity and duration of the exercise. The greater the exercise intensity, the greater is the reliance on CHO as a fuel. In low-intensity exercise, at less than 50% of $\dot{V}_{O_{2max}}$, fat is the predominant fuel, accounting for more than half of the total energy production, with oxidation of blood glucose and muscle glycogen contributing about equally to the remainder. At about 60–65% of $\dot{V}_{O_{2max}}$, the contributions of fat and CHO are roughly equal, and above this level of exercise CHO is the major fuel.

In moderate-intensity exercise corresponding to about 70–75% of $\dot{V}_{O_{2max}}$, which can usually be sustained for 2–4 h and is approximately the intensity at which the faster marathon runners are working, muscle glycogen will be the major fuel. At higher exercise intensities, the rate of CHO utilization increases still further, and once the muscle begins to rely on anaerobic glycolysis to supplement the energy produced by oxidative metabolism, the rate of glycogen utilization increases sharply.

Although the total amount of glycogen stored in all the body's muscles is about 300–400 g, only a part of this will be available during exercise. Unlike the glycogen stored in liver, muscle glycogen cannot contribute directly to the blood glucose pool, as discussed above. As glucose units are split off from glycogen, a phosphate group is added to each glucose molecule and these phosphorylated sugars cannot cross the cell membranes. In liver, but not in muscle, a phosphatase enzyme releases free glucose, which can then leave the cell. The CHO stored in inactive muscle can be made available if it is released in the form of pyruvate, lactate, or alanine which can freely cross cell membranes and which can then be used by active muscle as a fuel or taken up by the liver for gluconeogenesis. This does not, however, happen to any great extent in resting muscle.

Even when the exercise intensity remains constant, the pattern of substrate utilization changes with time. As exercise progresses, the glycogen stores in the working muscle become depleted, and the muscle is forced to rely on other fuels to an increasing extent (Fig. 2.3). Since the 1960s the muscle biopsy technique has been used to follow the changes in muscle glycogen occurring during exercise. The glycogen content of the quadriceps muscles falls progressively during exercise at 70% of $\dot{V}_{O_2max}$, and the point of exhaustion coincides with the time when the muscle glycogen is almost completely depleted. This is certainly true of exercise carried out in cool or temperate conditions, but may not apply in warm weather when there seems to be plenty of glycogen left in the muscles at the point of fatigue. The decline in the muscle glycogen content is paralleled by its decreased contribution to energy provision (Fig. 2.3). The rate of energy production is maintained by a corresponding increase in the oxidation of free fatty acids, which are taken up from the plasma. As exercise progresses, the plasma free fatty acid concentration rises due to an increased rate of breakdown of triglyceride in the adipose tissue. This is a result of an increase in the circulating level of catecholamines (adrenaline and noradrenaline), which stimulate the process of lipolysis, and a decrease in the

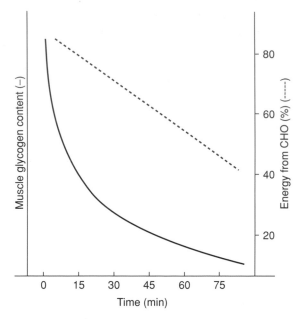

Fig. 2.3 Changes in muscle glycogen content and in the contribution of carbohydrate to energy metabolism in prolonged exercise.

circulating level of insulin, which inhibits lipolysis. The rate at which muscle uses fatty acids is determined largely by their availability, so the increased plasma concentration has the effect of causing the muscle to use more fat. This increased rate of fat oxidation has the effect of reducing CHO oxidation by the muscle, so it seems to be the increased supply of fatty acids rather than the falling glycogen concentration which shifts the muscle's choice of fuel towards fat.

In prolonged cycling exercise at about 70% of $\dot{V}_{O_2max}$, fatigue is generally associated with the depletion of glycogen in the quadriceps muscles. Once this point is reached, the individual is unable to continue working at the same exercise intensity, although it is possible to continue if the work intensity is reduced. Fat oxidation, even though supplemented by the oxidation of glucose derived from the blood, is unable to support the desired rate of energy production. A good example is the marathon runner who "hits the wall": fat oxidation can supply enough energy for a walking pace, but running pace is not possible without a supply of carbohydrate.

In some situations, the output of glucose by the liver fails to keep pace with the rate of utilization by muscle, and the blood glucose concentration begins to fall. Although a low blood glucose level (hypoglycemia, usually defined as a blood glucose concentration of less than 2.5 mmol·l^{-1}) is not in itself usually the factor limiting exercise performance, it is essential that the supply of glucose to the brain is maintained.

The metabolic response to exercise is influenced by many factors, some of which have important implications for performance. The need for glycogen to be available as a fuel when exercise of moderately high intensity is performed means that the athlete engaged in endurance training must ensure an adequate dietary intake of CHO. The body does not have the metabolic capacity to convert its fat stores to CHO. If the muscle glycogen is not replaced between training sessions, the muscle will be forced to rely on fat as a fuel; although the muscle will adapt by increasing its capacity to oxidize fat, it will not be possible to sustain the training intensity and performance will deteriorate. In competition, where the role of CHO is even more crucial, increasing the muscle glycogen content by consumption of a high-CHO diet will increase endurance capacity. The need to ensure an adequate muscle glycogen store prior to competition is well recognized in some sports, such as marathon running, but many sportsmen pay little attention to this aspect of their preparation for competition.

Summary

Muscle metabolism is fueled by a variety of substrates, according to the intensity and duration of exercise, and the characteristics of the athlete's preparation and environment. Limitations to exercise metabolism include inadequate supplies of substrates that can provide the muscle fiber with a sufficiently rapid supply of energy. In future chapters in this book, dietary strategies aimed at enhancing the availability of muscle substrates will be discussed. Although the major focus is on practices to enhance the availability of muscle CHO availability (see Chapters 7, 8, & 9), other strategies include enhancement of the muscle creatine phosphate content (Chapter 12) or the muscle's ability to utilize the considerable stores of body fat (Chapter 12). These strategies will form the key planks of an athlete's sports nutrition plan, and must be adapted to suit the specific physiological needs and practical opportunities of the athlete's training and competition schedule.

Reading list

Bangsbo, J., Gollnick, P.D., Graham, T.E., Juel, C., Kiens, B., Mizuno, M. & Saltin, B. (1990) Anaerobic energy production and O$_2$ deficit–debt relationships during exhaustive exercise in humans. *Journal of Physiology* **422**, 539–559.

Bergstrom, J., Hermansen, L., Hultman, E. & Saltin, B. (1967) Diet, muscle glycogen and physical performance. *Acta Physiologica Scandinavica* **71**, 140–150.

Boobis, L.H. (1987) Metabolic aspects of fatigue during sprinting. In: *Exercise: Benefits, Limits and Adaptations* (eds D. Macleod, R. Maughan, M. Nimmo, T. Reilly & C. Williams), pp. 116–140. E. & F.N. Spon, London.

Cain, D.F. & Davies, R.E. (1962) Breakdown of adenosine triphosphate during a single contraction of working muscle. *Biochemistry and Biophysics Research Communications* **8**, 361–366.

Hirvonen, J., Rehunen, S., Rusko, H. & Härkönen, M. (1987) Breakdown of high-energy phosphate compounds and lactate accumulation during short supramaximal exercise. *European Journal of Applied Physiology* **56**, 253–259.

Hultman, E., Bergstrom, J. & Anderson, N.M. (1967) Breakdown and resynthesis of phosphorylcreatine and adenosine triphosphate in connection with muscular work in man. *Scandinavian Journal of Clinical and Laboratory Investigation* **19**, 56–66.

Hultman, E., Spriet, L.L. & Söderlund, K. (1987) Energy metabolism and fatigue in working muscle. In: *Exercise: Benefits, Limits and Adaptations* (eds D. Macleod, R. Maughan, M. Nimmo, T. Reilly & C. Williams), pp. 63–80. E. & F.N. Spon, London.

Nilsson, L.H. (1973) Liver glycogen content in man in the postabsorptive state. *Scandinavian Journal of Clinical and Laboratory Investigation* **32**, 317–323.

Noakes, T.D. (1985) *Lore of Running*. Cape Town, Oxford.

EXPERT COMMENT 1 Muscle fiber types and fuel use. Mike Gleeson

Human muscles contain fibers with different contractile and metabolic characteristics, ranging from those with high oxidative capacity (slow-twitch Type I fibers) to those with substantially lower oxidative capacity, but higher glycolytic capacity and slightly higher content of glycogen and phosphocreatine (fast-twitch Type II fibers). Type I fibers are slower contracting than Type II fibers due to the lower activity of myosin ATPase in the Type I fibers. The recruitment pattern of the different fiber types is influenced by both exercise intensity and duration. At low to moderate exercise intensities (e.g. in cycling and running), the Type I fibers are the first to be activated and are kept activated at even higher exercise intensities. With increasing rates of work, there is a recruitment of the fast-twitch motor units, with recruitment of Type IIa fibers being followed by Type IIb. It is believed that fibers of all types are recruited at exercise intensities demanding more than about 80% of the maximum oxygen uptake ($\dot{V}_{O_{2max}}$). During very prolonged submaximal exercise, there is a time-dependent increase in the recruitment of Type II fibers, which appears to be related to the need to replace the power contribution from Type I fibers as the latter fatigue due to glycogen depletion.

Because the pattern of recruitment of Type I and Type II fibers is different during exercise and also because the metabolic capacities of the fiber types are different, the proportion of the different fiber types in the locomotor muscles will influence the metabolic response to exercise. For example, if we were to measure the depletion of glycogen content in different fiber types after 60 min of exercise at about 70% $\dot{V}_{O_{2max}}$, then we would see that glycogen content has fallen substantially in most Type I fibers, but that relatively large amounts still remain in the Type II

fibers. We can put this down to the fact that relatively few Type II fibers will have been recruited at this moderate exercise intensity. In contrast, if we were to look at what happens after 10 min exercise at 90% $\dot{V}_{O_{2max}}$, then we would see that glycogen depletion is now greater in the Type II fibers than in the Type I fibers (although, even at exhaustion, the glycogen content remaining in both fiber types is substantial). In the latter situation, both fiber types are recruited, but the activity of phosphorylase (the enzyme that breaks down glycogen) is much higher in the Type II fibers. The relatively higher rate of glycolysis and lower oxidative capacity in the Type II fibers results in a higher rate of lactate production in these fibers. In the Type II fibers there will also have been a greater contribution to ATP resynthesis from phosphocreatine breakdown than in the Type I fibers. One consequence of these differences is that the Type II fibers fatigue more rapidly than the Type I fibers.

Different individuals can possess quite different fiber type compositions in the muscles they predominantly use in the exercise activity. For example, elite sprinters are commonly found to have at least 60% Type II fibers in their leg muscles, whereas in elite marathon runners around 80–90% of their leg muscle fibers may be Type I. It follows that if two individuals with the same $\dot{V}_{O_{2max}}$, and same leg muscle mass, but very different fiber type compositions, run at the same relative submaximal exercise intensity (say 75% $\dot{V}_{O_{2max}}$), the metabolic responses will not be exactly the same. The individual with the higher proportion of Type I fibers will oxidize more fat, use up less muscle glycogen, and produce less lactate. Given this information, you should be able to work out which individual to put your money on in a contest of endurance if you know their muscle fiber composition.

Athlete

Dede was a heptathlete participating in national and international meets. Her status in the sport qualified her to participate in a USA Track and Field Development Program for elite heptathletes. She started the development program at the age of 24, was 180 cm in height, weighed 76 kg and had 17% body fat measured by dual energy X-ray absorptiometry. Her goal was to qualify for the US Olympic heptathlon team.

Reason for consultancy

Dede had attended the annual development program summit meetings for 6 years. At the start of the development program, Dede had minimal interest in dietary advice and considered her eating patterns to be adequate. Prior to each meeting she completed 4 days of training diet records and a questionnaire regarding eating practices during training and at competitions. At the summit meetings Dede attended the group nutrition education session and had an individual consultation. On one such occasion she decided to actively seek some specific advice. This was precipitated by a recognition that her training program was not being optimized. Dede now trained 6 days a week and was finding it difficult to recover between morning and afternoon training sessions and to maintain energy levels for her strength training workouts.

Existing dietary patterns

Dede completed a workout each morning from 7.30 to 9.30 AM, without eating anything before the session. She ate breakfast around 10 AM and lunch at noon, about 2 h before her afternoon workout. Three days a week she did a weight training workout between breakfast and lunch. Dinner was eaten after the evening workout, around 6 PM, followed by snacks during the evening. Dede made an effort to drink fluids throughout the day. She did not take any vitamin supplements. A typical day's eating plan is listed below.

Professional assessment

Mean daily intake from this self-reported eating plan was assessed to be ~ 10 500 kJ (2500 kcal); 314 g carbohydrate (4.1 g·kg body mass^{-1}); 119 g protein (1.6 g·kg BM^{-1}); 86 g fat (31% of energy). These eating patterns failed to provide the dietary reference intake (DRI) for calcium (reported intake estimated at 780 mg·day^{-1} vs. goal of 1000 mg) and were low in dietary fiber intake (14 g·day^{-1} vs. DRI of 20–30 g). Dede's reported energy intake was ~ 2100 kJ (500 kcal) below the estimated level for her energy needs, although this problem may be partly explained by under-reporting on food records. Although her intake of protein met the guidelines for an athlete undertaking heavy training, her intake of carbohydrate was well below the targets suggested for refueling between daily training sessions (5–7+ g·kg^{-1}). In particular, Dede's intake of fruits and vegetables was well below the recommended daily intake. Although food intake was spread over the day, more attention could be focused on promoting a good fuel supply for each of her daily training sessions, as well as her multi-event competition schedule.

Intervention

The following suggestions were made to increase her daily carbohydrate and fiber intake, and to meet the DRI for calcium. The timing of carbohydrate intake was specifically organized to promote fuel intake before, during, and after training sessions. This pattern would also be useful in the competition setting.

1 Eat a carbohydrate-rich snack before the morning training session—for example, fruit juice and a breakfast/cereal bar, or cereal or yoghurt.

2 Add a piece of fruit to breakfast, and to snacks eaten in the evening.

3 Add salad to lunch—for example as extra sandwich fillings.

4 Choose wholegrain breads and breakfast cereal.

5 Encourage fluid intake over the day, and during training sessions. Use a sports drink to provide fuel during the training session.

6 Consider a snack straight after the morning training session—fruit-flavored yoghurt and cereal bar or fruit, if unable to go straight to lunch.

Outcome

Dede failed to make selection for the 1996 Olympic team. However, she took notice when a successful team member provided a testimonial in the post-Olympic summit meeting about the positive effects of following the dietary advice provided in a previous development program. Subsequently she set to work on improving her own eating patterns in the following years. She increased her daily energy intake to ~ 13 400 kJ (3200 kcal), principally by increasing her intake of fruits and carbohydrate-rich snacks eaten before and after training sessions. She was reluctant to increase her intake of vegetables or switch permanently to wholegrain cereal choices. However, she took a multivitamin mineral supplement to better look after her vitamin needs, and improved her fiber intake to ~ 30 g·day^{-1}. Overall her meal spacing and fluid intake were improved. This assisted her to train with greater energy and attention to skill. Her body mass gradually increased to 80 kg, without a change in body fat levels, as her muscle mass increased through consistent attention to her strength training program. In her final year in the development program she qualified for the US heptathlon team for the 2000 Olympic Games.

Breakfast	Lunch	Dinner	Snacks
1.5 cups sugared breakfast cereal with 1% fat milk	Tuna sandwich One oatmeal raisin cookie	1.5 cups sugared breakfast with 1% fat milk 250-g steak $^{1}/_{2}$ cup macaroni and cheese One or two vegetables	Three oatmeal raisin cookies Half a glass of 1% fat milk

Chapter 3
Protein and amino acid requirements of athletes

Introduction

Foods with a high protein content have long been seen as a natural part of the diet of athletes, and the idea that a high-protein diet will help the athlete prepare for competition is an attractive one. Our understanding of the role of protein in exercise has changed dramatically over the last few centuries, ranging from the belief that it was the major fuel for muscle contraction (encouraging the intake of large amounts of protein by athletes) to the belief that exercise does not change the body's need for protein (distracting scientists from being interested in protein). This chapter will consider the recent evidence for special requirements of protein and amino acids arising from high-level exercise as well as the ability of athletes to meet these demands from their typical eating patterns.

General overview of protein metabolism

Amino acids are a family of chemicals with a common structure that includes an amine ($-NH_2$) group and a carboxyl ($-COOH$) group. A total of 20 different amino acids are present in the body. A 70-kg athlete typically has a body pool of ~ 12 kg of amino acids, with the vast majority of this existing in the form of protein (amino acid polymers) and a small amount (about 200 g) existing as free amino acids. Over the day, there is a constant process of protein turnover, with protein breakdown and protein synthesis occurring simultaneously, and amino acids continuously exchanging between the various amino acid pools. Skeletal muscle accounts for the largest reservoir of body protein as well as a significant proportion of the free amino acid pool. All body proteins have structural roles (e.g. skin) or functional and regulatory roles (e.g. enzymes and hormones), and most serve both roles.

Figure 3.1 summarizes daily protein turnover. New amino acids can enter the free amino acid pool from three sources—from dietary intake, from the breakdown of body protein, and from new synthesis within the body. Some amino acids cannot be manufactured within the body and must be recycled from body protein or consumed as dietary sources. These are known as the essential amino acids (see Table 3.1). On the other hand, amino acids leave the free amino acid pool via secretion into the gut, incorporation into new proteins, oxidation as a fuel source, or incorporation into body fat or carbohydrate stores. There is a huge amount of cycling between body pools and net changes can reflect a change in breakdown rates as well as a change in synthesis rates. In general, however, there is a limited capacity to store new proteins, and protein intake in excess of requirements is deaminated, with the nitrogen being incorporated into urea and excreted primarily in the urine, and the carbon skeleton being oxidized or stored as fat or carbohydrate.

Although the overall structure of the body is fairly stable, many of the component tissue proteins

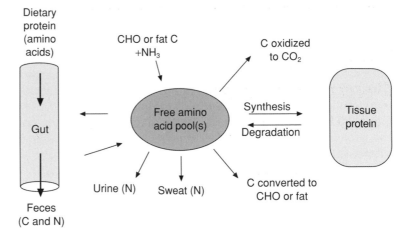

Fig. 3.1 Simplified diagram of protein metabolism. Nitrogen status (balance) measures involve quantifying the difference between nitrogen intake and excretion, while protein turnover measures estimate the various processes involved in protein synthesis and degradation.

Table 3.1 Essential and non-essential amino acids: these essential amino acids cannot be synthesized and must be supplied in adequate amounts in the diet.

Essential	Non-essential
Isoleucine	Alanine
Leucine	Arginine
Lysine	Asparagine
Methionine	Aspartate
Phenylalanine	Cysteine
Threonine	Glutamate
Tryptophan	Glutamine
Valine	Glycine
	Histidine
	Proline
	Serine
	Tyrosine

have a relatively short life span in the body. Most structural proteins and enzymes are synthesized and degraded at high rates, and as much as 20% of the basal rate of energy expenditure is the result of protein turnover. This process is obviously important in the repair of damaged tissue and in wound healing, but is also an ongoing process in healthy tissue.

The half-life of some proteins is extremely short—less than 1 h for some enzymes in the liver. Changes in the amount of these enzymes is an important factor in the control of their activity, and a high rate of turnover is therefore essential if the tissue is to be responsive to changes in metabolic requirements. In the liver, a high rate of turnover of the enzymes that regulate fuel homeostasis allows regulation to occur rapidly in response to feeding and to short-term fasting. Some proteins are much more stable, with half-lives measured in days and weeks rather than hours. Skeletal muscle adapts to training and detraining with a time course that can be measured in days, giving some indication of the rate of turnover of the enzymes involved in the process of adaptation.

Measuring protein turnover

The classical way to measure net protein turnover is to monitor the balance between the nitrogen consumed (from dietary protein) and the nitrogen excreted (mostly in urine). A positive nitrogen status (intake is greater than excretion) signals that there is a net gain of body protein, while negative nitrogen status signals a net loss of body protein. A long-term negative status should be avoided since it means that the body is losing protein that would otherwise have a structural or functional role. Unlike the case for fat and carbohydrate, the body has little capacity to store protein simply as an energy reserve. Positive nitrogen status, representing a gain in body protein, occurs during growth and pregnancy, but is also desired by athletes who wish to increase their muscle mass to enhance their size and strength. Unfortunately, reliable measurements of nitrogen balance are difficult and expensive to achieve. There is generally an overestimation of nitrogen status because there is a trend to overestimate nitrogen intake (the true amount absorbed from food) and to fail to collect total nitrogen losses (in sloughed skin, sweat, feces, etc.). There are also some discrepancies in the calculation and assumptions of nitrogen balance, which are affected by energy balance, and appear to take time to equilibrate when there is a change to a very high or very low protein intake. Data from existing nitrogen balance studies therefore need to be examined with care.

Metabolic tracer techniques offer a newer way to monitor protein turnover. Here, individual amino acids are "labeled" and their uptake, oxidation, or incorporation into various amino acid/protein pools can be tracked. The benefits of this new knowledge must also be balanced against problems such as expense, and some doubts as to the validity of various assumptions. For example, it may not be suitable to assume that the behavior of a single amino acid reflects the fate of all amino acids or total body protein pools. Nevertheless this technique has greatly added to our understanding of protein metabolism during and after exercise.

The effect of exercise on protein metabolism

Muscles consist largely of protein (although water is the largest component, accounting for about 75% of the total mass), and the functional properties of the muscles depend on their protein composition. It is also readily apparent that regular exercise has a number of highly specific effects on the body's protein metabolism. Strength training results in increases in muscle mass, indicating an increased formation of actin and myosin, and it is tempting to assume that this process is dependent on protein availability. Endurance training has little effect on muscle mass, but does increase the muscle content of mitochondrial proteins, especially those involved in oxidative metabolism. Hard exercise also results in an increased level of muscle damage, usually at the microscopic level, and there is clearly a role for protein in the repair and recovery processes.

The changes that comprise the adaptive response to exercise are selective, and are specific to the training stimulus. They are also dependent on the availability of an adequate intake of protein in the diet, but apparently cannot be accelerated by increasing protein intake above normal levels. Exercise also has a number of acute effects on protein metabolism, and the response to a hard bout of exercise represents a challenge to the muscle that is similar in many ways to the responses that follow infection or injury.

Effects of an acute bout of exercise on protein metabolism

Skeletal muscle has the capacity to metabolize a number of amino acids, particularly the branched-chain amino acids leucine, isoleucine, and valine. This includes the degradation of the branched-chain acids to form the chemical intermediates that take part in the tricarboxylic acid (TCA) cycle of oxidative metabolism. Although the majority of substrate used to fuel submaximal exercise comes from fat and carbohydrate stores, there is a small contribution from protein sources (3–6%) to the total energy cost of the exercise bout. This can be tracked directly by measuring the oxidation of a specific amino acid, typically leucine, or indirectly by measuring plasma urea concentrations. Such measurements typically show that the rate of leucine oxidation increases with the intensity and duration of exercise, and is greater in situations of glycogen depletion or low carbohydrate availability. Thus protein metabolism during bouts of prolonged endurance exercise is affected by the type of exercise and the dietary strategies used by the athlete. There are concerns, however, that the use of leucine as a tracer may not represent the overall rate of amino acid oxidation. The effects of protein ingestion following a bout of endurance exercise on protein synthesis has not been well studied, largely because of the limitations of the methodology. It appears that the response varies according to the intensity of the exercise, but may also vary according to the protein subfraction—for example, the responses of the mitochondrial proteins may be different from those of muscle fiber proteins.

By contrast, resistance training does not appear to increase leucine oxidation, perhaps reflecting the fact that such high-intensity exercise is fueled by non-oxidative pathways using high-energy phosphate and glycogen sources. Studies using new techniques have been able to monitor fractional rates of muscle protein breakdown and synthesis in response to resistance training. During the hours following the bout of exercise, there is an increase in protein breakdown but also an increase in protein synthesis. If subjects exercise but remain fasted, the net effect is catabolic (breakdown is greater than synthesis), but less negative than with fasting alone. In other words, resistance training helps to enhance protein status or reduce the catabolic state achieved by fasting and rest. However, when subjects consume a source of protein containing essential amino acids (~ 7 g essential amino acids or ~ 20 g high-quality protein) and a substantial source of carbohydrate (~ 50–100 g), there is a net anabolic effect (synthesis exceeds breakdown). This interaction occurs when the protein–carbohydrate feeding occurs after exercise, but according to very recent research, it may be even more pronounced when the feeding occurs immediately before the resistance training bout. These new data show potentially exciting ideas for sports nutrition strategies, but it must be remembered that these studies deal with the microresponse to an acute bout of exercise. We have yet to find evidence that the immediate muscle protein response to exercise is extended beyond the first few hours or will lead to a significant improvement in muscle size and strength in the long term.

Chronic effects of exercise on protein metabolism—the effect of training

The outcome of a training program is the result of the cumulative effects of a series of workouts. The net effect of a resistance training program is an increase in muscle size and strength, resulting from the series of transient increases in muscle protein balance following each exercise session. After the first few months or years of such a program, however, there is usually little further change in muscle mass. Endurance exercise appears to stimulate increases in mitochondrial proteins, but again, there is little change in muscle mass, and there may even be a decrease in the total muscle protein content.

There is some evidence that repeated bouts of exercise cause an adaptation to the protein response to exercise. For example, studies show that experienced strength training athletes achieve nitrogen balance at lower protein intakes than novice trainers. Further studies are needed to confirm these findings and translate them into protein requirements for athletes. It is likely that protein requirements are elevated at the onset of a training program or after a sudden increase in training volume and intensity, but that this increase in requirement is transient.

Recommendations for protein intakes by athletes

The requirement for dietary protein is influenced in part by the type of protein that is consumed. The body has an absolute requirement for nitrogen in the form of the amino groups that make up part of the structure of amino acids, and these can be used in the manufacture of the non-essential amino acids. The essential amino acids, which cannot be synthesized by humans, must be obtained from the diet. Different proteins contain different proportions of the various amino acids, and each of the essential amino acids must be supplied in an amount that meets the needs. In general, foods from animal sources contain substantial amounts of all the essential amino acids, but foods from other sources do not generally contain these amino acids in the same proportions as are found in animal tissues. However, various foods from plant sources can combine with each other to "complement" the amino acid profile of the total meal (see Table 3.2). Vegetarian eaters need to plan menus to achieve such mixing and matching of foods, although it is now recognized that this can occur over a day rather than at the same meal.

The protein requirements of the general population have been the subject of extensive investigation, and it is now generally accepted that a daily requirement of about 0.6 g of protein per kilogram body mass per day will meet the needs of most of the adult population, provided that a variety of different protein sources make up the diet and that the energy intake of the diet is adequate to

Type	Examples
Dairy products	Milk, yoghurt
Eggs	Boiled eggs, omelet
Meat and meat products	Steak, ham
Poultry	Chicken, turkey
Fish	Tinned salmon, fish fillets
Grains plus legumes	Mexican beans and rice, peanut butter sandwich, cereal with soy milk
Grains plus nuts or seeds	Muesli mix with cashews and oats, almonds in rice salad
Legumes plus nuts or seeds	Trail mix with peanuts
Grains plus dairy products	Cheese sandwich, yoghurt on breakfast cereal
Legumes plus dairy products	Milk-based pea soup

Table 3.2 Protein-containing foods or combinations that will supply all the essential amino acids in adequate amounts.

Population	Recommended protein intake ($g \cdot kg^{-1} \cdot day^{-1}$)
Sedentary populations	
Children	1.0
Adolescents	1.0–1.5
Adults	0.8–1.0
Pregnant women	+ 6–10 $g \cdot day^{-1}$
Breastfeeding women	+ 12–16 $g \cdot day^{-1}$
Athletic populations	
Recreational athletes	0.8–1.0
(four or five times a week for 30 min)	
Endurance training athletes	1.2–1.6
moderate intensity	1.2
extreme volume (e.g. cycling tour)	1.6
Resistance training athletes	1.2–1.7
novice	1.5–1.7
steady state	1.0–1.2
Adolescent athletes during growth spurt	1.5

Table 3.3 Recommended daily intakes for protein in various populations.

meet the energy expenditure. Protein requirements are increased during times of growth such as adolescence and pregnancy. Nutrition experts in various countries have interpreted these results into a range of recommended daily allowances or intakes, with some differences between countries due to differences in the way that the safety margin has added to the daily requirement. Table 3.3 summarizes the general recommendations made for various groups of sedentary people.

It is now recognized that protein requirements are increased by exercise, but few countries have included special recommendations for the protein requirements of athletes in their dietary recommendations. The exception appears to be the Dutch Nutrition Board which has set a specific guideline that physically active individuals should achieve a protein intake of 1.5 $g \cdot kg^{-1} \cdot day^{-1}$—well above the intake recommended for the sedentary population. Despite the lack of official recommendations, experts in sports nutrition have interpreted the result of various nitrogen balance studies to produce some guidelines for protein intakes by various athletic groups. These are also included in Table 3.3. These guidelines represent a departure from the early views of sports scientists, but they fail to meet the enthusiasm of many resistance training athletes who feel that optimal gains in muscle mass and strength are achieved only with very large intakes of protein (see Expert Comment 1).

Is there a need for high-protein diets and protein supplements?

If athletes have increased requirements for protein compared to their sedentary counterparts, it is tempting to consider that high-protein diets and special protein supplements are needed. However, an athlete's energy intake provides the factor that underpins their success in meeting many of their nutrition goals. With a moderate to high energy budget, high protein intakes can be achieved even within the boundaries of the typical ratios of protein in Western eating patterns. The following examples illustrate this point.

From a diet containing 12–15% of energy from protein:

70-kg athlete (typical male)
   12 MJ (3000 cal) = 90–112 g protein = 1.3–1.6 g·kg^{-1}
   20 MJ (5000 cal) = 150–188 g protein = 2.1–2.7 g·kg^{-1}
60-kg athlete (typical female)
   8 MJ (2000 cal) = 60–75 g protein = 1–1.3 g·kg^{-1}
   12 MJ (3000 cal) = 90–112 g protein = 1.5–1.9 g·kg^{-1}.

Thus, even without focusing on protein-rich foods or expensive protein products, most athletes have the potential to meet their protein requirement. Special dietary advice and menu planning may be needed to help some athletes meet these needs within their overall sports nutrition goals (see Chapter 13). This will be especially important for athletes with restricted energy budgets, limited finances, or practical constraints on eating.

Recommendations about timing of protein intake

Recent attention has focused on the timing of protein intake in relation to training rather than on the amount required. In the recovery period, muscle glycogen synthesis is a priority, but synthesis of new proteins should perhaps be seen as being of equal or even greater importance. Because little attention has been paid to this area until recently, we do not yet know how dietary or other factors may be manipulated to influence these processes. The supply of essential amino acids and the hormonal environment are the two obvious factors that may be important. Nutritional status can influence the circulating concentration of a number of hormones that have anabolic properties, the most obvious and important example being insulin. The diet can also supply amino acids for incorporation into proteins. A fall in the intracellular amino acid concentration will restrict the rate of protein synthesis, and there is some evidence that the muscle amino acid concentration does fall after exercise. Ingestion of protein or amino acids immediately after exercise, and even before exercise, can promote muscle protein synthesis, but no long-term studies have yet been conducted to establish whether these effects result in an improved adaptation of the muscle to the training stimulus. These ideas are discussed in more detail in Chapters 9 and 13.

Protein intakes of athletes

There have been a large number of studies of protein intake in different athletic groups, using a variety of different methods of assessment. These studies have found a wide range of values for the habitual protein intakes reported by athletes within groups and between groups. The general finding is, as predicted from the examples above, that athletes typically ingest sufficient protein to meet their needs, provided that adequate energy and a variety of different foods is consumed.

Notwithstanding the differences between and within groups, there are some interesting trends in the protein intakes reported by athletes. Mean protein intakes of groups of male endurance and team athletes are generally ~ 90–150 g per day, providing 12–16% of energy intake and an intake of 1.2–2.0 g·kg^{-1}·day^{-1}. Groups of female endurance and team athletes generally report a lower mean intake of protein: ~ 60–90 g per day, representing 1.1–1.7 g·kg^{-1}·day^{-1}. Lower intakes of protein are generally due to lower energy intakes rather than a lower contribution of protein to total energy intake. Protein intakes reported by strength training athletes are generally higher in absolute amounts, and in terms of the percentage contribution to energy intake—daily intakes of 150–250 g of protein, representing 14–20% of energy, are common. Sometimes, however, because of the large body size of these athletes, protein intakes expressed per kg body mass are similar to or even lower than those reported by endurance athletes. Very high values for protein intake are sometimes encountered, especially in body builders. Individual values as high as 4.0 g·kg^{-1}·day^{-1} have been reported in the precompetition period, providing 30–60% of total energy intake.

Concerns as to the adequacy of protein intake are generally found in athletes with low energy intakes. However, athletes who follow extreme dietary practices or restricted eating may also have a low protein intake. This is particularly the case with athletes who consume a diet extremely high in carbohydrate. Because of the common association between protein and fat in the diet, attempts to eliminate fat from the diet will often result in severe reductions in protein intake. Some distance runners habitually eat diets containing 85% carbohydrate: inadequacies of both essential fatty acids and the essential amino acids must be a real possibility in this situation. This is also the case for athletes with disordered eating practices who consume so-called vegetarian diets, which are really badly constructed diets in which animal protein is avoided but not replaced with suitable plant protein sources. Athletes whose diets are restricted in terms of energy, variety, or budget may need counseling in food choices to ensure that their protein requirements are met, but the use of high-protein supplements is seldom or never justified. Being a vegetarian or a vegan is in no way incompatible with success in sport, and many elite athletes, especially in endurance sports, eat a diet from which animal products are largely or even completely absent (see Chapter 13).

The recognition that the protein requirements of youngsters are higher, on a body mass basis, than those of adults, raises some special concerns as to the adequacy of dietary protein intake in the adolescent athlete. Published studies suggest that most young athletes achieve a dietary protein intake of about 1.6 g·kg^{-1}·day^{-1}, and that even in those sports where energy intake is commonly restricted there is no good evidence of an inadequate intake. It is equally clear, however, that there is a limited amount of information available on the protein requirements of the growing athlete who is engaged in intensive training: it is possible that there are substantial increases in the requirement during periods of rapid growth, as during the adolescent growth spurt. Special attention must be paid to the dietary intake of athletes who are training hard at this time, especially in sports where restriction of energy intake is commonly practiced to reduce or restrict body fat mass (e.g. gymnastics). Where energy, and especially carbohydrate, intake is inadequate, protein oxidation by the exercising muscles is increased, so the adequacy of protein intake cannot be considered independently of the overall diet.

Are very high protein intakes harmful?

Excess protein in the diet is not beneficial, but neither is it normally harmful as the excess amino acids will be used as an energy source and the nitrogen and sulphur content excreted. Although many people are concerned about possible harmful effects of the excess nitrogen on the kidneys, there is no evidence of any harmful effects in normal individuals even when extremely high intakes are sustained over prolonged periods. Anyone with a history of liver problems or impaired renal function, however, should be advised to take care to ensure that the handling capacity of these tissues is not exceeded. Possibly the most common problem associated with high protein intakes is the unnecessary expense. Since protein-rich foods, particularly from animal sources, are often among the most costly items in a shopping basket, athletes may be spending their sometimes limited resources on unnecessary food choices. Of particular concern is the expense of protein supplements including products supplying individual amino acids. While some sports foods or supplements may be useful to meet sports nutrition goals when everyday foods are impractical to consume, there is rarely a need to supply protein sources alone. Rather, multinutrient foods and sports foods are generally a lower-cost option that meets a range of sports nutrition goals. These ideas are covered in more detail in Chapters 12 and 13.

Reading list

Lemon, P.W.R. (2000) Effects of exercise on protein metabolism. In: *Nutrition in Sport* (ed. R.J. Maughan), pp. 133–152. Blackwell Science, Oxford.

Tarnopolsky, M. (2000) Protein and amino acid needs for training and bulking up. In: *Clinical Sports Nutrition* (eds L. Burke & V. Deakin), pp. 90–123. McGraw-Hill, Sydney, Australia.

Tipton, K.D. & Wolfe, R.R. (2001) Exercise, protein metabolism and muscle growth. *International Journal of Sports Medicine and Exercise Metabolism* **11**, 109–132.

Wagenmakers, A.J.M. (2000) Amino acid metabolism in exercise. In: *Nutrition in Sport* (ed. R.J. Maughan), pp. 119–132. Blackwell Science, Oxford.

EXPERT COMMENT 1 Is there really a case for very high protein intakes by athletes? Peter W.R. Lemon

For most of the 20th century scientists generally agreed that protein needs are largely unaffected by exercise. This opinion appears to have arisen from several early studies indicating that carbohydrate and fat contributed most of the fuel for muscle contraction. As a result, the vast majority of exercise metabolic studies during the first three-quarters of the 20th century ignored protein and focused on these two macronutrients. However, beginning in the 1970s a few published studies on prolonged moderate-intensity (endurance) exercise suggested that protein may contribute as much as 10% of exercise fuel, and since then more have followed. Apparently, exercise protein use is inversely related to carbohydrate availability. Consequently, dietary carbohydrate is critical for endurance athletes not only because it is a major exercise fuel source but also because it spares valuable muscle protein toward the later stages of prolonged exercise efforts when carbohydrate stores become very low. If dietary protein is inadequate this increased protein use during exercise could impair muscle recovery, reduce muscle size and function, and perhaps with time even affect health adversely. Based on studies utilizing a variety of measurement techniques (including nitrogen balance and metabolic tracers), regular endurance exercise training appears to increase dietary protein need by about 40–75%. This means that the recommended protein intake for most endurance athletes should be about 1.1–1.4 g per kilogram body mass per day. Interestingly, most dietary surveys indicate this intake of protein is common for endurance athletes. Therefore, it appears one can consume adequate protein by altering food selections without relying on special supplementation.

For the other end of the exercise continuum—heavy resistance (strength) exercise—dietary protein needs are even greater (protein intake recommendations of 1.5–1.8 $g \cdot kg^{-1} \cdot day^{-1}$). The mechanism of increased need here has little to do with exercise fuel use but rather involves providing the necessary amino acids to facilitate the increased muscle protein synthetic rate stimulated by this type of exercise. Although lower protein intakes will reduce muscle size and strength gains there is little good evidence that protein intakes of more than 1.8 $g \cdot kg^{-1} \cdot day^{-1}$ will provide any further stimulation. Nonetheless, most strength/power athletes are convinced that much more dietary protein is advantageous and many consume diets that contain more than 2.5 $g \cdot kg^{-1} \cdot day^{-1}$. More scientific study of these very high protein intakes is necessary because they could be beneficial for other reasons. For example, some other factor present in meat/fish when combined with regular strength training could enhance protein synthesis above that seen with training alone. Possible candidates include creatine, conjugated linoleic acid, specific amino acids, or some other, as yet unknown, constituent. If so, this could explain the differing opinions of the athletes and the scientists.

Finally, although adverse effects of high protein intakes are often suspected, few data support these claims, especially when intakes are less than 2.0 $g \cdot kg^{-1} \cdot day^{-1}$. Potential risks arising from very high intakes of protein include stress on the kidneys to excrete the additional nitrogen load, as well as the additional loss of body water in this process. Of course, challenges to hydration occur in most sports and can be managed by monitoring losses and matching fluid intake accordingly. Although very high protein intakes are not recommended, even they seem to be handled well by healthy individuals as indicated by the fact that significant renal or other health problems have not surfaced in older body builders who have consumed extremely high protein intakes for, in some cases, more than 20 years. Toxic effects from very high intakes of specific amino acids are also possible, and for this reason, megadoses of these preparations should be avoided.

CASE STUDY 1 Body builder with concerns about protein intake. Melinda M. Manore

Athlete
Pete was a 31-year-old male drug-free bodybuilder, with a considerable training history. Prior to his 5 years as a professional body builder, he had spent 9 years training as an amateur lifter. His immediate focus was an international bodybuilding competition in 8 weeks' time. He weighed 95 kg and did two daily workouts of strength training that rotated muscle groups, with a rest day every 5th day. His aerobic training was minimal.

Reason for consultancy
Pete consulted with a nutritionist for two reasons: (i) he wanted to decrease body fat (current level 9%) to 6% body mass, without losing lean tissue or body mass; and (ii) he was consuming ~ 6300–8400 kJ·day^{-1} (~ 1500–2000 kcal·day^{-1}) of medium-chain triglycerides (MCTs) as a dietary supplement to maintain body weight and was unsure of the health risks of this practice. He had been told that MCTs would help him burn fat.

Existing dietary patterns
Pete ate well, but reported rapid loss of weight if he did not use the MCT supplement and eat large amounts of protein. Pete's dietary goals were to consume a high carbohydrate and protein diet, while eating minimal dietary fat. To achieve these dietary goals, he consumed the same types of foods each day. He ate few processed foods, did not eat out, and prepared all of his meals at home. He avoided eating red meat (personal preference) and simple sugars. He ate large quantities of grains/cereals, vegetables, fruit, lean fish and chicken and egg whites, and moderate amounts of low-fat milk. He supplemented his diet with protein powder, MCTs and micronutrient supplements. A sample daily intake is outlined below.

Professional assessment
Mean daily intake from this self-reported eating plan was assessed to be ~ 20 920 kJ (5000 kcal); 450 g carbohydrate (4.7 g·kg body mass^{-1}); 250 g protein (2.6 g·kg^{-1}); 280 g fat (47% of total energy intake; 22 g·day^{-1} from diet and the rest

from MCTs). The recommended intakes for all micronutrients were met from dietary sources. Pete was assessed to be extremely disciplined, but willing to follow dietary advice.

Intervention
In order to reduce his daily intake of MCTs (by ~ 4200 kJ or 1000 kcal), increase his carbohydrate intake, and modify his protein intake while reducing body fat, the following suggestions were made.

1 Add 1 h of aerobic exercise to the morning or evening workouts to help increase oxidation of body fat. Increase energy intake as necessary to prevent loss of weight or lean tissue loss.

2 Replace ~ 1000 kcal·day^{-1} (4200 kJ) of MCT with glycogen-loading carbohydrate-based products (~ 700–800 kcal·day^{-1}). Make use of these products after morning and afternoon workouts, and use sport drinks to improve carbohydrate intake and replace fluids lost during workouts. Note that additional losses can be expected due to addition of aerobic exercise in program.

3 Stop using the protein powder, since this is an expensive source of protein in a diet that is already well supplied with protein from meat, milk, and egg whites. Replace with a liquid meal supplement, which is a more appropriate product to supply a compact form of energy from both carbohydrate and protein.

4 Stop using the vitamin and mineral supplementation, since dietary sources of micronutrients are easily able to meet recommended intakes.

Outcome
Pete immediately implemented the diet and exercise suggestions; his body mass was maintained but percentage body fat decreased from 9 to 7%. Total energy intake was maintained at ~ 23 000 kJ (5500 kcal·day^{-1}); carbohydrate intake increased (800 g·day^{-1}–8.4 g·kg body mass^{-1}); fat intake decreased to 29% of energy (22 g·day^{-1} from diet; 154 g·day^{-1} from MCT); and protein decreased to ~ 2 g·kg^{-1}. He successfully competed in his event and was happy with his new eating plans.

Breakfast	Mid-morning	Lunch	Mid-afternoon	Dinner
Two large bowls cooked oatmeal with blueberries and skimmed milk	Rice	Large salad (lettuce, tomatoes, green beans, carrots), no-fat dressing	Rice	Brown rice
Six cooked egg whites	2 scoops MCTs	2 tbspn MCTs	Sweet potatoes	Large salad
2 scoops MCTs	Fruit	Baked potato	Sword fish	(similar to lunch)
Protein powder	Vegetables	Egg whites	Vegetables	Baked sword fish
	Egg whites	Two chicken breasts	2 scoops MCTs	Egg whites
				Broccoli
				2 scoops MCTs

Chapter 4
Micronutrients: vitamins and minerals

Introduction

For normal health to be maintained, a wide range of vitamins, minerals, and trace elements must be present in adequate amounts in the body tissues, and the dietary intake must be sufficient to meet the requirement for these micronutrients. Many vitamins and minerals play key roles in energy metabolism or the production of body tissues, and the adverse effect of deficiencies of these components is well recognized and easily demonstrated. Marginal deficiency states may have little effect on the sedentary individual for whom performance is not critical, but small impairments of exercise capacity may have profound consequences for the serious athlete. Regular intense exercise training may also increase micronutrient requirements, either by increasing rates of utilization or by increasing losses from the body. Consequently, athletes are greatly interested in answers to the following questions.

1 To what extent are requirements for micronutrients increased by regular exercise? Should there be special guidelines for intakes of micronutrients by athletes?

2 How should optimal status with regard to micronutrients be measured in athletes? Do athletes have poorer micronutrient status than non-athletes?

3 Do micronutrient intakes above the recommended daily intakes further enhance exercise performance?

This chapter will explore the roles of micronutrients in the health and performance of the athlete, with the focus on situations in which there is a risk of inadequate intake, and the evidence for benefits arising from intakes above recommended daily intakes.

Vitamins

Biological functions of vitamins

Vitamins are organic compounds that are needed by the body in small amounts to enable key reactions of daily living to occur. Since these compounds cannot be manufactured by the body, they must be provided by dietary sources. Table 4.1 summarizes information about the various water-soluble and fat-soluble vitamins, including dietary sources and important biological functions related to physical activity. Many vitamins, particularly from the B group, act as cofactors for reactions involved in energy metabolism—for example, gly-colysis, the tricarboxylic acid cycle, the beta-oxidation of fatty acids, and oxidative phosphorylation. Vitamin C activates an enzyme regulating the synthesis of carnitine, which transports fatty acids into the mitochondria for oxidation. Other B vitamins act as cofactors for the synthesis of heme, which is involved in oxygen transport in blood and muscles. A severe deficiency of these vitamins will interfere

Table 4.1 Major biological functions of the vitamins in exercise. Vitamin K is not included in this table, as no specific role for this vitamin in exercise has been identified.

Vitamin	Metabolic role	Food sources
Fat soluble		
A	Antioxidant function	Liver, dairy products, fish
		Pro-vitamin A (carotenes) found in green, yellow, and orange fruits and vegetables
D	Calcium homeostasis	Butter, fish oils, eggs
E	Antioxidant, prevention of free radical damage	Nuts, seeds, vegetable oils, margarine
Water soluble		
Thiamin (B_1)	Carbohydrate metabolism	Breakfast cereals and bread, yeast extracts, liver
Riboflavin (B_2)	Mitochondrial electron transport (as FAD)	Dairy products, breakfast cereals and bread, yeast extracts, liver
Niacin (B_3)	Multiple metabolic pathways (as NAD and NADP)	Meats and dairy products, breakfast cereals and breads, yeast extract
Pyridoxine (B_6)	Amino acid synthesis	Protein-rich foods, wholegrain cereals and breads, bananas
Folate	Red blood cell synthesis	Green leafy vegetables, oranges, liver
		Breakfast cereals and breads
Pantothenic acid	Oxidative metabolism (as CoA)	Widely distributed in food
Biotin	Biosynthetic reactions	Liver, meat, egg yolks, nuts
B_{12} (cyanocobalamin)	Red blood cell synthesis	Animal foods
Ascorbic acid (C)	Antioxidant, catecholamine synthesis, tissue repair	Citrus, tropical, and berry fruits, tomatoes, green leafy vegetables

with the activity of these enzymes, and therefore reduce body function and health. Indeed, most of the vitamins were first recognized because of the deficiency syndromes that result when they are not present in the diet in adequate amounts. Marginal deficiency states may have a small impact on function, which is barely noticed by sedentary individuals, but of critical importance for high-performance athletes for whom success is decided by fractions of seconds and meters. Various depletion studies have shown that inadequate vitamin status is associated with impaired capacity for exercise, especially when there is a compromised status of more than one micronutrient. With this knowledge, it is intuitively attractive to believe that supplying additional amounts of these vitamins may be beneficial in "supercharging" energy turnover or other key functions in exercise metabolism.

Dietary intakes and vitamin status of athletes

Although an increased rate of flux through the various pathways involved in exercise metabolism may increase the utilization of some vitamins, studies have not been conducted to define with any degree of accuracy the vitamin requirements of highly active people. Indeed, the setting of recommended dietary intakes and allowances involves the addition of a "safety" margin for individuals with higher requirements, which could be expected to cover the needs of athletes. Of course, these deliberations could be rendered moot by the potential of the dietary patterns of athletes to provide generous amounts of vitamins and other micronutrients. With regular strenuous training, there must be an increased total food intake to balance the increased energy expenditure: without this, hard training cannot be sustained for long. Provided that a reasonably varied diet is consumed, a high-energy diet can be expected to provide vitamins in amounts well in excess of these recommended intakes. Even taking into the account the inaccuracies of dietary survey techniques (see Chapter 10), studies of athletes from a variety of sports typically report intakes of vitamins from food sources alone that easily meet the recommended daily intakes or allowances.

It is difficult to precisely determine the vitamin status of an individual. A diagnosis of vitamin deficiency is best made from a variety of sources of information, including an assessment of dietary intake, some biochemical or hematological measurements (see Expert Comment 1), and clinical signs and symptoms. Individually, each of these parameters must be judged cautiously in making a judgement of vitamin status. However, together they help to build a reasonable picture of an adequate or inadequate status. Most studies using biochemical measures of vitamin status do not reveal differences between the results of athletes and sedentary controls. This suggests that athletic training, *per se*, does not increase the risk of micronutrient deficiency, or at least does not increase the requirement disproportionately in relation to the effect on energy intake. However, these data need to be interpreted with care because of the insensitivity of most indices to states of marginal inadequacy. In other words, these results do not entirely exclude minor but functionally important differences between athletes and controls, or the possibility that an inadequate status may be present in some individuals in the group. Nevertheless, the available information suggests that frank vitamin deficiencies are rare among athletes, just as they are among the general population.

Athletes may put themselves at risk of inadequate vitamin intake by either restricting intake of energy, or failing to include a variety of nutrient-rich foods in their eating patterns. Energy restriction is common among athletes who are concerned about body weight and body fat levels. Many athletes follow weight-loss programs, fad diets and disordered eating practices for prolonged periods in an attempt to reach a perceived ideal body size and physique. Poor practical nutrition skills, inadequate finances, and an overcommitted lifestyle that limits access to food and causes erratic meal schedules may also restrict dietary variety. The best management is to educate the athlete with regard to the quality and quantity of their food intake (see Chapter 13). However, a low-dose, broad-range multivitamin/mineral supplement may be useful when the athlete is unwilling or unable to make dietary changes, or when the athlete is traveling to places with an uncertain food supply and eating schedule.

Evidence that vitamin supplementation enhances performance

Athletes often see dietary supplements as a form of "insurance policy". Even when there is no evidence that a deficiency may exist or that intakes above the normal level may be beneficial, they feel they should take vitamin supplements "just in case". This practice is generally harmless, except perhaps in the financial sense, but there are some concerns over the possible harmful effects of excessive intakes of the fat-soluble vitamins (A, D, E, and K) over long periods. The water-soluble vitamins are simply excreted if consumed in amounts in excess of the requirement, but the fat-soluble vitamins can accumulate in the body tissues and may reach toxic levels.

Whether supplementation with vitamins enhances athletic performance and recovery has been the subject of a number of studies. However, these studies have failed to find any sound evidence that vitamin supplementation provides a benefit to the performance of sport or exercise activities, except in cases where it was used to correct a pre-existing deficiency. Early studies that showed beneficial effects of supplementation on performance were usually poorly designed, often with no proper control group against which to compare the effects of supplementation. These studies should be regarded as a testament to the power of the placebo effect rather than evidence of the beneficial effects of supplementation.

Vitamins of special interest to athletes: antioxidant vitamins

Athletes engaged in very hard physical training and sedentary individuals participating in unaccustomed exercise show signs of muscle damage in the postexercise period, and there is evidence of free radical-induced damage to muscle membranes and subcellular structures. There is some evidence for an adaptive increase in antioxidant status in response to regular exercise, and this may help protect against further damage. Supplementation of the diet with antioxidant nutrients (particularly vitamins C and E) has been proposed as a possible way of further reducing the harmful effects of exercise. Some studies suggest that the severity of muscle damage—as assessed by circulating levels of muscle-specific proteins that have leaked out into the blood—can be reduced by supplementation with large doses of antioxidant vitamins but the evidence is not entirely convincing, and further information is required before any specific recommendations can be made.

There is little evidence that any favorable changes to antioxidant status transfer into a performance benefit, although it is possible that true changes occurring over the relatively short periods of most studies are too small to be detected. Another dimension to the antioxidant story is also emerging which suggests that small levels of oxidants in cells play an important role in body function—for example to act as signals for pathways promoting adaptive change, or as part of the immune system function (see Expert Comment 3). Therefore, any antioxidant supplementation needs to be carefully applied in case it interferes with positive oxidant-mediated function. In the absence of clear recommendations regarding antioxidant needs, athletes are advised to consume a diet that is rich in food sources of antioxidants (see Table 4.1). Supplementation may be most justified in situations where there is a sudden increase in training stress—for example, a sudden increase in training load, or exposure to altitude or a hot environment.

Minerals

Biological functions of minerals and evidence for benefits of supplementation

At least 20 different minerals are required in adequate amounts to sustain normal function of tissues and cells. Many of these are required in only trace amounts, but others must be supplied in greater quantities. Deficiencies of all of these elements are theoretically possible, but in practice, deficiencies are generally uncommon, with the possible exceptions of iron, calcium and, in some parts of the world, iodine. Since iron and calcium play an important role in the health and performance of athletes, and

high-level training may have an effect on iron and calcium status, these minerals will be considered separately. Otherwise, dietary surveys and mineral status studies generally show that athletes consume adequate intakes of minerals and trace elements, and show similar biochemical and hematological status to their sedentary counterparts.

The major electrolytes—sodium, potassium, and chloride—all play important roles in water homeostasis and in the distribution of water between the intracellular and extracellular spaces. Sodium is important for regulation of blood pressure, but this is more of an issue for the recreational athlete—and indeed for those in the population who take no exercise—than for the elite performer. The role of sodium and potassium will be considered in some detail in Chapter 5.

Magnesium plays a number of vital roles in the regulation of energy metabolism, acting as a cofactor and activator for a number of enzymes. Magnesium is also involved in calcium metabolism and in the maintenance of electrical gradients across nerve and muscle cell membranes. Magnesium homeostasis in athletes has received recent attention due to the potential for increased magnesium losses and requirements in those undertaking regular exercise. For example, magnesium is lost in sweat in concentrations that may be higher than those in the blood, leading to concern about magnesium deficiency in athletes training and competing in hot climates, where large amounts of sweat are lost from the body. Magnesium deficiency is often proposed as a cause of exercise-induced muscle cramps, even though there is no experimental evidence to support this hypothesis. In some countries, including Germany, this idea is so fixed that sports drinks intended for athletes invariably have added magnesium, even though the same products are sold in other countries without the addition of magnesium salts. Experimental magnesium deficiency results in a variety of symptoms, but these do not include muscle cramp.

Zinc is also involved as a cofactor in many enzyme reactions, and has many other roles, including an important function in the promotion of tissue repair processes. More recently, zinc supplementation has been promoted on the basis of a potential role in enhancing immune function and increasing resistance to minor illness and infection. Most of the body zinc content of about 2 g is present in muscle (60%) and bone (30%), and measurements of zinc levels in blood may not be very meaningful. Low concentrations are present in sweat, and exercise may stimulate urinary loss. This increased loss associated with exercise may account for the concern of many athletes, but there is no evidence that these losses are sufficient to cause concern. Small amounts of zinc are present in many foods, including both animal and vegetable products, and no benefit of regular supplementation for health or for performance has been established. Copper is another divalent cation with important biological functions including modulation of enzyme activity and also a role in the synthesis of hemoglobin, catecholamines, and some peptide hormones. Once again, deficiencies are rare as copper is found in a wide range of foods, including shellfish, liver, wholegrain cereals, legumes and nuts.

Selenium has an antioxidant function, since it forms an integral part of the glutathione peroxidase enzyme, which helps to protect cells against the damage that can result from free radicals. There is some evidence that selenium plays a role in protecting against some cancers. In regions of the world where the soil is low in selenium, vegetables will have a low selenium content and deficiencies are possible. However, these regions are generally well recognized, with appropriate measures for fortification in place. Most people now eat foods produced in diverse geographical locations, so the risk of specific deficiencies is much less than in former times when most fresh produce was grown locally.

An adequate dietary iodine intake is essential for synthesis of the thyroid hormones thyroxine (T4) and triiodothyronine (T3), and thyroid deficiency was once common in parts of the world where the availability of iodine is low. Recognition of the role of iodine led to iodization of salt in these regions. In most countries, intakes are well in excess of requirements, and there is no evidence to suggest a greater requirement in physically active individuals.

A variety of other elements, including cobalt, molybdenum, manganese, chromium, and phosphorus, play important metabolic roles and are required in the diet in small amounts. Deficiencies of all of these elements are sufficiently rare that the possibility of their being encountered in athletes is negligible. However, many of these elements, including cobalt, chromium, and phosphate, are used as supplements by athletes, despite a lack of evidence either for an increased requirement or for a beneficial effect of specific supplementation on performance.

Minerals of special interest to athletes: iron

Iron deficiency anemia is regarded as the most commonly occurring nutritional deficiency in the world. In developing countries or among high-risk groups, iron deficiency can affect 30–40% of the population, whereas the prevalence of iron deficiency anemia in the general community is typically 1–3%. Since the 1970s, athletes have come under scrutiny as one such high-risk group. In early studies of long-distance runners, exercise scientists commented on some confusing hematological findings. These athletes were found to have reduced hemoglobin concentrations in their blood (a sign of anemia); this characteristic seemed unfavorable for the performance of events that rely on the delivery of oxygen to working muscles. Later, this phenomenon was found to be a false or dilutional anemia, resulting from the acute increase in plasma volume that accompanies heavy aerobic training. Termed "sports anemia", it is not considered a pathology or disadvantage to performance, and does not respond to iron supplementation therapy. Of course, a low blood hemoglobin concentration may result from deficiency of other micronutrients such as vitamins B_{12} or folate, and should be investigated.

The body's iron is found in three main pools: storage iron (ferritin and hemosiderin found predominantly in the spleen, liver, and bone marrow); transport iron (transported by the protein carrier, transferrin); and oxygen transport iron (hemoglobin in the blood and myoglobin in the muscle). The majority of iron in the body is carefully recycled, with iron from destroyed red blood cells (erythrocytes) being salvaged for storage or reincorporation into new blood cells. Iron status is a result of the balance between the small amounts of dietary iron that are absorbed each day and the sum of the small

Table 4.2 Stages of iron drain (adapted from Deakin 2000).

Stage	Characteristics	Diagnostic criteria from blood measures		
		Hemoglobin (g·100 ml^{-1})	Ferritin (ng·ml^{-1})	Transferrin saturation (%)
Normal iron status	Iron status measurements within normal reference ranges. Normal appearance of erythrocytes	> 12.0 (F) > 16.0 (M)	> 30 (F) > 110 (M)	20–40 (M, F)
Iron depletion	Normal hematocrit, normal hemoglobin, low serum ferritin, normal to high transferrin saturation	As above	< 30 (M, F)	20–40 (M, F)
Iron deficiency	Low serum ferritin, low serum iron and serum transferrin. Reduced transferrin saturation. Normal hemoglobin	As above	< 12 (M, F)	< 16 (M, F)
Iron deficiency anemia	Low hemoglobin, change in erythrocytes (small and pale), low hematocrit, low serum iron, low transferrin saturation	< 12.0 (F) < 14.0 (M)	< 10 (M, F)	< 16 (M, F)

iron losses from skin, sweat, and the gastrointestinal and urinary tracts. Important functions of iron and iron-related compounds in the body are:

• transport of oxygen in the blood (hemoglobin) and muscle (myoglobin);

• as a component of enzyme systems such as the electron transport chain, and enzymes involved in DNA synthesis; and

• as a catalyst in the production of free oxygen radical species.

Iron drain is thought to progress through a number of stages with different functional and diagnostic criteria (see Table 4.2). The end stage of iron deficiency anemia is detected by blood iron status measures that are below population reference standards and also below the "normal or usual" concentrations for an individual. At this stage, there is inadequate iron available in the bone marrow for the normal manufacture of hemoglobin and erythrocytes, leading to the production of red blood cells that are small and pale. Anemia causes a reduction in exercise performance. In cases of severely reduced hemoglobin levels, individuals may report breathlessness on even the mildest exertion, and may be unable to carry out everyday activities and work tasks. Impaired functioning of iron-related enzymes may result in reductions in brain function, temperature control, and immunity, which exacerbate the symptoms of impaired exercise tolerance.

Although the effects of gradually reduced hemoglobin on performance have not been systematically studied, it is believed that even a small decline in hemoglobin levels (e.g. 1–2 g·100ml^{-1}) will reduce the competition performance of athletes. Since the range of "normal" hemoglobin levels is reasonably wide, it is possible that an athlete may show a level that is within reference standards, but is below the level that is "usual" for them and is required for their optimal performance. Although a low hemoglobin level may be relatively easy to detect, it is difficult to confirm optimal iron status from a single blood test. Fluctuations in iron status measures may occur without any change in true iron status. For example, concentrations of all parameters are increased by hemoconcentration (for example, in the severely dehydrated athlete) just as parameters are diluted when there is an increase in blood volume. Ferritin levels are increased in response to acute stress—such as a strenuous training session, infection or illness, further confusing the picture in athletes in training.

Therefore, it is valuable to standardize the time and conditions of iron status monitoring, and to establish a history of iron status results from the individual athlete to establish a feel for what is normal and "optimal" for them. Athletes often believe that the "more is better" principle applies to hemoglobin levels *per se* and may undertake specialized training, such as altitude training, to stimulate the production of erythrocytes. However, in the absence of hemoconcentration due to dehydration, very high hemoglobin levels are usually explained by genetic individuality or drug use (e.g. erythropoietin (EPO)).

The most contentious issue about the iron status of athletes is whether iron depletion, in the absence of anemia, reduces exercise performance. Low serum ferritin levels have become synonymous with reduced iron status, and the effect on performance has been investigated mostly by studying the effects of iron supplementation on the performance of individuals with low ferritin levels. In general, there is little evidence that low ferritin levels, in the absence of anemia, are associated with reduced performance of a single exercise task, or that iron supplementation enhances the performance of athletes with moderately low serum ferritin but normal hemoglobin levels. Studies in which a performance improvement was seen after iron supplementation in subjects with low ferritin levels also show an increase in hemoglobin levels in response to the therapy, suggesting that the subjects had suboptimal hemoglobin levels prior to the supplementation. However, studies have failed to address the complaint commonly made by athletes with reduced iron stores that they fail to recover between a series of competitions or training sessions.

Therefore, at the present time there is no evidence to suggest that a moderately reduced ferritin level *per se* is detrimental to performance, or that endurance athletes should receive routine iron supplementation. However, low ferritin levels may become progressively lower and eventually lead to problematic iron deficiency. For this reason, it makes sense to routinely assess the iron status of athletes with high risk of iron deficiency and implement a treatment plan where iron status is declining.

Causes of iron deficiency

Athletes are often considered a high-risk group for iron deficiency, but the causes of iron deficiency in athletes are the same as those in sedentary populations: iron requirements and/or losses exceed iron intake over a sufficiently lengthy period of time. Iron requirements are increased during periods of growth, reflected by the higher recommended dietary allowances for iron during adolescence and while pregnant. Iron needs are higher in females of reproductive age than in males because of the need to replace the monthly menstrual blood losses. Given the individual characteristics of athletes it is not possible to make general recommendations as to iron requirements of people who exercise, but there is a general appreciation that there is an increase in iron requirements and iron turnover in those who undertake prolonged and heavy training. Even though the small losses from mechanical trauma and gastrointestinal blood loss might seem inconsequential, they may lead to iron drain over a prolonged period unless there is a compensatory increase in iron intake or absorption. Of course, iron losses may also occur due to medical problems that cause substantial or prolonged blood loss such as tumors, gastrointestinal ulcers, surgery, or severe bruising. Risk factors for poor iron status, including an overview of the dietary patterns that lead to inadequate intake of available iron, are summarized in Table 4.3.

Prevention and treatment of iron deficiency and anemia

Evaluation and management of iron status should be undertaken on an individual basis by a sports medicine expert, and preferably by a team including the physician and dietitian. Cases of frank iron deficiency anemia warrant immediate iron therapy supported by a long-term management plan. Low iron status, indicated by serum ferritin levels lower than 20 ng·ml^{-1}, should be considered for further assessment and treatment, and the prevention and treatment of iron deficiency may also include iron supplementation. The long-term management plan should be based on dietary counseling to increase the intake of bioavailable iron, and appropriate strategies to reduce any unwarranted iron loss should also be implemented.

Iron is found in a range of plant and animal food sources in two forms: as heme iron, found only in flesh- or blood-containing animal foods, and organic iron which is found in both animal foods and plant foods. Whereas heme iron is relatively well absorbed from single foods and mixed meals (15–35% bioavailability), the absorption of nonheme iron from single plant sources is low and variable (2–8%). The bioavailability of non-heme iron is affected by the presence of enhancing or inhibiting factors in foods eaten at the same meal. Inhibiting factors include phytates (found in wholegrain cereal foods and soy protein), polyphenols (found

Table 4.3 Factors indicating high risk of iron drain or iron deficiency in athletes. (Adapted from Burke, in press.)

Predictors of increased iron requirements
Recent growth spurt in adolescents
Pregnancy (current or within the past year)

Predictors of increased iron losses or iron malabsorption
Sudden increase in training load, particularly involving running on hard surfaces
Gastrointestinal malabsorption problems (e.g. Crohn's disease, ulcerative colitis, parasite infestation)
Gastrointestinal bleeding due to chronic use of some anti-inflammatory drugs, ulcers, or other problems
Heavy menstrual blood losses
Excessive blood losses such as frequent nose bleeds, recent surgery, substantial contact injuries
Frequent blood donation

Predictors of inadequate intake of bioavailable iron
Chronic low energy intake (< 8400 kJ or 2000 kcal·day^{-1})
Vegetarian eating—especially poorly constructed diets ignoring alternative food sources of iron (e.g. legumes, nuts, and seeds)
Fad diets or erratic eating patterns
Restricted variety of foods in diet, and failure to promote mixing and matching of foods at meals (especially fruit and vegetables containing vitamin C)
Heavy reliance on convenience foods and micronutrient-poor sports foods (high-carbohydrate powders, bars, and gels)
Very high carbohydrate diet with high fiber content and infrequent intake of meats/fish/chicken
Natural food diets: failure to consume iron-fortified cereal foods such as commercial breakfast cereals and bread

---

in tea and red wine), calcium (found in milk and cheese), and peptides from plant sources such as soy protein. Enhancing factors include vitamin C (found in citrus, tropical, and berry fruits, and some vegetables), peptides from meat/fish/chicken, alcohol, and some foods with a low pH due to fermentation or the presence of citric or tartaric acids. Until recently, the absorption of heme iron was considered to be relatively unaffected by other dietary compounds, but updated study techniques have shown that other meal components such as calcium and plant peptides may reduce heme iron bioavailability. The absorption of both heme and non-heme iron is increased as an adaptive response in people who are iron deficient or have increased iron requirements. It should be noted that iron bioavailability studies have not been undertaken on special groups such as athletes. The general assumption is that observations of iron absorption characteristics can be applied across populations of healthy people.

Assessment of total dietary iron intake is not necessarily a good predictor of iron status. After all, the mixing and matching of foods at meals plays an important role by determining the bioavailability of dietary iron intake. In a mixed diet, where lean meats are consumed regularly, heme iron may provide around half of the absorbable iron. However in many Western countries, cereal products such as bread and breakfast cereals are the single greatest source of total dietary iron due to the fortification of these products with additional iron and the frequency with which they are consumed. Dietary strategies to increase intake of bioavailable iron, particularly in conjunction with other goals of sports nutrition, are explored in more detail in Chapter 13.

Minerals of special interest to athletes: calcium

Bone is a dynamic tissue, continually undergoing remodeling through the simultaneous processes of bone resorption and rebuilding. Osteoporosis, or low bone density, is now widely recognized as a problem for both men and women, and an increased bone mineral content is one of the benefits of participation in an exercise program. Regular exercise results in increased mineralization of those bones subjected to stress and an increased peak bone mass may delay the onset of osteoporotic fractures. Exercise may also delay the rate of bone loss. The specificity of this effect is demonstrated by the increase in forearm bone density observed in the dominant arm of tennis players. Calcium plays a permissive role in bone status, meaning that an inadequate calcium intake can interfere with optimal bone health, while high calcium intakes do not stimulate additional bone growth.

Interest in the calcium status of female athletes has intensified with recent studies reporting low bone density and an increased risk of stress fractures in various groups. However, these problems do not simply arise from inadequate calcium intake. Rather, there is a complex interrelationship between hormonal status, particularly of the female sex hormone estrogen, and bone health. Athletes often experience disturbances to regular menstrual function. Secondary amenorrhea (cessation of the normal menstrual cycle) is the most widely publicized form, but primary amenorrhea (failure to start menstruating) is commonly encountered in sports such as gymnastics where girls train intensively from early ages. Alterations in the luteal phase of the menstrual cycle may precede secondary amenorrhea and may also cause significant disruption to hormonal patterns. Since this will not be noticed unless blood tests are taken, the female athlete may not be aware of the early signs of menstrual dysfunction.

The prevalence of menstrual dysfunction in female athletes is uncertain as it is hard to compare reports that have studied athletes of different caliber, or that have used different definitions to describe menstrual dysfunction. Nevertheless, it appears that problems occur more frequently than in the general female population, and that athletes in "weight-conscious" sports are most at risk. Despite a number of interesting hypotheses, there is no single cause that can explain menstrual disturbances in athletes. Low body fat levels *per se* do not seem to predict amenorrhea, as was originally proposed. Many athletes are able to maintain regular cycles while at low body fat levels, while other athletes and non-athlete counterparts may become amenorrheic at relatively higher body fat levels. Rather, a number of risk factors seem to be involved and individual athletes may be susceptible to certain factors or combinations of these factors. A more complex scenario involving a cluster of proposed risk factors is the "energy drain" syndrome. This syndrome describes the female athlete who consumes a diet that is restricted in energy intake and variety, while undertaking a heavy exercise load. This athlete is exposed to a chronic energy deficit,

psychological stress and/or perhaps a struggle to achieve or maintain body fat below the level that is genetically determined as "natural" for them.

Of course, observations of impaired menstrual function in female athletes are not new. In fact, they have been reported for at least 30 years. However, it is only recently that the negative outcome of altered menstrual function has been recognized: the alteration of steroid hormone profiles in female athletes has a detrimental effect on bone health.

Education is needed to raise the awareness of athletes about the problems associated with amenorrhea or other forms of menstrual dysfunction. Many athletes, particularly female endurance athletes, consider amenorrhea to be a "normal" condition for heavily training athletes. Although it might be "normal" in the sense that it is widely prevalent among some athletic groups, it is clearly not a healthy or desirable state. As part of this education process, sports medicine experts have described the syndrome as the "female athlete triad". This describes the common presentation of disordered eating, menstrual dysfunction, and reduced bone health among female athletes. Of course, each of these problems is multifactorial, and does not always occur in the presence of the other problems. Nevertheless, the female athlete triad has drawn the attention of doctors, coaches, and athletes towards the importance of early intervention and management of any symptoms. Reduced bone density in athletes or failure to optimize peak bone mass may be a risk factor for the development of stress fractures during their athletic career, and more importantly, the earlier onset, or increased risk of osteoporosis in later life. In the case of stress fractures, many factors can combine to cause excessive loading on the bone. The role of reduced bone density in athletes in later osteoporosis remains speculative since it will take extensive longitudinal studies into middle age and beyond to determine its significance.

Of course, factors other than hormonal status and exercise can affect bone mineral status. These include dietary factors, such as intakes of calcium, protein, and phosphorus, as well as genetic or familial predisposition, and smoking. Population guidelines for calcium intake recognize increased calcium requirements during periods of growth, as well as during pregnancy and breastfeeding. The recommended intakes proposed by some countries also include increased calcium intake for postmenopausal women, recognizing that higher calcium intakes are needed to maintain calcium balance in a lower estrogen state. Note that some calcium balance studies suggest that calcium intakes of 1500 mg·day^{-1} might be needed in such situations. Presumably the recommended dietary intake guidelines for postmenopausal women should be extended to athletes who have developed a low estrogen status as evidenced by menstrual dysfunction.

Typically, dairy products provide around 50–70% of the calcium intake in Western diets. In many dietary surveys of female athletes, it has been reported that they consume significantly less calcium than the recommended intakes. Dietary restriction or disordered eating may not only be a risk factor for the development of menstrual dysfunction, but is also likely to be associated with suboptimal intakes of calcium. Restriction of energy intake is a common cause of inadequate consumption of calcium. Many athletes also restrict their intake of dairy foods because of false beliefs that these foods are fattening, or cause "allergies" or "mucus". It is rare to find true situations where all dairy foods must be avoided on medical grounds. Some athletes have cultural, religious, or environmental beliefs that prevent them from consuming dairy foods. In this case, fortified soy products provide an alternative source of calcium; moderate sources of calcium include canned fish eaten with bones, and some vegetables. It is useful to provide dietary advice for athletes in which high calcium eating is matched with other dietary goals—for example, finding low-fat calcium choices, or mixing a calcium-rich food into a high-carbohydrate meal. These ideas are discussed in further detail in Chapter 13.

It is often difficult to work with athletes who suffer from disordered eating, amenorrhea, impaired bone status, or combinations of these problems, and there is no single management plan. Rather, these athletes need individualized assessment and therapy, involving input from appropriate experts. Assessment is necessary to determine the factors underlying each problem, and the overall threat to the athlete's health and performance. Ideally, the athlete should aim to return to menstrual health and an optimum diet, even though this may not be possible, at least in the short term. The role of estrogen replacement therapy and calcium supplementation as interim or long-term interventions requires further research (see Expert Comment 4). There is some doubt about the degree of reversibility of bone loss, and in particular the restoration of strong bone formation, particularly in cases of long-term loss. Early intervention and prevention are clearly the preferred options.

Summary

Vitamins and minerals play a key role in optimizing the health and performance of the athlete. In many cases there may be an increased requirement for a particular micronutrient, arising from the commitment to a regular exercise schedule. However, there are no fixed guidelines for recommended intakes of vitamins and minerals by athletes. Rather, it is suggested that a moderate to high energy intake, coupled with a variety of nutrient-rich food choices, will enable the athlete to achieve intakes of vitamins and minerals that are in excess of both the population recommended dietary intakes, and their increased requirements. Studies fail to provide evidence that vitamin supplementation enhances exercise performance, except in cases where there was a pre-existing deficiency. Nevertheless, there is interest in the possible role of antioxidant vitamins in the prevention of damage arising from excessive production of free oxygen radicals. With regard to minerals, some athletes are at risk of suboptimal intakes of iron and calcium, which may have detrimental effects on either immediate performance or long-term health. The prevention and management of such problems requires input from experts in sports medicine and nutrition.

Reading list

Aulin, K.P. (2000) Minerals: calcium. In: *Nutrition in Sport* (ed. R.J. Maughan), pp. 318–325. Blackwell Science, Oxford.

Burke, L.M. Nutrition for training and performance. In: *Physiological Bases of Sports Performance* (eds M. Hargreaves & J. Hawley). McGraw-Hill, Sydney (in press).

Deakin, V. (2000) Iron depletion in athletes. In: *Clinical Sports Nutrition* (eds L. Burke & V. Deakin), 2nd edn, pp. 273–311. McGraw-Hill, Sydney, Australia.

Eichner, E.R. (2000) Minerals: iron. In: *Nutrition in Sport* (ed. R.J. Maughan), pp. 326–338. Blackwell Science, Oxford.

Fogelholm, M. (2000) Vitamins: metabolic functions. In: *Nutrition in Sport* (ed. R.J. Maughan), pp. 266–280. Blackwell Science, Oxford.

Fogelholm, M. (2000) Vitamin, mineral and antioxidant needs of athletes. In: *Clinical Sports Nutrition* (eds L. Burke & V. Deakin), 2nd edn, pp. 312–340. McGraw-Hill, Sydney, Australia.

Kerr, D., Khan, K. & Bennell, K. (2000) Bone, exercise, nutrition and menstrual disturbances. In: *Clinical Sports Nutrition* (eds L. Burke & V. Deakin), 2nd edn, pp. 241–272. McGraw-Hill, Sydney, Australia.

Yeager, K.K., Agostini, R., Nattiv, A. & Drinkwater, B. (1993) The female athlete triad: disordered eating, amenorrhea, osteoporosis. *Medicine and Science in Sports and Exercise* 25, 775–777.

EXPERT COMMENT 1 Assessing vitamin status in athletes: do they achieve their vitamin requirements? Mikael Fogelholm

An organism has an adequate nutritional status when its cells, tissues and anatomical systems can undertake all nutrient-dependent functions. The metabolic functions of vitamins of particular interest to athletes include the production of energy and their role in neuromuscular functions (skills). Inadequate intake of vitamins will impair these functions. However, the relation between vitamin supply and functional capacity is "bell-shaped", meaning that the output (functional capacity) is not improved after the "minimal requirement for maximal output" is reached. In fact, overvitaminosis may in some cases reduce the output below the maximal level. How, then, does an athlete (or his or her coach) know whether vitamin intake is adequate, but not too high? And what does the available scientific literature tell about athletes' vitamin status?

Assessment of dietary intakes provides only rough estimates of "usual" intakes of foods and nutrients. Although a low intake of a certain vitamin is an indicator of possible dietary deficiency, it is not very specific in ascertaining individuals or populations with adequate dietary intake. Moreover, uncertainty about the specific nutritional requirements of individuals and inaccuracies related to dietary assessment preclude the use of dietary intakes as a sole indicator of vitamin status. Nevertheless, the available research data show that vitamin intakes reported by athletes are generally higher than the intake in untrained individuals.

Vitamin status may also be assessed by biochemical methods. Blood samples (serum or plasma) are easy to collect and analyse, and therefore suitable for large studies. Some water-soluble vitamins respond quickly to dietary intake and positive correlations between dietary intake and plasma concentration of, for instance, ascorbic acid have been reported. All publications with data on plasma ascorbic acid levels in athletes indicate adequate status. In fact, the levels reported in many studies are associated with a saturated body pool. Plasma vitamin E levels may also be used as an indicator of vitamin status, but the concentration should be adjusted for variations in low density lipoprotein (LDL)-cholesterol concentration. The available research data do not indicate that vitamin E status is compromised in athletes.

Because serum and plasma concentrations are rather insensitive to marginal situations of micronutrient deficiency, further work has been done to identify other body compartments that would better represent the body's micronutrient status. Vitamin C concentrations in mononuclear leukocytes (a type of white blood cell) appear to be a more sensitive indicator of vitamin C status than plasma vitamin C levels. Unfortunately, although these methods are interesting, they are still not used routinely. Therefore, little is known about these status measures in athletes.

Another useful way to monitor vitamin status is to measure the activity of a vitamin-related enzyme in an appropriate body tissue. Enzyme activation coefficients (ACs) in red blood cells are used as indicators for thiamine (enzyme: transketolase, TK), riboflavin (glutathione reductase, GR) and vitamin B_6 (aspartate aminotransferase, AST) status, with high ACs indicating inadequate nutritional status. Again, this measurement has not been used in many studies of athletes, and the available results do not give a clear-cut picture on differences between athletes' and controls' ACs. However, all differences reported are small and most probably without any functional significance. It should be noted that erythrocyte levels of TK, GR and AST are not *in vivo* saturated by their cofactor in people with adequate vitamin intake. Consequently, after pharmacological supplementation, their basal activity increases and activation coefficient decreases. However, these changes are not associated with improved physical performance.

Should athletes have their vitamin status assessed regularly, and if so, by which methods? Unfortunately, there are no methods that are routinely available, simple, reliable, cheap, sensitive, and specific at the same time. Therefore, assessment of vitamin status, for screening purposes, is not justified, unless there are specific reasons to suspect deficiency of a certain vitamin. Fortunately, a well-chosen diet seems to ensure adequate vitamin status in athletes, even (perhaps that should be especially) when energy turnover is high.

EXPERT COMMENT 2 Should athletes routinely receive iron injections or iron supplements? Louise M. Burke

A rapid reversal of iron depletion and an increase in iron stores can be achieved via intramuscular injections of iron. This is sometimes provided in cases of extreme iron depletion which carries a significant penalty to the individual involved, or where oral iron intake is not tolerated. However, in some athletic circles iron injections have become popular as a "high-tech" method of iron supplementation. Sometimes they are used even in cases where iron deficiency has not been properly diagnosed, but where the athlete reports fatigue or simply falls into a high-risk group for iron deficiency. Iron injection does not provide a superior technique of iron repletion *per se,* particularly as a significant proportion of the iron remains in the buttock, unabsorbed. Since it carries a risk of anaphylactic shock as well as iron overload, it should not be regarded as the first choice of treatment or a benign therapy. Iron injections will not increase hemoglobin levels or other iron parameters in people who are not otherwise suboptimal in iron status.

Oral iron supplements provide part of the usual therapy recommended to treat iron deficiency and anemia. Most authorities recommend that such therapy should be prescribed on a case-by-case basis, as part of a treatment plan involving strategies to reduce or prevent unusual iron losses, and dietary counseling to maximize the intake of bioavailable iron. The recognized therapy is a daily dose of 100 mg elemental iron (which may be equal to 500 mg of ferrous sulphate), taken on an empty stomach. Many people take a vitamin C supplement or juice with their supplement to enhance the absorption of this organic iron. A 3-month period of supplementation is needed to restore depleted iron stores. In some cases, when it is not possible to enhance dietary iron intake sufficiently, it may be necessary to continue iron supplementation at a lower dose, or to reduce frequency of supplement use to 1–2 times weekly to prevent ongoing iron drain.

Although iron supplements are available as over-the-counter medications, there are dangers in self-prescription as a tonic or long-term supplementation in the absence of medical follow-up. Iron supplementation is not a replacement for medical and dietary assessment and therapy, since it fails to correct underlying problems that have caused iron drain. In many cases a diet that is inadequate in iron will also fail to meet other sports nutrition goals. Chronic supplementation with high doses of iron carries a risk of iron overload disease (hemochromatosis), especially in males for whom the genetic traits for this problem are more prevalent. Iron supplements can also interfere with the absorption of other minerals such as zinc and copper. Some individuals suffer from gastrointestinal side-effects arising from the use of iron supplements.

EXPERT COMMENT 3 Does antioxidant supplementation reduce muscle damage from oxygen free radicals?
Priscilla M. Clarkson

Overexertion exercise can result in damage to muscle fibers, and some evidence points to oxygen free radicals as playing a role in the damage process. During aerobic production of ATP, most of the oxygen consumed is reduced and combines with hydrogen to form water. However, about 4–5% of the oxygen is not completely reduced and forms oxygen free radicals that can attack cell membrane lipids and result in lipid breakdown called lipid peroxidation. Strenuous endurance exercise that relies heavily on aerobic metabolism will increase the production of oxygen free radicals. Also, exercise that places high forces on the muscle can result in damage to cell proteins, leading to an increase in macrophages and white blood cells as part of the repair process. These cells release free radicals, which can result in more damage if left unchecked. To counter the increases in free radicals, the body contains an elaborate antioxidant defense system that depends on dietary intake of antioxidant vitamins (e.g. vitamins C, E, and beta-carotene) and minerals (e.g. selenium) as well as the endogenous production of numerous antioxidant compounds (e.g. glutathione) and enzymes (e.g. superoxide dismutase) that are involved in the quenching of free radicals.

There is little evidence that antioxidant supplements will reduce muscle damage. While vitamin C supplements of 200–300 mg·day^{-1} for 3–4 weeks have been reported to reduce indices of muscle damage, including reduced muscle soreness after the exercise, not all studies confirm this, and most studies of vitamin C supplementation have not found that the supplements reduced muscle damage. Few studies have investigated the efficacy of combinations of these vitamins, and the results of these studies are equivocal.

Perhaps the reason that antioxidant supplementation has not proven as effective as was predicted is that the body, given adequate antioxidants in the diet, is designed to be able to mount its own defense system in response to exercise stress. This makes teleological sense, since the body is intended to perform high-intensity exercise for purposes of survival. Moreover, exercise training has been found to be associated with an enhanced antioxidant defense system. Many studies have reported that trained subjects have increased levels of antioxidant compounds and enzymes in the blood, and muscle biopsies of trained subjects also showed higher amounts of antioxidants. In response to exercise, there was evidence of less lipid peroxidation in trained subjects, independent of supplementation.

There appears to be a balance where any increase in free radicals with exercise is checked by the body's natural antioxidant defenses. A diet rich in antioxidant nutrients should be sufficient to quench free radicals produced during training, making antioxidant supplements unnecessary. Athletes who worry that their diet is not sufficient often take antioxidant supplements as an insurance policy. While supplementation of antioxidant vitamins near to or slightly above the recommended levels is not harmful, there is a growing body of evidence that free radicals may be necessary to stimulate the process of adaptation. An increase in free radicals during exercise may act as signals for cellular adaptation to training by influencing gene expression. If this proves to be the case, then megadoses of antioxidant supplements may ultimately prove to be counter indicated for athletes.

Bone health and bone mineral content are influenced by many different factors. Environmental factors such as physical activity, dietary calcium intake, and hormonal status interact with each other and their combined effects determine the extent to which bone density genotype influences the peak bone density achieved in young adulthood.

Adolescents

A positive calcium balance, defined as calcium intake exceeding calcium loss, is necessary for bone growth and peak bone mass to be achieved. Studies of the effects of dietary calcium intake on bone mass in women have shown that adequate amounts of calcium during adolescence or early adulthood result in higher bone mass during adulthood and the early postmenopausal period, than when low intakes are consumed during these critical times. Hormonal status during adolescence is another important factor in achieving peak bone mass. This is a question of a sufficient energy consumption to balance energy needs, and a gain in body weight in order to achieve menarche at a proper time. Extended periods of amenorrhea, due to insufficient energy intake together with strenuous physical training, may result in low bone density at multiple skeletal sites including those subjected to impact loading during exercise. Early identification of low bone mineral density (BMD) and treatment is critical to protect young amenorrheic athletes from developing premature osteoporosis. The preferred treatment would be to encourage changes that lead to the resumption of normal menses—for example, improved nutrition including calcium-fortified foods, weight gain and a decrease in training load. However there are reports indicating that this loss of BMD may be irreversible in spite of any treatment. As an example, the (US) recommended dietary allowance (RDA) for calcium intake during adolescence and early adulthood is 1200 mg per day.

Young adults

Gain in bone mass in healthy young women occurs mainly before the third decade of life. Thereafter, a slow but progressive age-related bone loss occurs. During this period calcium intakes have less effect than circulating hormone levels in creating a positive effect on bone maintenance. Changes in lifestyle, involving a modest increase in physical activity and calcium intake preferably through consumption of dairy products, together with significant estrogen levels, may significantly reduce the risk for development of early osteoporosis. There is no evidence that exercise alone or exercise plus additional calcium intake can prevent the rapid decrease in bone mass in the immediate postmenopausal years and it is not a substitute for hormone replacement therapy. The RDA for calcium intake by young adults is 1000 mg per day.

Older adults

Bone loss is widely accepted as a normal part of the aging process. Bone mass in the elderly reflects the accumulation and maintenance of bone tissue achieved during growth and maturation, and the rate and duration of bone loss thereafter. Genetic, endocrine, and lifestyle factors contribute to the final picture. Nutritional factors including calcium intake, as well as daily physical activity, may slow the rate of mineral loss from the skeleton. Due to an age-related decrease in calcium absorption from the small intestine and decline in exposure to sunlight, medication with vitamin D may be undertaken to enhance bone formation and mineralization. The RDA for calcium intake by older adults is 800 mg per day.

Athlete

Susan was a 19-year-old long-distance runner (53 kg) on the cross-country team at her college. One of the first things she had undertaken on starting college 6 months previously was to decrease her fat intake by eliminating meat, fish, and poultry from her diet. This was done to prevent the "freshman 15"—the typical weight gain of about 15 pounds (7 kg) that frequently occurs in the first year of college. She was now in the competitive season of cross-country (spring) and was undertaking daily training sessions, except on days spent traveling to meets and during competition. She had recently noticed problems with her sleep patterns and an overwhelming feeling of fatigue—as well as a deterioration in performance. Her coach suggested that decreasing her weight by 2–3 kg might improve her running times.

Reason for consultancy

Susan was referred to the sports medicine clinic where she was diagnosed with iron deficiency anemia. Her blood iron parameters were as follows: ferritin = 5 ng·ml^{-1};% transferrin saturation = 10%; total iron binding capacity (TIBC) = 513 µg·100 ml^{-1}; serum iron = 28 µg·100 ml^{-1}; hemoglobin = 11 g·100 ml^{-1}. Susan also reported that her menstrual periods were irregular and that iron supplements upset her stomach.

Current dietary patterns

Susan reported restrictive eating patterns, with an avoidance of fats and oils, limited intake of dairy products and avoidance of meat, fish, or poultry. Following the coach's advice that a lower body weight would improve her running performances, she had further reduced her energy intake to produce a 2-kg weight loss over the previous month. Susan ate in the cafeteria in her college dormitory, but skipped breakfast to allow a longer sleep in. A typical day's diet is outlined below.

Professional assessment

Mean daily intake from this self-reported eating plan was assessed to be ~ 8400 kJ (2000 kcal); 300 g carbohydrate (5.7 g·kg body mass^{-1}); 45 g protein (0.8 g·kg^{-1}); 70 g fat (31% of energy). Intakes of minerals (iron, calcium, and zinc) were assessed to be below recommended daily allowances. Whereas Susan's protein intake failed to meet the guidelines for an athlete undertaking endurance training, her intake of fat intake was higher than she expected. Susan had previously tried iron supplements but refused to continue this medication due to side-effects including stomach discomfort. In addition to the problem of poor iron status, Susan needed to address her menstrual dysfunction.

Intervention

Dietary goals were set to normalize Susan's eating patterns and her weight, gradually improve her iron status via an increased intake of well-absorbed iron, and increase her intake of protein and calcium. An increase in food variety was negotiated, and Susan agreed to include low-fat sources of fish and chicken but declined to eat red meat. In addition, carbohydrate intake was to be maintained, but provided by foods with greater nutrient density (whole fruits, vegetables, and wholegrain cereals). Better intake of carbohydrate and fluid in conjunction with training was encouraged to promote better energy levels and reduce these factors as a source of fatigue. The following dietary suggestions were made.

1 Eat breakfast each morning from foods providing carbohydrate, protein, and micronutrients (iron-fortified breakfast cereal, skimmed milk, orange juice, coffee made with milk).

2 Consume two servings of fish or chicken each day, one serving of beans or legumes and two or three additional servings of low-fat dairy foods such as milk or yoghurt. Recognize that these foods are important to increase intakes of iron, zinc, calcium, and protein, with fish and chicken providing a small to moderate source of iron, in the well-absorbed heme form.

3 Eat a snack 1–2 h before her afternoon workout (fruit, raisins, bagel, yogurt, or sports bar). Include more whole fruits, vegetables, and wholegrain cereal foods at meals or snacks in preference to high-sugar snacks and desserts.

4 Complement iron-rich cereal foods (iron-fortified cereal, wholegrain pasta) with a vitamin C source (fruit or fruit juice) or animal flesh (chicken or fish) to enhance the absorption of iron from the meal.

5 Plan 1 rest day each week. Use sports drinks before, during, and after workouts, especially on hot days, to provide fluid and fuel.

Outcome

Susan began eating breakfast, added a snack before workouts, and included some white meat and dairy foods in meals each day. After 3 months her weight had stabilized and she felt better. Reassessment of iron status showed an improvement, although her hemoglobin level was still low. Susan was advised to maintain these dietary changes and have iron and menstrual status rechecked in a further 3 months. Follow-up with her physician was recommended to monitor menstrual irregularity.

Breakfast	Lunch	Dinner	After-dinner snacks
Coffee with dairy whitener and sugar	Large salad (lettuce, tomatoes, cucumber, low-fat cheese) Fat-free dressing Breadsticks Diet Coke	Spaghetti with tomato pasta sauce Garlic bread Salad with fat-free dressing Diet coke	Any of the following: cheese pizza diet Coke popcorn jelly beans; low-fat ice cream or cookies

CASE STUDY 2 Low calcium diet. Linda Houtkooper

Athlete

Emily was a 20-year-old female collegiate Division I swimmer. Emily undertook nine pool training sessions each week: six afternoon sessions of 2^1/$_2$ hours, and three 1^1/$_2$ hour morning practices. Pool training was supplemented twice a week with a 45-min session of weight training. Emily was 163 cm in height and weighed 57 kg.

Reason for consultancy

Emily's mother had been recently diagnosed with osteoporosis while going through menopause. Conscious of the importance of family history in the development of health problems, Emily was concerned that her own diet might be inadequate in nutrients important to healthy bones.

Current dietary patterns

Emily was a picky eater. She occasionally drank milk, but only if flavored with chocolate syrup, and avoided most dairy foods in the fear that they would promote weight gain. Her diet was based on fruits and refined grain-based foods. Dinner was her largest meal of the day, and was the only meal at which she consciously included protein-rich food choices. Emily took a multivitamin supplement but no mineral supplements. She carried a water bottle with her and drank throughout the day, paying special attention to drinking during practice. A typical day's intake during training periods is outlined below.

Professional assessment

Mean daily intake from this self-reported eating plan was assessed to be ~ 9600 kJ (2300 kcal); 369 g carbohydrate (6.5 g·kg body mass^{-1}); 63 g protein (1.1 g·kg^{-1}); 67 g fat (26% total calories). These dietary patterns failed to provide the dietary reference intakes (DRI) for adequate intake of calcium (300 mg vs. DRI 1000 mg), or of vitamin D. Emily's reported intake was at the low end of the recommended range for energy, protein, and carbohydrate. She also ate less than the recommended number of servings of vegetables. She was conscious of meeting her fluid needs each day, particularly during training sessions. She was motivated to improve her diet in order to help prevent osteoporosis.

Intervention

In order to increase Emily's calcium and vitamin D intakes as well as introduce a greater variety of food choices the following recommendations were made.

1 Eat a low-fat granola bar and half a cup of calcium-fortified juice before morning practice.

2 Replace granola bar at breakfast with a bowl of calcium-fortified cereal and low-fat milk, and continue to enjoy fruit at this meal.

3 At lunch, replace butter on bagel with peanut butter or lean meat and include one cup of calcium-fortified juice.

4 Add stir-fried vegetables to white rice, or salad to bagel.

5 Add a glass of 1% milk with chocolate syrup at dinnertime.

Outcome

Emily was able to increase her dietary intake of calcium to 1300 mg, which exceeds the DRI (1000 mg). Her total energy intake increased slightly to ~ 10 460 kJ (2500 kcal), while increasing intakes of carbohydrate to 429 g (7.5 g·kg body mass^{-1}) and protein to 81 g (1.4 g·kg body mass^{-1}). To her surprise, Emily found herself more energized during practice, as a result of an increased intake of carbohydrate, and better patterns of refueling over the day. Emily was pleased to find that she was able to easily meet her daily calcium requirements.

Breakfast	Lunch	Snacks (AM and PM)	Dinner
Banana	White rice	Low-fat granola bar	Skinless grilled chicken
Low-fat granola bar	Bagel with butter	Box of raisins	Mixed greens salad with Italian dressing
	Apple juice		Banana
	Piece of fruit		
	Large bottle of apple juice		

Chapter 5
Fluids and electrolytes

Introduction

Most athletes and coaches are aware that dehydration—a reduction in the body's water content—will result in a loss of performance. It is equally clear, however, that this knowledge does not always translate into behaviors designed to prevent or limit the risk of dehydration. Many recent major sports events—the 2002 Soccer World Cup, the 1996 Olympic Games, the 1998 Commonwealth Games —have been held in hot humid climates; these events are often organized in the summer months, and are often scheduled for the hottest part of the day. There no longer remains any doubt that exercise performance is impaired in most types of activity in these conditions, yet the athlete has no choice but to compete. All athletes will be affected, but the athlete who has prepared by a period of acclimatization to these conditions, and who has a clear rehydration strategy, is likely to be least affected. Although these preparations are not a substitute for talent, training, or motivation, they are prerequisites if the individual is to realize his or her potential.

Daily fluid needs

Water is often referred to as the "silent nutrient", reflecting the extent to which its presence and availability are taken for granted. As with all nutrients, however, a regular intake of water is required for the body to maintain health, and both deficiency symptoms and overdosage symptoms can be observed. Water is the largest single component of the normal human body, accounting for about 50–60% of total body mass. Lean body tissues contain a constant fraction—about 75%—of water by mass, whereas adipose tissue has little water content. The fraction of body mass that is accounted for by fat therefore largely determines the normal body water content: the higher the body fat level, the lower the fraction of total mass that is accounted for by water. For a healthy lean young male with a body mass of 70 kg, total body water will be about 42 l. The turnover rate of water exceeds that of most other body components: for the sedentary individual living in a temperate climate, daily water turnover is about 2–4 l, or about 5–10% of the total body water content. In spite of its abundance, however, there is a need to maintain the body water content within narrow limits, and the body is much less able to cope with restriction of water intake than with restriction of food intake. In the absence of strenuous exercise, a few days of total fasting has little impact on functional capacity, provided fluids are allowed, and even longer periods of abstinence from food are well tolerated. In contrast, except in exceptional circumstances, cessation of water intake results in serious debilitation after times ranging from only an hour or two to a few days at most.

Several factors will influence the body's water losses and thus determine the requirement for fluid intake. Among the most important of these are the ambient climatic conditions and the level of physical activity. Body size is, of course, also important: both body composition and volume, which is closely related to body mass and which defines the amount of metabolically active tissue, and body surface area, which is a function of the square of body mass and which represents the surface available for heat exchange with the environment, are important. There also appears to be a large interindividual variability in water intake and loss even after accounting for body size, but the reasons for this have not been thoroughly studied. All of these factors will combine to determine the physiological requirement for water.

The requirement for water is set by the total water losses occurring by various routes, for in all cases except the very short term, the water intake must equal the loss (Fig. 5.1). The only significant additional factor influencing the water requirement is the electrolyte content, and to a lesser extent the protein content, of the diet, which will influence the volume of urine that must be excreted. The water formed by the oxidation of foodstuffs will make some small contribution to meeting the daily water losses, but water in drinks and in foods will meet most of the demand. The water losses from the body are highly variable and include a number of significant losses as well as a number of minor ones. Losses in urine, feces, sweat, expired air and through the skin are the major avenues of water loss; smaller losses occur through blood loss, and in semen, tears, etc., but these are normally trivial.

The regulation of body water and electrolyte concentrations involves a number of neural and hormonal mechanisms which influence both intake and loss. Superimposed on these physiological control mechanisms are the various social and other factors that act to increase or restrict fluid intake.

Basal water requirements

The extent of the daily water loss and intake will vary from individual to individual, but a general example for a sedentary individual is outlined in Fig. 5.1. Body size is clearly a factor having a major influence on water turnover, but the total body water content will also be markedly affected by the body composition. It is expected therefore that there will be differences between men and women and

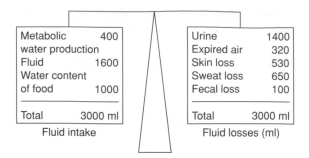

Fluid intake		Fluid losses (ml)	
Metabolic water production	400	Urine	1400
Fluid	1600	Expired air	320
Water content of food	1000	Skin loss	530
		Sweat loss	650
		Fecal loss	100
Total	3000 ml	Total	3000 ml

Fig. 5.1 Schema of daily fluid balance (intake and loss) for a typical 70-kg sedentary man.

between adults and children. Unless otherwise specified, the values given here will relate to the average 70-kg male with a moderate body fat content.

Environmental conditions will affect an individual's water requirements by altering the losses that occur by the various routes. Water requirements for sedentary individuals living in the heat may be two- or threefold higher than the requirement when living in a temperate climate, even when this is not accompanied by pronounced sweating. Transcutaneous and respiratory losses will be markedly influenced by the humidity of the ambient air, and this may be a more important factor than the ambient temperature. Respiratory water losses are incurred because of the humidification of the inspired air. These losses are relatively small in the resting individual in a warm, moist environment (amounting to about 200 ml per day), but will be increased approximately twofold in regions of low humidity, and may be as high as 1500 ml·day^{-1} during periods of hard work in the cold dry air at altitude. To these losses must be added insensible loss through the skin (about 600 ml·day^{-1}) and urine loss, which will not usually be less than about 800 ml·day^{-1}.

The water content of food ingested will also be influenced greatly by the nature of the diet, and water associated with food may make a major contribution to the total fluid intake. Some additional water is obtained from the oxidation of nutrients, and this will depend on the total metabolic rate, but will also be influenced to a lesser extent by the nature of the substrate being oxidized. If we assume an energy expenditure of 3000 kcal·day^{-1}, composed of 50% carbohydrate, 35% fat, and 15% protein, this will give about 400 ml of water per day. Reducing the energy expenditure to 2000 kcal but keeping the same diet composition will give about 275 ml of water. The contribution of water of oxidation to water requirements is thus appreciable when water turnover is low, but becomes a rather insignificant fraction of the total when water losses are high.

Control of water balance

Water intake and excretion are driven by a complex interaction of neural and hormonal factors which respond to a number of different inputs. Under normal conditions, the blood volume and the osmolality of the extracellular fluid are maintained within narrow limits: a rise or fall of about 5 mosmol·l^{-1} in the plasma osmolality is sufficient to switch the kidney from maximum conservation of water to maximum urine output. Sodium, as the major ion of the extracellular space, accounts for about 50% of the total plasma osmolality, with the result that maintenance of osmotic balance is closely coupled to the intake and excretion of both sodium and water. The profound diuresis that ensues when plasma osmolality falls normally prevents water overload, but cases of hyponatremia (low plasma sodium levels) have been reported. These normally occur when a conscious effort is made to override the physiological signals and ingest large volumes of plain water or other low-electrolyte fluids. Some degree of hyponatremia may be a normal accompaniment of the consumption of large volumes of beer, which is essentially sodium free.

The kidneys can conserve water or electrolytes by reducing the rate of loss, but can do nothing to restore a deficit, which can only be corrected by fluid intake. The subjective sensation of thirst initiates the desire to drink and hence plays a key role in the control of fluid balance. Thirst, whether measured as a perceived response or as the outcome (i.e. the volume of fluid consumed), appears to be relatively insensitive to acute changes in hydration status in humans, but the overall stability of the total water volume of an individual indicates that the desire to drink is a powerful regulatory factor over the long term. The absence of a sensation of thirst should not be taken as an indication that the body is fully hydrated.

Thirst may not be a direct consequence of the physiological need for water intake, but can be initiated by a number of unrelated factors, including habit, ritual, taste or desire for nutrients, stimulants, or a warm or cooling effect. A number of the sensations associated with thirst are learned, with drinking behavior being initiated by signals such as dryness of the mouth or throat, while distention of the stomach can stop ingestion before a fluid deficit has been restored. However, the underlying regulation of thirst is controlled separately by both the osmotic pressure and the volume of the body fluids, and as such is regulated by the same mechanisms that affect water and solute reabsorption in the kidneys and control central blood pressure.

The thirst control centers in the brain play a key role in the regulation of both thirst and diuresis. Receptors in these centers respond directly to changes in plasma osmolality and blood pressure and volume, while others are stimulated by the fluid balance hormones which also regulate renal excretion. The level of neural activity in the thirst control centers regulates the relative sensations of thirst and satiety, and can also influence urine output. Input from the higher centers of the brain, however, can override these physiological mechanisms. A rise of between 2 and 3% in plasma osmolality from the normal level of about 285–290 mosmol·l^{-1} is sufficient to evoke a profound sensation of thirst coupled with an increase in the circulating concentration of antidiuretic hormone (ADH). The mechanisms that respond to changes in intravascular volume and pressure are less sensitive, reflecting the large variations in blood volume and pressure that occur during normal daily activity.

When a water deficit has been incurred, the normal drinking response in humans involves a period of rapid ingestion during which 50% or more of the total intake is consumed, followed by a longer period during which intermittent consumption of relatively small volumes of drink occurs. The initial alleviation of thirst occurs before significant amounts of the beverage have been absorbed and entered the body pools. This indicates a role for receptors in the mouth, esophagus, and stomach, which are thought to respond to the volume of fluid ingested; distension of the stomach also tends to reduce the perception of thirst. These preabsorptive signals appear to be behavioral, learned responses and may be subject to disruption in situations which are essentially novel to the individual. This may partly explain the inappropriate voluntary fluid intake in individuals exposed to an acute increase in environmental temperature or to exercise-induced dehydration. In the longer term, a fall in plasma osmolality and increase in the extracellular volume inhibit the sensation of thirst.

Impact of physical activity on water balance

Exercise elevates the metabolic rate, and only about 25% of the energy made available by the metabolic pathways is used to perform external work, with the remainder being dissipated as heat (see Fig. 5.2). When the energy demand is high, as occurs during exercise, this results in high rates of heat production. The normal resting oxygen consumption is about 4 ml·kg body mass^{-1}·min^{-1}: for a 70-kg individual, this gives a resting rate of heat production of about 60–70 W (the equivalent of a small electric light bulb). Running a marathon in 2 h 30 min requires an oxygen consumption of about 4 l·min^{-1} to be sustained throughout the race for the average runner with a body mass of 70 kg. The accompanying rate of heat production is now about 1100 W (1.1 kW), and body temperature begins to rise rapidly. To limit the potentially harmful rise in core temperature, the rate of heat loss must be increased accordingly. Maintenance of a high skin temperature will facilitate heat loss by radiation and convection, but these mechanisms are effective only

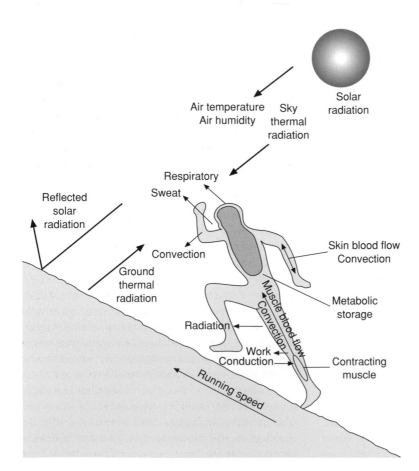

Fig. 5.2 Avenues of heat gain or heat loss in the exercising individual.

when the ambient temperature is low and the rate of air movement over the skin is high. At high ambient temperatures (above about 35°C), skin temperature will be below ambient temperature, and the only mechanism by which heat can be lost from the body is evaporation. Evaporation of 1 l of water from the skin will remove 2.4 MJ (580 kcal) of heat from the body. For the 2 h 30 min marathon runner with a body mass of 70 kg to balance the rate of metabolic heat production by evaporative loss alone would therefore require sweat to be evaporated from the skin at a rate of about $1.6\ l\cdot h^{-1}$; at such high sweat rates, an appreciable fraction drips from the skin without evaporating, and a sweat secretion rate of about $2\ l\cdot h^{-1}$ is likely to be necessary to achieve this rate of evaporative heat loss. This is possible, but would result in the loss of 5 l of body water, corresponding to a loss of more than 7% of body weight for a 70-kg runner. Water will also be lost by evaporation from the respiratory tract. During hard exercise in a hot dry environment, this can amount to a significant water loss, although it is not generally considered to be a major heat loss mechanism in humans.

In most activities, the energy demand varies continuously: average sweat losses for various sporting activities are well categorized (Table 5.1), but average values often conceal the responses at the extremes of the range. Even at low ambient temperatures high sweat rates are sometimes observed when the energy demand is high as in marathon running, so it cannot be concluded that dehydration is a problem only when the ambient temperature and humidity are high. The sweat loss is, however, closely related to the environmental conditions, and substantial fluid deficits are much more common in the summer months and in tropical climates. Body mass losses of 6 l or more are reported for marathon runners in warm weather competition. This corresponds to a water deficit of about 8% of body mass, or about 12–15% of total body water. In spite of the large variation between individuals, sweating rate has been found to be related to running speed in a heterogeneous group of marathon runners; there was, however, no relationship between total sweat loss and running speed.

It is well established that women tend to sweat less than men under standardized conditions, even

Table 5.1 Rates of sweat loss measured in different sports and exercise activities. These average values do not reveal the large variability between individuals (data taken from Rehrer & Burke 1996).

Sport	Gender	Environment (°C)	Sweat loss (ml·h⁻¹)
10-km run	F	19–24	1490
10-km run	M	19–24	1830
Marathon	M	6–24	540–1520
40-km cycle	F	19–25	750
40-km cycle	M	19–25	1140
Soccer	M	10	1000
		25	1200
Soccer	F	26	800
Netball	F	16–22	900–1000
Basketball	F	20–25	900
	M	20–25	1600
Rowing	F	10	780
		32	1390
	M	10	1165
		30	1980
Rugby	M	18–23	1600–2200
Cricket	M	23	500
		33	700–1400

after a period of acclimatization. It is likely, however, that a large part of the apparent sex difference can be accounted for by differences in training and acclimatization status. There is a limited amount of information on the effects of age on the sweating response, and again levels of fitness and acclimatization are confounding factors, but the sweating response to a standardized challenge generally decreases with age. These observations should not, however, be interpreted as suggesting an inability to exercise in the heat, nor should they be taken to indicate a decreased need for women or older individuals to pay attention to fluid intake during exposure to heat stress. There are some differences between children and adults in the sweating response to exercise and in sweat composition. The sweating capacity of children is low, when expressed per unit surface area, and the sweat electrolyte content is low relative to that of adults, but the need for fluid and electrolyte replacement is no less important than in adults. Indeed, in view of the evidence that core temperature increases to a greater extent in children than in adults at a given level of dehydration, the need for fluid replacement may well be greater in children.

Dehydration is harmful to athletic performance, and both endurance sports and high-intensity events are adversely affected. It is commonly stated that exercise performance is impaired when an individual is dehydrated by as little as 2% of body mass, and that losses in excess of 5% of body mass can decrease the capacity for work by about 30%. An examination of the original data (derived from a total of 13 trials involving three subjects) on which this statement was based, however, shows that the conclusion is much less robust than it might appear: there was no good relationship between the extent of dehydration incurred by sauna exposure and the degree of impairment of the capacity to perform a high-intensity exercise test lasting about 6 min, and a large variation in response between and within individuals was observed. Nonetheless, there is convincing evidence that prior dehydration will impair the capacity to perform high-intensity exercise as well as endurance activities. It has been shown that prolonged exercise, which resulted in a loss of fluid corresponding to 2.5% of body weight, resulted in a 45% fall in the capacity to perform high-intensity exercise. There is equally convincing evidence the prevention of dehydration by administration of fluids can improve exercise performance, and the evidence to support this will be discussed later.

Fluid losses are distributed in varying proportions among the plasma, extracellular water, and intracellular water. The decrease in plasma volume which accompanies dehydration may be of particular importance in influencing work capacity; blood flow to the muscles must be maintained at a high level to supply oxygen and substrates, but a high blood flow to the skin is also necessary to convect heat to the body surface where it can be dissipated. When the ambient temperature is high and blood volume has been decreased by sweat loss during prolonged exercise, there may be difficulty in meeting the requirement for a high blood flow to both these tissues. In this situation, skin blood flow is likely to be compromised, allowing central venous pressure and muscle blood flow to be maintained but reducing heat loss and causing body temperature to rise.

The preferential loss of water from the extracellular space reflects the relatively high sodium and

Table 5.2 Concentration ($mmol \cdot l^{-1}$) of the major electrolytes in sweat, plasma, and intracellular water. These values are taken from a variety of sources.

	Sweat	Plasma	Intracellular
Sodium	20–80	130–155	10
Potassium	4–8	3.2–5.5	150
Calcium	0–1	2.1–2.9	0
Magnesium	< 0.2	0.7–1.5	15
Chloride	20–60	96–110	8

chloride concentration in sweat. Electrolyte losses in sweat are a function of sweating rate and sweat composition, and both of these vary over time as well as being substantially influenced by the exercise intensity, the environmental conditions, and the physiology of the individual. Added to this variability is the difficulty in obtaining a reliable estimate of sweat composition, and these methodological problems have contributed at least in part to the diversity of the results reported in the literature (see Expert Comment 1). In spite of the variability in the composition of sweat, however, it is invariably isotonic with respect to plasma, and the major electrolytes are sodium and chloride, as in the extracellular space (Table 5.2). It is usual to present the composition in $mmol \cdot l^{-1}$, and the extent of the sodium losses in relation to daily dietary intake, which is usually expressed in grams, is not widely appreciated. Loss of 1 l of sweat with a sodium content of 50 $mmol \cdot l^{-1}$ represents a loss of 2.9 g of sodium chloride; the athlete who sweats 5 l in a daily training session will therefore lose almost 15 g of salt. Even allowing for a reduced sweat sodium concentration and a decreased urinary output when sodium losses in sweat are large, this amount is large in comparison to the reported normal intakes, and it is clear that the salt balance of individuals exercising in the heat is likely to be precarious. The possible need for supplementary salt intake in extreme conditions is something that the athlete training hard in warm conditions must consider.

It was mentioned earlier that there appear to be few reliable measurements of water turnover in normal healthy individuals. There are formidable obstacles that tend to confound the results of measurements of the various components of water intake and water loss. Intake is usually estimated from weighed or measured food and fluid intake diaries, but the data are complicated by uncertainties in the water content of foodstuffs, and are subject to the usual reliability issues. Measurement of the various avenues of water loss is beset by similar problems. Advances in the application of isotopic tracer methodology have recently permitted the non-invasive measurement of water turnover, using deuterium as a tracer for body water. The principle of the measurement and the practicalities are both relatively straightforward. Body water is labeled with deuterium, and the water turnover is measured over a period of a few days from the rate of decrease in the tracer concentration in body water. The measurement can be made conveniently on blood or urine samples. Collection of 24-h urine output allows non-renal losses (consisting mainly of sweat and transcutaneous losses, respiratory water loss, and fecal loss) to be calculated by difference.

Application of this method to two groups of subjects, including runners and matched sedentary individuals, showed a higher rate of water turnover in the exercising group. Both groups had a similar total body water content, but the average daily water turnover over the 7-day measurement period in the active group was about 4.7 l per day, which was higher than that of the sedentary subjects (about 3.3 l·day^{-1}). It might have been expected that the runners would have a greater daily sweat loss than the sedentary group, but there was no significant difference between the groups in non-renal water losses. These results seem surprising, but may reflect the relatively low total exercise load of the runners and the temperate climate at the time of the study. The results also suggest that the runners were habituated to drinking a volume of fluid in excess of that required to match the sweat loss incurred during exercise, perhaps because they were conscious of the need for an increased water intake in active individuals. When the same methodology was applied to another physically active group, in this case cyclists covering an average daily distance of 50 km in training for competition, and another matched sedentary group, the water turnover rate was again higher in the cyclists than in the sedentary individuals. In this study, however, there was no difference between the groups in the daily urine output, indicating that the difference in water intake was largely accounted for by an increased sweat loss.

Measures of hydration status

Dehydration generally has a negative effect on physical performance as well as on overall health. A reliable marker of hydration status may therefore be of benefit to many individuals in many situations. A body water deficit of as little as 1–2% of total body water impairs exercise performance, so any marker that is to be of use in this situation would have to be capable of indicating such a deficit. Acute changes in body mass during exercise will generally be due to loss of body water in the form of sweat; respiratory water loss and substrate oxidation are relatively small. A 1-g change in mass represents a 1-ml change in water status. Over the course of a single bout of exercise, a reduction in body mass, measured nude and with skin toweled dry before and after exercise, will indicate a state of dehydration. However, food or fluid consumed during the exercise will confuse the picture. Urinary indices, including the volume, color, protein content, specific gravity, and osmolality of the urine, have been investigated as hydration status markers. Urine color, estimated from a color chart, has been demonstrated to provide a reasonable "in the field" estimate of hydration status in association with exercise.

Bloodborne indices, including hemoglobin and hematocrit, plasma osmolality and sodium concentration, plasma testosterone, adrenaline, noradrenaline, cortisol, and atrial natriuretic peptide, have been investigated as hydration status markers. These bloodborne indices have the disadvantage of being more invasive than many of the other measures described, and in an exercise setting some respond not only to hydration stresses but to exercise stresses too. Bioelectrical impedance analysis can give a rapid estimate of total body water, and its cellular divisions if a multifrequency device is utilized. Changes in hydration status may be detected if the procedure is carefully standardized in many ways but the precision and sensitivity of the method remain to be established.

Alterations in the response of pulse rate and systolic blood pressure to postural change have been demonstrated in clinical settings of dehydration and rehydration. However, these measures may not be sensitive enough to be of value in an exercise situation. A wide variety of indices have been investigated to establish their effectiveness as markers of hydration status in an exercise situation. An individual's choice of hydration status marker will be influenced by the sensitivity and accuracy with which they need to establish hydration status, together with the technical and time requirements and expense involved.

Water replacement in exercise

The major issues in fluid replacement are the optimization of hydration status prior to exercise, the provision of fluid and substrate (and possibly also other nutrients) during exercise, and rehydration and recovery after exercise. The kidneys effectively prevent attempts to increase the body water content prior to exercise, and although the addition of osmotically active substances such as glycerol to ingested fluids can decrease the fraction of ingested fluid that appears promptly in the urine, the effectiveness of this procedure in affecting the physiological responses to exercise is unclear.

Dilute glucose–electrolyte solutions are the most effective way of replacing water losses when rapid rehydration is desired: variations on this formulation are the basis of oral rehydration solutions for the treatment of infectious diarrhea and of sports drinks. The rate of gastric emptying of such solutions is slowed in proportion to the carbohydrate content, and concentrated solutions will be unable to deliver water at high rates. Intestinal water absorption is driven by osmotic gradients and by solvent drag resulting from active absorption of solute, especially glucose and sodium which are cotransported by an ATP-dependent mechanism. Hypotonic (200–250 mosmol·kg^{-1}) solutions containing glucose and sodium will maximize the rate of water absorption, but hypertonic solutions will cause a temporary secretion of water into the intestinal lumen, exacerbating any existing dehydration.

The ingestion of water or carbohydrate–electrolyte sports drinks during exercise has been shown to help reduce the fall in plasma volume that normally occurs: this in turn helps to maintain cardiac output by maintaining stroke volume and increases the skin blood flow, which helps promote heat loss and limit the rise in core temperature. Although ingestion of plain water can help to improve exercise performance, further benefits are observed if glucose or glucose plus electrolytes are added.

Rehydration is a vital part of the recovery process after exercise which has resulted in sweat loss. The usual recommendation to ensure adequate fluid replacement after exercise is to replace each kilogram of weight lost during exercise with 1 liter of fluid, but there is now compelling evidence, that it is necessary to ingest at least 50% more volume than the volume of sweat lost if euhydration is to be achieved. It is also essential to replace the electrolytes lost in sweat if the ingested fluid is to be retained rather than being lost in the urine. These issues are covered in detail in Chapter 9.

Electrolytes

Variations in the amount and type of food eaten have some effect on water requirements because of the resulting demand for excretion of excess electrolytes and the products of metabolism. An intake of electrolytes in excess of the amounts lost (primarily in sweat and feces) must be corrected by excretion in the urine, with a corresponding increase in the volume and osmolality of urine formed. The daily intake of electrolytes is subject to wide variation between individuals, with strong trends for differences between different geographical regions. Daily dietary salt (sodium chloride) intakes for 95% of the young male UK population fall between 3.8 and 14.3 g with a mean of 8.4 g; the corresponding values for young women are 2.8–9.4 g, with a mean value of 6.0 g. For the same population, mean urinary sodium losses were reported to account for about 175 mmol·day^{-1}, which is equivalent to about 10.2 g of sodium chloride.

There are also large differences between countries in the recommended intake of salt: the British advice is for a maximum of 6 g·day^{-1}, but in Germany, a maximum of 10 g·day^{-1} is recommended. In contrast, Sweden recommends a maximum of 2 g·day^{-1}, and Poland recommends a minimum of 1.4 g·day^{-1}. These differences in the recommendations by different expert committees reflect in part different interpretations with regard to the evidence linking salt intake and health, but also reflect regional consumption patterns. Water intake will reflect rather closely the patterns of salt intake. A high-protein diet also requires a greater urine output to allow excretion of water-soluble nitrogenous waste: this effect is relatively small compared with other losses, but becomes meaningful when water availability is limited.

Salt losses in sweat can be significant. The sweat that is secreted onto the skin contains a wide variety of organic and inorganic solutes, and significant losses of some of these components will occur where large volumes of sweat are produced. The electrolyte composition of sweat is variable, and the concentration of individual electrolytes as well as the total sweat volume will influence the extent of losses. The content of the major electrolytes is shown in comparison with their plasma and intracellular concentrations in Table 5.2. A number of factors contribute to the variability in the composition of sweat; methodological problems in the collection procedure, including evaporative loss, incomplete collection, and contamination with skin cells, account for at least part of the variability, but there is also a large biological variability. (see Expert Comment 1, p. 62)

The sweat composition undoubtedly varies between individuals, but can also vary within the same individual depending on the rate of secretion, the state of training, and the state of heat acclimatization. In response to a standard heat stress, the sweat rate increases with training and acclimatization and the electrolyte content decreases. These adaptations are generally considered to allow improved thermoregulation while conserving electrolytes. There are, however, some puzzling aspects: where the sweat rate is sufficient to keep the skin wet, further increases in the sweat rate will increase the amount of water which drips from the skin without evaporation but will not further increase the rate of evaporative heat loss.

In spite of the variations which do occur, the major electrolytes in sweat, as in the extracellular fluid, are sodium and chloride (Table 5.2), although the sweat concentrations of these ions are invariably lower than those in plasma. Contrary to what might be expected, there is some evidence that the concentration of sodium and chloride in sweat increases with increased flow, as a result of a reduced opportunity for reabsorption in the sweat duct. Acclimatization studies have shown that elevated sweating rates are accompanied by a decrease in the concentration of sodium and chloride in sweat in spite of the increased flow rate. The potassium content of sweat appears to be relatively unaffected by the sweat rate, and the magnesium content is also unchanged or perhaps decreases slightly. These apparently conflicting results demonstrate some of the difficulties in interpreting the literature in this area. Differences between studies may be due to differences in the training status and degree of acclimatization of the subjects used, as well as difference in methodology: some studies have used whole body washdown techniques to collect sweat, whereas others have examined local sweating responses using ventilated capsules or collection bags. There may be differences between the composition of sweat from a specific region, such as the hand and forearm, and the whole body sweat. The use of improved sweat collection techniques will begin to resolve these issues.

Because sweat is hypotonic with respect to body fluids, the effect of prolonged sweating is to increase the plasma osmolality, which may have a significant effect on the ability to maintain body temperature. A direct relationship between plasma osmolality and body temperature has been demonstrated during exercise. Hyperosmolality of plasma, induced prior to exercise, has been shown to result in a decreased ability to regulate body temperature; the threshold for sweating is elevated and the flow of warm blood to the skin is reduced. In short-term (30-min) exercise, however, the cardiovascular and thermoregulatory response appears to be independent of changes in osmolality induced during the exercise period. The changes in the concentration of individual electrolytes are more variable, but an increase in the plasma sodium and chloride concentrations is generally observed in response to both running and cycling exercise. Exceptions to this are rare and occur only when excessively large volumes of drinks low in electrolytes are consumed over long time periods.

The plasma potassium concentration has been reported to remain constant after marathon running, although others have reported small increases, irrespective of whether drinks containing large amounts of potassium or no electrolytes were given. Much of the inconsistency in the literature relating to changes in the circulating potassium concentration can be explained by the variable time taken to obtain blood samples after exercise under field conditions; the plasma potassium concentration rapidly returns to normal in the postexercise period. Laboratory studies where an indwelling catheter can be used to obtain blood samples during exercise commonly show an increase in the circulating potassium concentration in the later stages of prolonged exercise. The potassium concentration of extracellular fluid (4–5 mmol·l^{-1}) is small relative to the intracellular concentration (150–160 mmol·l^{-1}), and release of potassium from liver, muscle, and red blood cells will tend to elevate plasma potassium levels during exercise in spite of the losses in sweat.

The blood magnesium concentration is usually reported to be unchanged after prolonged moderate-intensity exercise, but a 20% fall in the serum magnesium concentration has been observed after a marathon race. A larger fall in the serum magnesium concentration has been observed during exercise in the heat than at neutral temperatures, supporting the idea that losses in sweat may be responsible. There are, however, reports that the fall in plasma magnesium concentration that occurs during prolonged exercise is a consequence of redistribution between tissues, with uptake of magnesium by red blood cells, active muscle, or adipose tissue, rather than a net loss from the body. Although the concentration of potassium and magnesium in sweat is high relative to that in the plasma, the plasma content of these ions represents only a small fraction of the whole body stores; only about 1% of the body stores of these electrolytes is lost when individuals are dehydrated by about 5–6% of body weight.

Practical implications for the athlete

Although the basic principles that govern fluid replacement strategies for athletes are well established, there are some real difficulties in putting these into practice. Athletes and their advisers want a prescription for the composition, amount, and timing of fluid intake that will cover all situations. Even within a single event, however, the requirement will vary so much between individuals, depending on the physiological and biochemical characteristics of the individual as well as on the training load and on other factors such as taste preference, that such recommendations can only be made on an individual basis. When the possible effects of different climatic conditions and different training and competition schedules are added, the problems in making a simple recommendation are multiplied.

These difficulties are immediately apparent when any of the published guidelines for fluid intake during exercise are examined. These guidelines are generally formulated to include the needs of most individuals in most situations, with the results that the outer limits become so wide as to be at best meaningless, and at worst positively harmful. The guidelines of the American College of Sports Medicine, expressed in their 1984 Position Statement on the prevention of heat illness in distance running, were an attempt to give athletes some indication of the amount of fluid they might need. The recommendation for marathon runners was for an intake of 100–200 ml every 2–3 km, giving a total intake of 1400–4200 ml at the extremes. Taking these extreme values, it is unlikely that the elite runners, who take only a little over 2 h to complete the distance, could tolerate a rate of intake of about 2 l·h^{-1}, and equally unlikely that an intake of 250 ml·h^{-1} would be adequate for the slowest competitors except perhaps when the ambient temperature was low. These same guidelines also recommended that the best fluid to drink during prolonged exercise is cool water: in view of the accumulated evidence, this recommendation seems even less acceptable now than it was in 1984 (see Chapter 10).

Because of the difficulty in making specific recommendations that will meet the needs of all individuals in all situations, the only possible way forward is to formulate some general guidelines and to indicate how these should be modified in different circumstances. Assuming that athletes are willing and able to take fluids during training, the recommendations for fluid use in training will not be very different for training and competition, except in events of very short duration. The sprinter or pursuit cyclist, whose event lasts a few seconds or minutes, has no opportunity or need for fluid intake during competition, but should take fluids during training sessions which may stretch over 2 h or more.

All athletes should aim to ensure that they begin exercise fully hydrated, and this includes those who may have had to meet weight categories and have undergone fluid restriction practices to do so. Attempts to overhydrate by the ingestion of saline or glycerol solutions have met with limited success, but the negative effects of beginning exercise in a state of fluid deficit are clear. The most effective drinks to be consumed during exercise will vary greatly between individuals, as will the amounts and timing of intake. In general, the aim should be to replace a substantial fraction of the fluid loss and to limit the extent of dehydration to no more than 1–2% of the pre-exercise body mass. The sweat rate can vary from a few hundred ml to more than 3 l per hour, depending on the climatic and exercise conditions and on the acclimatization status and physiological characteristics of the individual. Only by self-monitoring in the conditions of training and competition can athletes learn how much fluid they need and how much they can tolerate.

Fluids should contain some carbohydrate, and also some electrolytes, of which sodium is the main requirement. Information on sports drinks is covered in greater detail in Chapter 8. Although the optimum formulation of a sports drink will depend on the conditions, it is important that athletes choose a drink that is palatable under the conditions in which they will perform. Practicing drinking in training is an important skill that is often neglected.

Summary

Dehydration impairs performance and increases the risk of heat illness during exercise. Daily fluid losses are small in temperate conditions when no physical activity is performed, but sweat losses increase with ambient temperature and humidity and are greatly increased during hard exercise. Replacing losses by ingesting fluid during exercise improves performance and adding carbohydrate further improves performance. Sweat contains variable amounts of electrolytes, but sodium is the primary electrolyte lost. High sodium intakes may be necessary to replace losses in sweat. Carbohydrate and sodium should be added to drinks ingested during exercise, but the optimum formulation will depend on the exercise conditions and on the relative needs for carbohydrate supply and rehydration. Strategies for fluid intake before, during, and after exercise will be discussed in greater detail in Chapters 7–9 in the section on "Competition nutrition strategies".

Reading list

Maughan, R.J. (2000) Fluid and carbohydrate intake during exercise. In: *Clinical Sports Nutrition* (eds L. M. Burke & V. Deakin), 2nd edn, pp. 369–395. McGraw Hill, Sydney, Australia.

Maughan, R.J. & Murray, R. (eds) (2000) *Sports drinks: Basic Science and Practical Aspects*, p. 279. CRC Press, Boca Raton.

Nicholas, C.W., Williams, C., Lakomy, H.K.A., Phillips, G. & Nowitz, A. (1995) Influence of ingesting a carbohydrate-electrolyte solution on endurance capacity during intermittent, high-intensity shuttle running. *Journal of Sports Sciences* **13**, 283–290.

Rehrer, N.J. & Burke, L.M. (1996) Sweat losses during various sports. *Australian Journal of Nutrition and Dietetics* **53** (Suppl. 4), S13–S16.

EXPERT COMMENT 1 The composition of sweat. Susan M. Shirreffs

A wide range of values for all of the major sweat solute components has been reported, reflecting variations between individuals, differences due to the experimental conditions, and differences due to the method of collection. The sweat secreted onto the skin is the sum of the original tubular secretion in the gland, minus the substances that are reabsorbed further up the tubule. This means that the composition of the fluid that is secreted into the coil of the sweat gland may be substantially changed by the time it reaches the skin surface. The fluid secreted is initially isotonic with body fluids. Most of the major electrolytes (Na^+, Cl^-) are transported out of the duct back in to the extracellular fluid in excess of water. The final sweat secreted onto the skin is therefore hypotonic with respect to body fluids (approximately 150 mosmol·l^{-1}).

Due to the nature of the secretion and reabsorption processes in sweat production within the sweat gland and duct, sweat composition is influenced by sweat rate, at least within single ducts, such that a reduction in rate allows for greater reabsorption of electrolytes from the duct. This means that a higher sweat rate results in a lower concentration in the final sweat produced. There do, also, appear to be regional variations in sweat composition, as evidenced by the different values obtained when the composition of sweat obtained from different parts of the body is compared. The values obtained with this method also differ from those obtained by the whole body washdown technique.

Sweat production is influenced by a number of factors. In response to thermal stress, as opposed to, for example, mental stress, the hypothalamic temperature, together with skin temperature, seem to be the largest determinants. Despite the composition of human sweat being highly variable, both between individuals and within an individual over time, it is generally agreed that sodium is the major electrolyte lost in sweat. The sweat electrolyte composition of an individual (see Table 5.2) seems primarily to be related to sweat rate, but can be influenced by his or her training status as this affects sweat rate, extent of heat acclimatization, and diet.

Athlete

Sheila was a 26-year-old elite female heptathlete training to qualify for the US Olympic team. She was 170 cm in height and weighed 68 kg. During the precompetition phase of her training cycle she undertook two training sessions a day, each lasting 2–3 h, with 1 rest day each week.

Reason for consultancy

Sheila was a participant in a USA Track and Field elite heptathlete Development Program and attended the summit meeting training camps provided by this program. At one camp she consulted a dietitian, reporting problems with fatigue during her afternoon training sessions and on the second day of her 2-day competitions. This fatigue limited her training intensity and prevented her from performing at her best. Sheila thought she was getting adequate rest and was not overtraining. She wondered whether improving her diet would help to make her feel more energetic during intense training workouts and at competitions.

Current dietary patterns

Sheila's typical training diet included the following daily food choices:

large amounts of low-fat, high-protein foods including lean cuts of fish, red meats, chicken, and turkey;

nine servings of fruits and vegetables (serving = one piece of fruit, or $\frac{1}{2}$ cup cooked or chopped fruit or vegetable, or 1 cup of fresh vegetable greens);

10 servings of grains and cereals (serving = $\frac{1}{2}$ cup breakfast cereal or one slice bread);

1–2 cups of skimmed milk;

fluids when she was thirsty; water during training workouts and at competitions.

Professional assessment

Mean daily intake from this self-reported eating plan was assessed to be slightly below recommended levels for energy intake, although under-reporting needed to be taken into account since she appeared to be weight stable. Her intake of protein appeared to be adequate (achieving at least 1.2 g·kg body mass^{-1}). However, her carbohydrate intake (5 g·kg body mass^{-1}) was estimated to be well below the recommended range (7–10 g·kg body mass^{-1}) and fat intake was low (~ 20% of her energy intake). Food intake was well spread throughout the day. Sheila did not drink beverages with her meals and relied only on her thirst to determine whether she needed to drink fluids. She did not monitor her hydration status.

Intervention

In order to ensure adequate energy intake and to increase fluid intake throughout the day, particularly before, during and after competitions, the following recommendations were made.

1 Continue eating large amounts of fluid-rich fruits and vegetables.

2 Measure body weight before and after workouts and when possible at competitions. Drink enough fluids (approximately 1.0–1.5 l·kg body water weight loss^{-1}) to attain preworkout or precompetition body weight.

3 Regularly check urine color to assess hydration status using the marker of a clear, pale yellow color as a sign of adequate hydration.

4 Drink a sports beverage in addition to water during training workouts in order to help maintain the drive to drink fluid, add variety to fluid choices to encourage more fluid intake, and obtain some additional energy.

5 Develop and follow a plan for drinking fluid before, during, and after competitions. Use a written nutrition planner to make a practical plan for what to drink and eat during each of the 2 days of competitions.

Outcome

Sheila was able to periodically check her weight before and after training workouts to assess the amount of her fluid loss. She started drinking a sports beverage, plus water at workouts, which helped her drink more fluid and keep better pace with fluid losses. She also quickly developed the habit of monitoring her urine color and used it as a marker for deciding whether she needed to drink more fluids. With these strategies in place, she reported an improvement in her energy levels at afternoon practices. Making changes during competition was a more difficult process. Sheila found it difficult to regularly check her weight on competition days, and found it hard to know how much to drink during breaks between competition events. However, with the help of the nutrition planner and more practice, she was gradually able to develop a competition hydration strategy. Implementing her plan was a challenge but she adopted good habits with help from her coach and a friend. As a result of her efforts, her energy level was more sustained during training and her performance improved. Sheila qualified to become a member of the 2000 US Olympic heptathlon team.

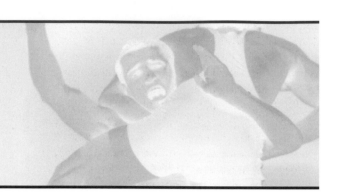

Chapter 6
Alcohol and sport

Introduction

Alcohol and sport are closely linked through sponsorship and advertising, with many sporting organizations, teams, and events being supported by companies who make beer and other alcoholic drinks. While a small number of athletes drink alcohol in the belief that it may improve their sports performance, alcohol consumption by athletes generally occurs in a social environment. However, these social occasions are often embedded in the culture that surrounds participation in sport. This chapter will review the effect of alcohol on sports performance, particularly binge drinking patterns that typify the alcohol intake of many athletes, and will provide some guidelines for sensible use of alcohol by sportspeople.

Alcohol use by athletes

How many athletes regularly consume alcohol and how much do these athletes drink? It is hard to find reliable answers to these questions. First, because alcohol intake typically provides only a minor contribution to daily energy intake (usually less than 5% of the total energy intake of adults), it is often excluded or forgotten in the results of dietary surveys of athletes. Second, experts in dietary survey research tell us that what people report about their use of alcohol is particularly unreliable. Athletes

may either under-report their true use of alcohol if they feel they will be judged poorly because of it, or they may exaggerate their intake if they feel it is something to brag about.

In general, dietary surveys of athletes which include information about alcohol intake suggest that it contributes 0–5% of total energy intake in the everyday diet. However, these figures may provide a misleading view of the drinking habits of athletes. After all, many athletes only consume alcohol on a few occasions each week or month, but they consume it in large amounts at these times. This pattern was demonstrated in a dietary survey of Australian Football players whose mean daily intake of alcohol was reported to be a modest 20 g or two standard drinks. However, almost all this intake occurred during postmatch celebrations or commiserations, with the mean intake in this situation being 120 g (range 27–368 g), and alcohol providing a mean contribution of 19% of total energy intake on match day (range 3–43% of total energy intake). These self-reports of excessive alcohol intake after the game were confirmed when blood alcohol levels (BALs) were estimated at a training session on the morning after a game: 34% of players registered a positive BAL, with 10% of players showing a level above the legal limit for driving a motor vehicle. Binge drinking episodes are frequently the topic of stories or media reports about the off-field exploits of athletes. These appear to occur most often after a session of sport, at sport-related social events, or in the company of other athletes. Postexercise drinking is subject to many rationalizations and justifications by athletes including "everyone is doing it", "I only drink once a week" and "I can run/sauna it off the next morning". In some cases these episodes are romanticized and the drinking prowess of the athletes is admired (see Expert Comment 1).

Whether total alcohol intake, or episodes of heavy alcohol intake, by athletes are different from those of the general population is not known. Various theories have been proposed to explain likely associations between sport and alcohol use. On one hand it has been suggested that athletes might have a lower intake due to increased self-esteem, a more rigid lifestyle, and greater interest in their health and performance. Alternatively, alcohol has been associated with the rituals of relaxation and celebration in sport, and with risk taking, which may be higher among athletes. Several studies in different countries have reported that athletes report greater intakes of alcohol than sedentary people, with team sport players recording higher intakes than other types of athletes.

While there is some evidence that many athletes consume alcohol in excessive amounts, on at least some occasions, further studies are needed to fully determine the alcohol intake and patterns of use by athletes. Information on the attitudes and beliefs of athletes about alcohol is also desirable, since it would allow education programs to specifically target current drinking practices that are detrimental to the athlete's performance or health.

Metabolism of alcohol

The metabolism of alcohol (ethanol) occurs primarily in the liver, where it is oxidized first to acetaldehyde and then to acetate. The first step is catalysed by a number of hepatic enzymes, the most important of which is the NAD-dependent alcohol dehydrogenase:

$$CH_3CH_2OH + NAD^+ \rightarrow CH_3CHO + NADH + H^+$$

Aldehyde dehydrogenase catalyses the further oxidation of acetaldehyde to acetate:

$$CH_3CHO + NADH^+ + H_2O \rightarrow$$
$$CH_3COO^- + NADH + 2H^+$$

Table 6.1 A standard drink contains approximately 10 g of alcohol.

Drink	Amount (ml)
Standard beer (4% alcohol)	250
Low-alcohol beer (2% alcohol)	500
Cider, wine coolers, alcoholic soft drinks	250
Wine	100
Champagne	100
Fortified wines, sherry, port	60
Spirits	30

The NADH formed in these reactions must be re-oxidized within the mitochondria, but transfer of the hydrogen atoms into the mitochondria might be a limiting process that can interfere with carbohydrate metabolism. If the liver glycogen stores are low because of a combination of exercise and a low carbohydrate intake, the liver will be unable to maintain the circulating glucose concentration, leading to hypoglycemia.

Acetaldehyde, which is thought to be responsible for many of the adverse effects of alcohol, is metabolized within the liver. The rate at which ethanol is cleared by the liver varies widely between individuals, and the response of the individual will depend on the amount of ethanol consumed in relation to their habitual intake. There is conflicting information about whether the rate of metabolism of alcohol is increased by exercise. Table 6.1 summarizes the amount of alcohol contained in some standard servings of alcohol drinks.

Effects of acute alcohol ingestion on exercise

In previous times, some athletes deliberately consumed alcohol immediately before or during an event in the hope of improving their performance. Alcohol was believed to decrease sensitivity to pain and increase confidence. Additional effects on the cardiovascular system were thought to reduce tremor and stress-induced emotional arousal, important issues during fine motor control sports. For this reason, although alcohol is no longer on the general doping list of the International Olympic Committee (IOC), it is still considered a banned substance in some sports such as shooting and fencing.

In modern sports practice, few athletes would intentionally consume alcohol during exercise as a performance aid. Even in sports like darts and billiards where participants popularly drink during competition, this practice is probably a reflection of the culture of games that are usually played in a hotel environment. Similarly, some people may undertake recreational exercise, such as snow- or water-skiing, with a positive blood alcohol level as a result of social activities between sessions of exercise. For these reasons it is useful to examine the effects of alcohol on exercise metabolism and performance. However such outcomes are hard to determine since alcohol has a variety of effects on different body tissues and there is great variability in individual responses to alcohol intake.

A position stand released in 1982 by the American College of Sports Medicine reviewed the acute effects of alcohol ingestion on metabolism and performance of exercise. The conclusion was that alcohol does not contribute significantly to energy stores used for exercise, and in situations of prolonged exercise it may increase the risk of hypoglycemia due to the suppression of glucose production by the liver. Increased heat loss may be associated with this hypoglycemia, as well as the cutaneous vasodilatation caused by exercise, causing an impairment of temperature regulation in cold environments.

Studies of the effects of alcohol on cardiovascular, respiratory, and muscular function have provided conflicting results. The outcomes vary according to the dose of alcohol consumed and there is considerable variability in the responses of different subjects. It is difficult to conduct alcohol studies according to the ideal protocols for scientific research since it is hard to provide a suitable placebo treatment—people can generally tell when they have consumed large amounts of alcohol, and their beliefs may bias their performance. Ethics committees are also reluctant to approve studies that may appear to encourage individuals to consume alcohol. Nevertheless, it has been generally concluded that the acute ingestion of alcohol has no beneficial

effects on muscle function, and alcohol may actually produce detrimental effects on exercise performance when consumed in large doses.

Studies of alcohol and fine motor control and skill show a detrimental effect of small to moderate amounts of alcohol on reaction time, hand–eye coordination, accuracy, balance, and complex skilled tasks. In fact there is no evidence to support the proposed beneficial effects of reduced muscle tremor. However, alcohol intake may result in a greater feeling of self-confidence in athletes, and this may, in turn improve performance, or the perception of performance, in some situations. There is good reason for the legal bans on driving motor vehicles after having consumed moderate to large amounts of alcohol since this will interfere with the judgement and skill involved in this activity. Skilled performance in sport is not so different in this respect from driving a motor car.

Effects of acute alcohol ingestion on postexercise recovery

Alcohol intake and binge drinking seem particularly linked with postcompetition activities, and perhaps even the social rituals following training or practice sessions in some sports. Athletes are likely to be dehydrated and to have eaten little on the day of competition. Therefore, alcohol consumed after exercise is more quickly absorbed and likely to have greater effects than under normal circumstances. It is important to examine the effects of alcohol on processes that are important in the recovery from exercise, and on the performance of subsequent exercise bouts.

Rehydration

Rehydration is an important component of postexercise recovery. The restoration of the fluid deficit caused by exercise is a balance between the amount of fluid that the athlete will drink after exercise, and their ongoing fluid losses. The palatability of drinks provided after exercise will help to determine total fluid intake, while replacement of sodium losses is a major determinant of the success in retaining this fluid (see Chapter 9). It has been suggested that beer may be an acceptable postexercise beverage since athletes will voluntarily consume it in large volume! However, beer does not provide a substantial sodium content (unless it is accompanied by the intake of salty foods). Furthermore, alcohol is known to have a diuretic action that is likely to promote increased urine losses.

A study by Susan Shirreffs and Ron Maughan examined the effect of alcohol on postexercise rehydration after subjects had lost fluid equivalent to 2% of body mass (BM). Subjects replaced 150% of this volume of fluid by consuming drinks containing 0, 1, 2, or 4% alcohol. The study found that total volume of urine produced during the 6 h of recovery was positively related to the alcohol content of the fluid. In the case of the 4% alcohol drink, subjects were still dehydrated at the end of the recovery period, despite having consumed 1.5 times the volume of their fluid deficit. Although individual variability must be taken into account, this study suggests that the intake of significant amounts of alcohol will interfere with rehydration.

In practical terms, low-alcohol beers (< 2% alcohol) or beer "shandies" (beer mixed in equal proportions with lemonade, to dilute the alcohol content and provide some carbohydrate) may not be detrimental to rehydration. In fact, these drinks might be useful in encouraging large fluid intakes in dehydrated athletes and the carbohydrate content of the lemonade may be useful for the replenishment of glycogen stores. However, wine and spirits with a more concentrated alcohol content are not advised, since effective fluid replacement will be reduced by the combination of a smaller fluid volume and a greater alcohol intake When rapid rehydration is required, the athlete should stick to a well-considered fluid intake plan that includes replacement of sodium (see Chapter 9).

Glycogen storage

Since alcohol has a number of effects on carbohydrate metabolism, it is possible that postexercise intake might impair the restoration of depleted glycogen stores. In the absence of carbohydrate intake, alcohol intake is known to impair the liver carbohydrate stores. Alcohol intake has been reported to impair muscle glycogen storage in rats following depletion by fasting or exercise; however, the effect in humans is not clear. Burke and colleagues undertook an investigation of the effects of alcohol intake on muscle glycogen storage in humans over 8 h and 24 h of recovery from a prolonged cycling bout. In these studies, athletes undertook three different diets following their glycogen-depleting exercise: a high-carbohydrate diet, an alcohol displacement diet (reduced carbohydrate + ~ 120 g alcohol) and an alcohol plus carbohydrate diet (~ 120 g alcohol added to the high-carbohydrate diet). Muscle glycogen storage was significantly reduced on the alcohol displacement diets when inadequate amounts of carbohydrate were consumed. On the other hand, when the high-carbohydrate diet was eaten, there was no clear evidence that alcohol intake caused a reduction in muscle glycogen storage. However, this may have been masked by the variability of the responses of different subjects.

The most important message of this study is that alcohol intake often has an indirect effect on postexercise refueling. Binge drinking is likely to prevent the athlete from consuming adequate carbohydrate intake—after all, athletes do not often eat much food or make good choices of high-carbohydrate food on such an occasion. Food intake may also be affected over the next day as the athlete sleeps off his or her hangover.

Other effects

Many sporting activities are associated with muscle damage and soft tissue injuries, either as a direct consequence of the exercise, or as a result of accidents or the tackling and collisions involved in contact sports. Standard medical practice is to treat soft tissue injuries with vasoconstrictive techniques (e.g. rest, ice, compression, elevation). Since alcohol causes blood vessels to dilate it has been suggested that the intake of large amounts of alcohol might cause or increase undesirable swelling around damaged sites, and might impede repair processes. The evidence for this is mainly based on case studies and the subjective evaluation of physiotherapists who treat injured athletes, and there is a need for carefully controlled studies to investigate these observations. Until such studies are undertaken, it seems sensible for players who have suffered considerable muscle damage and soft tissue injuries to avoid any intake of alcohol in the immediate recovery phase (e.g. for 24 h after the event).

Since heat loss from the skin is another effect of cutaneous vasodilatation, athletes who consume large quantities of alcohol in cold environments may have problems with thermoregulation. An increased risk of hypothermia may be found in sports or recreational activities undertaken in cold weather, particularly hiking or skiing, where alcohol intake is an integral part of "après ski" activities.

However, it is likely that the major effect of excessive alcohol intake comes from the athlete's failure to follow guidelines for optimal recovery. The intoxicated athlete may fail to undertake sensible injury management practices or to report for treatment. In cold environments they may fail to seek suitable clothing or shelter, or to notice early signs of hypothermia. Studies which measure the direct effect of alcohol on thermoregulation and soft tissue damage are encouraged.

Accidents and high-risk behavior

Alcohol impairs judgement and reduces inhibitions. As a result, intoxicated athletes frequently undertake high-risk behavior, leading to an increased risk of accidents that may lead to injury and an inability to train or compete. Alcohol consumption is a major factor in road accidents, and is frequently involved with drowning accidents, spinal injuries, and other problems in recreational water activities. As outlined in Expert Comment 1, athletes are not immune to the social and behavioral problems following excess alcohol intake. Further research is needed to investigate whether athletes, or some groups of athletes, are more likely to drink excessively or suffer a greater risk of alcohol-related problems. However, it appears that athletes should at least be included in population education programs related to drink-driving and other high-risk behavior.

Effect of previous day's intake (hangover) on performance

Some athletes will be required to train (or even compete again) on the day after a competition and its post-event drinking binge. In some cases, athletes may choose to drink heavily the night before a competition, as a general part of their social activities, or in the belief that this will help to "relax" them prior to the event. The effect of an "alcohol hangover" on performance is widely discussed by athletes, but has not been well studied. Two studies have looked at "next day" performance in athletes who consumed large amounts of alcohol. Although the study design was not ideal in either study, they reported a reduction in some but not all aspects of exercise performance in the hungover athletes. Research in other areas of industrial work (e.g. machine handling and flying) suggests that impairment of psychomotor skills may continue during the hangover phase. This is likely to be an issue in team and court sports that demand tactical play and a high skill level.

Effects of chronic alcohol intake on issues of sports performance

Athletes who frequently consume large amounts of alcohol face the large number of health and social problems associated with problem drinking. Early problems to affect sports performance include inadequate nutrition and a generally poor lifestyle (e.g. inadequate sleep and recovery). Since alcohol is an energy-dense nutrient (providing 7 kcal or 27 kJ per gram), weight gain is a typical problem arising from frequent episodes of heavy alcohol intake. The accompanying factors of erratic eating patterns and choice of high-fat foods can lead to excess energy consumption. A common story, particularly in team sports, is that athletes gain significant amounts of body fat during the off season due to increased alcohol intake coupled with reduced exercise expenditure. Many players need to spend a significant part of their preseason (and even early season) conditioning to reverse the problems of being overfat and unfit. Clearly this is a disadvantage to performance and to the longevity of a sports career.

Guidelines for sensible use of alcohol by athletes

It is important for athletes to set themselves a sensible plan regarding alcohol intake. The following guidelines are suggested.

1 It is an athlete's personal decision about whether to consume alcohol or not. Alcohol is not an essential component of a diet. However, there is no evidence of impairments to health and performance when alcohol is used sensibly.

2 Community guidelines in various countries provide messages about intakes of alcohol that are "safe and healthy". In general, they suggest that mean daily intake of alcohol intake should be less than 40–50 g (4–5 standard glasses) for males, and perhaps 20–30 g (2–3 standard glasses) for females. Binge drinking is discouraged. Since individual tolerance to alcohol is variable, it is difficult to set a precise definition of "heavy" intake or an alcohol "binge". However, intakes of about 80–100 g (8–10 standard glasses) at a single sitting are likely to constitute a heavy intake for most people.

3 Alcohol is a high-energy (and nutrient-poor) food and should be restricted when the athlete is attempting to reduce body fat.

4 Drinking large amounts of alcohol on the night before competition is unwise. However, it appears unlikely that the intake of one or two standard drinks will have negative effects in most athletes.

5 The intake of alcohol immediately before or during exercise does not enhance performance. In many athletes it may impair performance, particularly of psychomotor skills and judgement. Therefore the athlete should not consume alcohol deliberately to aid performance, and should be wary of exercise that is conducted in conjunction with the social intake of alcohol.

6 Excess intake of alcohol is likely to interfere with recovery after exercise. It may directly impair rehy-

dration, glycogen recovery, and repair of soft tissue damage. More importantly, the athlete is unlikely to remember to undertake strategies for optimal recovery when they are intoxicated. Therefore, the athlete should attend to these strategies first before any alcohol is consumed. In the case of the athlete who has suffered a substantial soft tissue injury, no alcohol should be consumed for 24 h after the event.

7 The athlete should rehydrate with appropriate fluids in volumes that are greater than their existing fluid deficit. Low-alcohol beers and beer–soft drink mixes may be suitable and seem to encourage large volume intakes. However, drinks containing more than 2% alcohol are not recommended during rehydration. Better choices include sports drinks, fruit juices, soft drinks (all containing carbohydrate), and water (when refueling is not a major issue). Sodium replacement via sports drinks, oral rehydration solutions, or salt-containing foods is also important to encourage the retention of these rehydration fluids.

8 Before consuming any alcohol after exercise, the athlete should consume a high-carbohydrate meal or snack to aid muscle glycogen recovery. Food intake will also help to reduce the rate of alcohol absorption and thus reduce the rate of intoxication.

9 Once postexercise recovery priorities have been addressed, the athlete who chooses to drink is encouraged to do so "in moderation". Drink-driving education messages in various countries provide guidelines for sensible and well-paced drinking.

10 Athletes who drink heavily after competition or at other times should take care to avoid driving and other high-risk activities.

11 It is difficult to change the attitudes and behaviors of athletes with regard to alcohol. However, coaches, managers, and sports medicine staff can encourage guidelines such as these. Importantly, they should reinforce these messages with an infrastructure that promotes sensible drinking practices. For example, alcohol should be banned from locker rooms, and replaced with snacks or meals appropriate to postexercise recovery strategies. In many cases, athletes drink in a peer group situation and it may be easier to change the environment in which this occurs than the immediate attitudes of the athletes.

Summary

Alcohol is strongly linked with modern sport. The alcohol intakes and drinking patterns of athletes are not well studied, but it appears that some athletes undertake binge drinking practices, often associated with postcompetition socializing. There is no evidence that alcohol improves sports performance; in fact there is evidence that intake during or immediately before exercise, or large amounts consumed the night before exercise, may actually impair performance. There are considerable differences in the individual responses to alcohol intake. Recovery after exercise is likely to be impaired, particularly by the failure of the intoxicated athlete to follow guidelines for optimum recovery. Athletes are not immune to alcohol-related problems, including the greatly increased risk of motor vehicle accidents following excess alcohol intake. Not only should athletes be targeted for education about sensible drinking practices, they might also be used as spokespeople for community education messages.

Athletes are admired in the community and may be effective educators in this area. Alcohol is consumed in greater or lesser amounts by the vast majority of adults around the world, and merits education messages about how it might be used to enhance lifestyle rather than detract from health and performance.

Reading list

American College of Sports Medicine. (1982) Position statement on the use of alcohol in sports. *Medicine and Science in Sports and Exercise* **14**, ix–x.

Burke, L.M. & Maughan, R.J. (2000) Alcohol in sport. In: *Nutrition in Sport* (ed. R.J. Maughan), pp. 405–414. Blackwell Science, Oxford.

O'Brien, C.P. (1993) Alcohol and sport: impact of social drinking on recreational and competitive sports performance. *Sports Medicine* **15**, 71–77.

Shirreffs, S.M. & Maughan, R.J. (1997) Restoration of fluid balance after exercise-induced dehydration: effects of alcohol consumption. *Journal of Applied Physiology* **83**, 1152–1158.

EXPERT COMMENT 1 Alcohol—the problem of post-event intake. Louise M. Burke

Steve Prefontaine (American middle distance runner), Ben Alexander (Australian Rugby League player), Darren Millane (Australian Rules Football player). These are just a few examples of elite athletes who finished their sporting careers, suddenly and drastically, as a result of being killed in accidents while intoxicated. The list is tragically long. In fact, we are probably unaware of the real numbers because such circumstances are often covered up by the "codes" that operate in sport. However, the list pales in comparison to the number of athletes who have to live with the consequences of alcoholic binges—drink-driving convictions, episodes of domestic violence, public brawling, or other publicly embarrassing behavior, as well as health problems. There is some camouflage in being "one of the lads". However these issues become less attractive when the athlete is aging—soccer provides many such examples.

Alcohol intake is often linked with the social routines of sport, particularly during post-event situations and postseason activities. However, the consumption of large amounts of alcohol after a competitive event or training session removes the athlete's focus from the strategies that are important in enhancing recovery or injury management. This may result in poor refueling and rehydration. An increased prevalence of sports-related injury has also been reported in athletes who binge drink. This may be a result of undertaking subsequent exercise sessions while "hungover", or alternatively may reflect poor handling of injuries in the early stages after the session in which they occur. Athletes and sports officials are not immune to the problems associated with alcohol abuse in the community. In fact there is some evidence that they are at greater risk.

A well-known side-effect of the consumption of large amounts of alcohol is an increase in risk-taking behavior. Therefore, the worst-case scenarios with alcoholic binges involve the outcomes of poor judgement. Alcohol intake is a high risk factor for death by drowning, diving incidents, spinal cord injuries, and motor vehicle or cycle accidents. It is often associated with activities that are considered unlawful, with consequences including jail time, a criminal record, or a blemish to the public character for which sponsors are paying large sums of money.

It is heartening to see evidence over the last 5 years that some sporting associations are paying attention to problem drinking behaviors among athletes. Previously, many sports have actively encouraged the environments in which this occurs, and tried to cover up the problems or minimize the consequences for the athletes involved. A better approach is to educate athletes about the reality of the problems, and to present models for sensible drinking practices. To date, alcohol awareness programs have been instigated into a variety of sporting organizations, including all codes of professional football in Australia, the Australian Institute of Sport, and the National Collegiate Athletic Association in the USA. However, these programs must often contend with a highly entrenched pattern of behavior and a sporting culture that does not want to recognize the problem. It will be interesting to judge the results of these and future alcohol education programs.

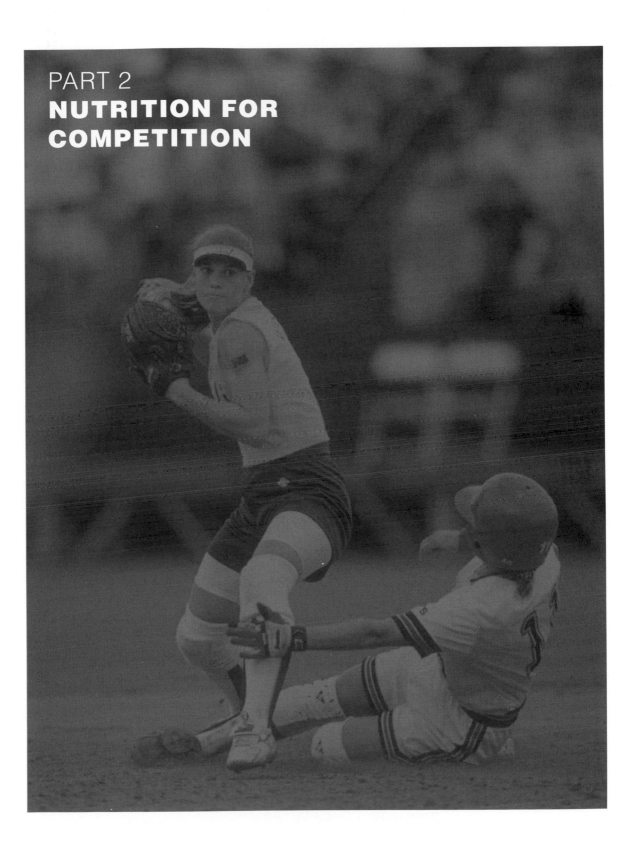

PART 2
**NUTRITION FOR
COMPETITION**

Chapter 7
Preparation for competition

Introduction

The goal of competition nutrition strategies is to combat factors that would otherwise cause fatigue or loss of performance during an event. Factors that can stop the athlete from performing optimally include depletion of glycogen stores in the active muscle, hypoglycemia (low levels of blood glucose) and other mechanisms of "central fatigue" involving neurotransmitters, hyperthermia, dehydration, hyponatremia (low levels of blood sodium), and gastrointestinal discomfort and upset. These factors vary according to the duration and intensity of the exercise, the environmental conditions, and the athlete's individual characteristics including their nutritional and training status. Competition nutrition includes special eating strategies undertaken before, during, and in the recovery from the event. In this chapter we will review the strategies undertaken in the hours or days prior to competition to prepare the athlete to perform at his or her best. Ideally, these will form part of a total nutrition plan that is developed to meet the challenges of the event within the practical opportunities provided to the athlete.

Hydrating before the event

Dehydration poses one of the most common nutritional problems occurring in sport. Chapter 8 will focus on strategies of fluid intake *during* exercise to replace sweat losses, and will note that on most occasions the athlete will be unable to match fluid losses, leading to a progressively increasing fluid deficit. Since some degree of dehydration during exercise is commonly experienced, it is critical for the athlete to start the session as well hydrated as possible. Therefore, athletes must ensure that they have fully replaced any previous fluid deficits, such as the dehydration incurred during a previous exercise session or in an attempt to "make weight" in a weight division sport. Sometimes the challenge comes simply from the fluid losses incurred as a result of living in a hot environment. The athlete needs to recognize such fluid deficits and drink appropriately during the hours leading up to the event to ensure that fluid balance is achieved prior to the start of the new event. Strategies for rapid rehydration are outlined in Chapters 9 and 13.

Some athletes attempt to "hyperhydrate" prior to a competition, especially when they expect that conditions in the event will lead to an inevitable and detrimental fluid deficit. Such dehydration can occur when an athlete's sweat rate is extremely high, when there is little opportunity to drink during the event, or when these factors are combined (see Expert Comment 1). However, even if the athlete is not aiming to "fluid overload", there can be good reasons to drink just before exercise. Effective rehydration during exercise depends on maximizing the rate of fluid delivery from the stomach to the intestine for absorption, with gastric stretching arising from the volume of stomach contents being one of the factors that stimulates high rates of gastric emptying. An effective way to optimize fluid delivery during exercise is to begin the session with a comfortable volume of fluid in the stomach, then adopt a pattern of periodic fluid intake during exercise to replace the partially emptied gastric contents. Obviously the athlete will need to experiment to determine what is a comfortable volume with which to prime gastric volume, and in particular how comfortable this feels once exercise has commenced. However, as a general rule of thumb, most athletes can tolerate a bolus of about 300–400 ml of fluid immediately before the event starts. Waiting to become dehydrated before beginning to drink is a recipe for disaster.

Fueling up for the event

Depletion of body carbohydrate (CHO) stores is a major cause of fatigue during prolonged exercise, so pre-event nutrition strategies should focus on optimizing CHO stores in the muscle and liver. Early studies using muscle biopsy techniques, combined with new techniques involving nuclear magnetic resonance spectroscopy, have enabled sports scientists to investigate the factors that enhance or impair storage of muscle glycogen. Typically, the resting values for muscle glycogen in trained muscle are 100–120 mmol·kg wet weight (ww)$^{-1}$, and this will fall to a greater or lesser extent during each training session, depending primarily on the duration and intensity of the session. In the absence of muscle damage, muscle glycogen stores can be normalized by 24 h of rest and an adequate intake of CHO: 7–10 g per kilogram body mass (BM). Such stores appear adequate for the muscle fuel needs of events of less than 60–90 min in duration; at least, studies in which muscle glycogen stores have been supercompensated have generally failed to show a performance enhancement for events of this type.

For many athletes, normalizing muscle glycogen stores prior to competition might be as simple as scheduling a day of rest or light training before the event, while continuing to follow high CHO eating patterns. However, not all athletes eat sufficient CHO in their typical or everyday diets to maximize glycogen storage. This applies particularly to female athletes who restrict their total energy intake to control body fat levels. These athletes may need education or encouragement to temporarily increase their energy intakes to make fueling up the chief dietary goal on the day before competition. Similarly, some athletes may need to reorganize their training programs to allow lighter training sessions on the day prior to their event. In particular, the athlete should avoid training sessions that cause significant muscle damage on the day before competition, since glycogen storage is impaired by this damage.

Carbohydrate loading for endurance events

Carbohydrate loading refers to practices that aim to maximize or supercompensate muscle glycogen stores prior to a competitive event that would otherwise deplete these fuel reserves. CHO loading protocols may elevate muscle glycogen stores to ~ 150–250 mmol·kg ww^{-1}—up to twice the normal level. This will be an important strategy for events lasting more than 90 min, which would otherwise be limited by the depletion of muscle glycogen stores. CHO loading protocols were an outcome of the first studies to use biopsy techniques to directly measure glycogen concentrations in the muscle. In a series of now classic studies undertaken in the 1960s, Scandinavian sports scientists showed that the capacity for prolonged moderate-intensity exercise was determined by the size of the pre-exercise muscle glycogen stores. Several days of low-CHO eating combined with regular training were found to deplete muscle glycogen stores, leading to a reduction in cycling endurance compared to that achieved on a normal CHO diet. However, the subsequent intake of a high-CHO diet for a few days caused a supercompensation of glycogen stores in the muscle that had previously been depleted, and an increase in the time to exhaustion during submaximal cycling. The activity of the glycogen synthase enzyme was identified as an important factor in glycogen synthesis. As a result of these studies, the sports world was introduced to the "classical" 7-day model of CHO loading, involving a 3–4-day "depletion" phase of hard training and low CHO intake, and finishing with a 3–4-day "loading" phase of high CHO eating and exercise taper. Early field studies of prolonged running events showed that CHO loading enhanced performance, not by allowing the athlete to run faster, but by prolonging the time that race pace could be maintained.

In the 1980s, sports scientists produced a "modified" CHO loading strategy after finding that well-trained athletes were able to supercompensate muscle glycogen stores without a depletion or 'glycogen-stripping" phase. Runners were found to be able to elevate their muscle glycogen stores with 3 days of taper and high CHO intake, regardless of whether this was preceded by a depletion phase or a more typical diet and training preparation. For well-trained athletes at least, CHO loading may be seen as an extended period (3–4 days) of "fueling up". This modified CHO loading protocol offers a more practical strategy for competition preparation, by avoiding the fatigue and complexity of extreme diet and training requirements associated with the previous depletion phase. However, although CHO loading is so well known that it has entered everyday language, even in its simplified form it seems difficult for athletes to master. At least one study has shown that in real life, athletes may not have the knowledge to plan a suitable exercise taper; furthermore, they fail to reach the daily CHO intake targets of $7–10 \text{ g·kg BM}^{-1}$ needed to maximize glycogen storage.

Theoretically, CHO loading could enhance the performance of exercise or sporting events that would otherwise be limited by glycogen depletion. An increase in pre-event glycogen stores can prolong the duration for which moderate-intensity exercise can be undertaken before fatiguing. In fact, a review of available literature on CHO loading found that it typically postpones fatigue and extends the duration of steady-state exercise by ~ 20%. CHO loading may also enhance the performance of a set amount of work (i.e. a set distance) by preventing the decline in pace or work output that would otherwise occur as glycogen stores decline towards the end of the task. Again, the literature

suggests that a performance improvement of 2–3% is achieved by CHO loading. Such an intervention would provide a substantial improvement in most simple endurance events such as marathons, prolonged cycling and triathlon races, and cross-country skiing events. However, shorter events of 45–90-min duration do not generally show significant performance benefits from CHO loading.

While it is relatively easy to measure performance in a predictable event like a marathon, complex and variable events such as tennis matches or football matches that last for 90 min or more of playing time are harder to study. These sports, mixing prolonged duration and intermittent high-intensity exercise, which is associated with an increased rate of glycogen utilization, might be expected to result in muscle glycogen depletion. Intuitively, supercompensation of muscle glycogen stores prior to the event should lead to enhanced performance. Some studies have shown that CHO loading strategies are of benefit to the performance of the movement patterns in a soccer-simulated trial, an indoor soccer match, and a real-life ice hockey game. However, other studies have failed to show significant improvement in the performance of skill-based tasks in a simulation of a soccer match.

It is likely that benefits of CHO loading are specific not only to the sport, but to the individual athlete, depending on the requirements of their position or style of play. Of course, the logistics of competition in many of these sports, where games may be played twice a week or even more frequently, prevent the athlete from undertaking a full CHO loading preparation before each event. Nevertheless, athletes in these sports should fuel up prior to each competition as completely as is practical, and should perhaps experiment with an extended preparation before the most important games, such as the final of a tournament.

It should be remembered that most studies of glycogen storage or CHO loading have been undertaken in male subjects. It is assumed that the findings of these studies also apply to female athletes, although one study reported that female athletes are less responsive to a CHO loading protocol; they failed to supercompensate muscle glycogen stores or show a performance benefit compared to male subjects. However, it is difficult to undertake gender comparison studies due to problems in matching males and females for important parameters such as aerobic capacity (relative vs. absolute values), and to control for the phase of the menstrual cycle in females. One of the confounding issues in studies of female athletes is their intake of smaller amounts of dietary CHO as a result of restricted energy intake. Although females may increase CHO intake to achieve a similar relative energy contribution, total CHO intake will be restricted if total energy intake is low. Without a substantial increase in the intake of substrate, a female athlete could not expect to increase muscle fuel stores nor gain the potential performance enhancement arising from increased fuel availability.

Gender differences in substrate utilization and storage are still being investigated. There is some evidence that the menstrual status of female athletes affects glycogen storage, with greater storage occurring during the luteal phase rather than the follicular phase. One study of CHO loading undertaken with well-trained female athletes during the luteal phase of their menstrual cycle found an increase in muscle glycogen stores compared with storage on a moderate CHO intake, and increased time to exhaustion during submaximal cycling. Other studies have shown that females are equally able to increase muscle glycogen stores with an increase in dietary CHO intake, provided that total energy intake is adequate. It is likely that inadequate CHO intake is a common cause of suboptimal fuel stores in athletes who are driven by body fat and body mass concerns.

The pre-event meal (1–4 hours pre-event)

The goals of the pre-event meal are to:
1 continue to fuel muscle glycogen stores if they have not been fully restored or loaded since the last exercise session;
2 restore liver glycogen content, especially for events undertaken in the morning where liver stores are depleted from an overnight fast;
3 ensure that the athlete is well hydrated;

4 prevent hunger, yet avoid the gastrointestinal discomfort and upset often experienced during exercise; and
5 include foods and practices that are important to the athlete's psychology or superstitions.

A CHO-rich meal consumed 4 h before exercise significantly increases the glycogen content of muscle and liver that has been depleted by previous exercise or an overnight fast. Compared to results achieved after an overnight fast, the intake of a substantial amount of CHO (~ 200–300 g) in the 2–4 h before exercise has been shown to prolong cycling endurance and to enhance performance of time trial undertaken at the end of a standardized cycling task. CHO availability is enhanced by increasing muscle and liver glycogen stores, as well as providing a later release of glucose from the gastrointestinal space. Since liver glycogen stores are labile and may be substantially depleted by an overnight fast, CHO intake on the morning of an event may be important for maintaining blood glucose levels via hepatic glucose output during the latter stages of prolonged exercise.

Thus, the pre-event menu should include CHO-rich foods and drinks, especially in situations where body CHO stores are still suboptimal, or where the event is of a sufficient duration and intensity to challenge these stores. In the field, it is not always possible to consume a substantial amount of CHO in the 4 h before a sporting event. For example, it is unlikely that an athlete will want to sacrifice sleep to eat a large meal before an early morning race start. An alternative plan is to consume a lighter meal or snack before the event, and consume CHO throughout the event to balance missed fueling opportunities. This strategy may also make sense for athletes who are at risk of gastrointestinal discomfort from an excessive volume of food intake. Foods with a low fat, low fiber, and low to moderate protein content are the preferred choice for the pre-event menu since they are less prone to cause gastrointestinal upsets. Liquid meal supplements or CHO-containing drinks and bars are also useful for athletes who suffer from pre-event nerves. Practical ideas for pre-event meals are discussed in more detail in Chapter 13. Above all, the athlete should practice their pre-event eating strategies during training and in less important competitions, and fine-tune a plan to meet their individual situation.

Is it bad to consume CHO in the hour before exercise?

Theoretically, CHO intake prior to exercise could provide a disadvantage rather than an advantage for exercise metabolism and performance. The elevation of plasma insulin concentrations following pre-exercise CHO feedings suppresses the release of fatty acids from adipose cells and thus decreases fat utilization, causing an increase in CHO oxidation and a decline in plasma glucose concentrations at the onset of exercise. These metabolic alterations have been observed even when CHO was consumed 4 h before exercise, and persisted despite the normalization of plasma glucose and insulin concentrations at the onset of exercise. However, they might be of greater magnitude if exercise is undertaken in the hour after eating a CHO-rich snack, and insulin is still elevated at the onset of the session.

Warnings to avoid CHO intake during the hour prior to endurance exercise became sports nutrition dogma following the results of a couple of studies published in the late 1970s. One investigation in particular found that athletes who consumed 75 g of glucose 30 min prior to exercise had a performance impairment in comparison to a trial undertaken after an overnight fast. The researchers observed a rapid drop in blood glucose concentration during the first 10 min of exercise after subjects had been fed CHO, but noted that this response was transient and was not associated with fatigue. Instead they attributed the reduction in endurance following CHO feeding to an accelerated utilization of muscle glycogen, although muscle glycogen content was not actually determined. However, reviews of the literature reveal that this is the only study to find a reduction in performance capacity after the ingestion of CHO in the hour before exercise. This must be balanced against the large number of other investigations of pre-exercise CHO feeding where the effect on performance has ranged from neutral to a significant improvement. In most cases, the decline in blood glucose observed during the first

20 min of exercise is self-corrected with no apparent effects on the athlete.

Nevertheless, it seems that there are a few athletes who have a negative response to CHO feedings in the hour before exercise. These athletes experience an exaggerated CHO oxidation and decrease in blood glucose concentrations at the start of exercise, suffering a rapid onset of fatigue and symptoms of hypoglycemia. Why some athletes experience such an extreme reaction is not known. One study found that risk factors for this problem include the intake of small amounts of CHO (< 50 g), increased sensitivity to insulin, a lower sympathetic-induced counter-regulation, and exercise intensity of low to moderate workload. Not all athletes who experience a major decline in blood glucose concentrations experience hypoglycemic symptoms; these is some evidence that sensitization to low glucose levels may adapt the athlete to an increased threshold before symptoms are reported. Nevertheless, these effects are so clear-cut that athletes at risk are easily identified. Preventative action includes a number of options such as experimenting to find the critical time before exercise that CHO intake should be avoided and ensuring that the pre-event snack/meal provides a substantial amount of CHO (> 70 g). The choice of low glycemic index (GI) CHO-rich options in the pre-event menu, which have an attenuated and sustained blood glucose and insulin response, may also be useful for some athletes, although a universal benefit is not supported (see Expert Comment 2). Athletes may also find it helpful to include some high-intensity sprints during the warm-up to the event to stimulate hepatic glucose output. To many sprints will reduce the muscle glycogen content so some care is necessary. Finally, the intake of CHO during the event should prevent any problems of hypoglycemia as well as providing an important strategy for the promotion of performance (see Chapter 8).

Summary

The importance of pre-event eating strategies will depend on the range and severity of physiological challenges that are likely to limit performance in the athlete's individual event. This is determined by characteristics of the event itself, as well as the degree to which the athlete has been able to recover since his or her last workout or competition event. Pre-event preparation should consider fluid balance, with strategies to rehydrate from previous dehydration associated with exercise or weight-making activities, as well as the potential for hyperhydration in preparation for events in which a large fluid deficit is unavoidable. Nutrition strategies should also include an increase in dietary CHO during the day or days prior to the event, as well as the extended fueling up known as CHO loading, which has been shown to enhance endurance and the performance of prolonged exercise events. The pre-event meal also provides an opportunity to refuel muscle and liver glycogen stores. There is some concern that pre-exercise CHO feedings may increase CHO utilization during exercise, but the intake of substantial amounts of CHO can offset the increased rate of substrate use. The choice of low GI CHO-rich foods in the pre-event menu may also sustain the delivery of CHO during exercise; however, this does not provide a guaranteed performance advantage, especially when additional CHO is consumed during the event. A variety of eating practices can be chosen by athletes to meet their competition preparation goals. These need to consider the practical aspects of nutrition such as gastrointestinal comfort, the athlete's likes and dislikes, and food availability. Above all, athletes should experiment with their pre-event nutrition practices to find and fine-tune strategies that are successful.

Reading list

Akermark, C., Jacobs, I., Rasmusson, M. & Karlsson, J. (1996) Diet and muscle glycogen concentration in relation to physical performance in Swedish elite ice hockey players. *International Journal of Sport Nutrition* 6, 272–284.

Balsom, P.B., Wood, K., Olsson, P. & Ekblom, B. (1998) Carbohydrate intake and multiple sprint sports: with special reference to football (soccer). *International Journal of Sports Medicine* 20, 48–52.

Bangsbo, J., Norregaard, L. & Thorsoe, F. (1992) The effect of carbohydrate diet on intermittent exercise performance. *International Journal of Sports Medicine* 13, 152–157.

Burke, L. (2000) Preparation for competition. In: *Clinical Sports Nutrition* (eds L. Burke & V. Deakin), 2nd edn, pp. 341–368. McGraw-Hill, Sydney, Australia.

Burke, L.M., Claassen, A., Hawley, J.A. & Noakes, T.D. (1998) Carbohydrate intake during prolonged cycling minimizes effect of glycemic index of preexercise meal. *Journal of Applied Physiology* 85, 2220–2226.

Foster, C., Costill, D.L. & Fink, W.J. (1979) Effects of pre-exercise feedings on endurance performance. *Medicine and Science in Sports* 11, 1–5.

Hawley, J.A. & Burke, L.M. (1997) Effect of meal frequency and timing on physical performance. *British Journal of Nutrition* 77 (Suppl.), S91–S103.

Hawley, J.A., Schabort, E.J., Noakes, T.D. & Dennis, S.C. (1997) Carbohydrate-loading and exercise performance: an update. *Sports Medicine* 24, 73–81.

Hitchins, S., Martin, D.T., Burke, L.M., Yates, K., Fallon, K., Hahn, A. & Dobson, G.P. (1999) Glycerol hyperhydration improves cycle time trial performance in hot humid conditions. *European Journal of Applied Physiology* 80, 494–501.

Rehrer, N.J., Van Kemenade, M., Meester, W., Brouns, F., & Saris, W.H.M. (1992) Gastrointestinal complaints in relation to dietary intake in triathletes. *International Journal of Sport Nutrition* 2, 48–59.

Sherman, W.M., Costill, D.L., Fink, W.J. & Miller, J.M. (1981) Effect of exercise-diet manipulation on muscle glycogen and its subsequent utilization during performance. *International Journal of Sports Medicine* 2, 114–118.

Tarnopolsky, M.A. (1999) *Gender Differences in Metabolism*. CRC Press, New York.

Thomas, D.E., Brotherhood, J.E. & Brand, J.C. (1991) Carbohydrate feeding before exercise: effect of glycemic index. *International Journal of Sports Medicine* 12, 180–186.

EXPERT COMMENT 1 Does hyperhydration using glycerol provide an advantage for exercise performance? Louise M. Burke

Some athletes try to hyperhydrate or "fluid overload" in the hours prior to the event to attempt to reduce the total fluid deficit incurred during the session. Drinking a large amount of fluid has been shown to increase total body water, expand plasma volume and, in some situations, enhance performance in a subsequent exercise trial. However, there are some shortcomings and possible disadvantages to simple fluid overloading techniques. First, having a large amount of fluid in the gut poses a risk factor for gastrointestinal upset during the event, especially when it involves high-intensity exercise, or a highly "joggling" form of exercise such as running. Second, it may lead to the significant interruption of having to urinate immediately before or in the early stages of the event. On rare occasions, if taken to extreme levels and in susceptible individuals, excessive fluid intake may lead to hyponatremia or "water intoxication". Clearly, fluid overloading just before an event is a strategy that may actually cause impairment of performance. It needs to be carefully practiced by an athlete before use in an actual competition.

A method of hyperhydration under current study involves the consumption of a small amount of glycerol (1–1.2 g·kg BM^{-1}) along with a large fluid bolus (25–35 ml·kg^{-1}) in the hours prior to exercise. Glycerol, a three-carbon alcohol, provides the backbone to triglyceride molecules and is released during lipolysis. Within the body it is evenly distributed throughout fluid compartments and exerts an osmotic pressure. When consumed orally, it is rapidly absorbed and distributed among body fluid compartments before being slowly metabolized via the liver and kidneys. When consumed in combination with a substantial fluid intake, the osmotic pressure will enhance the retention of this fluid and cause expansion of the various body fluid spaces. Typically, this allows a fluid expansion or retention of ~ 600 ml above a fluid bolus alone, by reducing urinary volume.

The effect of glycerol hyperhydration strategies on thermoregulation and exercise performance is at present unclear. Several studies investigating the effects on sports performance show different outcomes, although at least some of the inconsistency in the literature is due to differences in study methodologies. However, the most promising scenario involves the use of glycerol to maximize the retention of fluid bolus just prior to an event in which a substantial fluid deficit cannot be prevented. In some but not all studies of this type, glycerol hyperhydration has been associated with performance benefits. Two recent studies found that competitive athletes were able to do more work in a time trial undertaken in the heat following hyperhydration with glycerol, compared with a trial using a fluid overload with a placebo drink. Even if future studies confirm the beneficial effects of glycerol hyperhydration strategies it may require careful research to determine the mechanisms behind the effect. At present the theoretical advantages of increased sweat losses and greater capacity for heat dissipation, and attenuation of cardiac and thermoregulatory challenges, are not consistently seen.

Finally, glycerol hyperhydration strategies need to be fine-tuned, and perhaps individualized for specific situations. Side-effects from the use of glycerol include nausea, gastrointestinal distress, and headaches resulting from increased intracranial pressure. These problems have been reported among some, but not all, subjects in the current studies. Fine-tuning of protocols may reduce the risk of these problems, but some individuals may remain at a greater risk than others. At the present time, glycerol hyperhydration should remain an activity that is supervised and monitored by appropriate sports science/medicine professionals, and only used in competition situations after adequate experimentation and fine-tuning has occurred.

CHO-rich foods and drinks do not produce identical blood glucose and insulin responses; neither do they respond according to the stereotype that "simple" CHO types produce rapid and short-lived rises in blood glucose concentrations while "complex" CHO-rich foods produce a flatter and sustained blood glucose rise. The glycemic index (GI) provides a more realistic ranking of CHO foods based on a measurement of the actual blood glucose response to the food, compared to that of a reference food (glucose or white bread). It has been shown to provide a reliable and consistent measure of relative blood glucose response to CHO-rich foods and meals, and can be used to manipulate meals and diets to produce a desired metabolic or clinical outcome (e.g. in the treatment of diabetes, hyperlipidemias and, potentially, obesity).

Australian Diana Thomas and coworkers were the first to suggest the potential of the glycemic index in the arena of sports nutrition by undertaking a manipulation of the glycemic response to pre-exercise CHO-rich meals. A meal providing 1 gram of CHO per kg BM in the form of a low GI food (lentils), eaten 1 h prior to cycling at 67% of $\dot{V}o_{2max}$ was found to prolong time to exhaustion compared with the ingestion of an equal amount of CHO eaten in the form of a high GI food (potatoes). These results were attributed to lower glycemic and insulinemic responses to the low GI trial compared with the high GI meal, promoting more stable blood glucose levels during exercise and increased free fatty acid (FFA) concentrations. Reduced rates of CHO oxidation were observed with the low GI CHO trial, and although muscle glycogen was not measured, the authors suggested that glycogen sparing might have occurred.

This study suggested a way to eat CHO prior to exercise while moderating any harmful responses of pre-exercise CHO feedings. The results have been widely publicized and are largely responsible for the general advice that athletes should choose pre-exercise meals based on CHO-rich foods and drinks with a low GI. However, a number of other studies have failed to find clear benefits following the pre-exercise intake of low GI carbohydrates. The literature shows that CHO meals based on low GI foods achieve a lower postprandial blood glucose response, and a general reduction in the decline in blood glucose concentrations at the onset of exercise. There is some, but not complete, evidence that low GI meals provide a sustained source of CHO throughout the exercise and later recovery. However, most studies fail to show performance benefits arising from the consumption of a low GI pre-event meal, even when metabolism has been altered throughout the exercise.

An important factor in the interpretation of these studies, as with many areas of sports nutrition research, lies in the issue of defining and measuring "performance". The small number of studies that report a beneficial exercise outcome following the lowering of the GI of the pre-event meal have measured time to exhaustion at a fixed work rate as their interpretation of performance, but not all studies of this type report a benefit. It has been observed that "time to exhaustion" protocols have a high coefficient of variation with respect to time. Thus, a possible explanation for the failure of studies to find an improvement in *endurance* associated with improved metabolic characteristics during prolonged exercise is that small changes are masked by the inherent variability of the exercise task. Whether changes in endurance, if they exist, translate into improvements in competitive sports performance must also be questioned. It is important, if the results of studies are to be translated into practical advice for competitive athletes, that the study design and variables should be chosen to mimic the situation of sport as closely as possible. It is interesting to note that none of the studies that have used a time trial outcome to measure performance has shown enhancements as a result of lowering the GI of the pre-event meal.

Finally, a central issue that is overlooked in the debate is the overall importance of pre-exercise feedings in determining CHO availability during prolonged exercise. In endurance exercise events a typical and effective strategy used by athletes to promote CHO availability is to ingest CHO-rich drinks or foods during the event. Yet, in the typical pre-event meal study, athletes are expected to perform prolonged exercise while consuming water or nothing at all. We recently found that when CHO is consumed during exercise according to sports nutrition guidelines, the effects of the type of pre-exercise CHO intake on both metabolism and cycling performance are negligible.

Each athlete must judge the benefits and the practical issues associated with pre-exercise feedings in their particular situation. In cases where an athlete may not be able to consume CHO during a prolonged event or workout, they may find it useful to choose a menu based on low GI CHO foods to promote a more sustained release of CHO throughout exercise. However, there is no evidence of universal benefits from such menu choices, particularly where the athlete is able to refuel during their session or where their favored and familiar food choices happen to have a high GI. In the overall scheme, pre-event eating needs to consider a number of factors including the athlete's food preferences, the availability of menu choices, and gastrointestinal comfort.

CASE STUDY 1 Pregame meal. Melinda M. Manore

Team

The coaches of the collegiate male basketball team were working hard to educate their athletes about good nutrition, optimal body weight for performance, and what to eat prior to competition. All away games involved air travel, arrival at the hotel by 4 PM, dinner at 5 PM, and travel to the gym for warm-up and the game (8 PM). The opportunity to eat and the availability of foods were limited by travel arrangements and were dependent on the flights keeping to schedule. All of the players were over 90 kg and 190 cm.

Reason for consultancy

The coaches wanted advice about meal choices during the flight and the pregame meal, and courtside choices for intake during the game. Challenges included difficulty in maintaining body weight during the competitive season, and for two athletes, severe nervousness before difficult games, which interfered with their ability to eat. What could the players eat to give them energy without upsetting their stomach?

Current dietary patterns

Currently the athletes were given the responsibility for choosing their own meal patterns while traveling to the game. They usually bought food at the airport prior to the flight or between flights. On arrival at the hotel, they were allowed to order from the restaurant menu to choose a pregame meal. During the game, water and sport drinks were available. A typical day's diet for one of the athletes is outlined below.

Professional assessment

These athletes had no plan for food intake on travel days; rather, they ate what was available and quick to order. As a result of the reliance on "fast foods", fat intake was high, carbohydrate intake was often inadequate, and fluid intake was not undertaken in relation to actual requirements. A meal plan needed to be developed for the team, which included special advice and menu choices for the two athletes at risk of gastrointestinal problems. The use of specialized sports foods and supplements should be considered to meet practical needs.

Intervention

The dietitian developed a food plan for travel days and the pregame meal to be provided before all games—home and away. The goals of the plan were to maximize glycogen stores, provide adequate energy for athletes with high energy needs, and prevent hunger and weight loss. Foods that were easy to consume were provided as options for players at risk of poor appetite or gastrointestinal discomfort. Pregame meals eaten away from home were planned in advance with the hotel.

1 On travel days, breakfast was provided before leaving for the airport and special meals were requested for the flight. To supplement the airline meals, snacks packs were provided to each athlete along with a list of suggested items that could be purchased at the airport. Athletes were encouraged to use fruit juice and sport drinks on the plane to maintain hydration instead of caffeinated soft drinks.

2 The pregame menu was chosen from foods that are high in carbohydrate (grains, fruit, and starchy vegetables), with lean meats and moderate amounts of fat. Caffeinated beverages were not served at the pregame meal; again the emphasis was on hydrating with juices and sports drinks.

3 During the game sport drinks were provided. Athletes were encouraged to drink at every opportunity and to monitor changes in body weight as an indication of fluid losses.

4 High-carbohydrate beverages, liquid meal drinks and energy/sports bars were made available for athletes who were too nervous to eat.

Outcome

The new plan found the athletes arriving at the hotel having eaten good meals and snacks. The pregame menu was served as a group meal, with a varied menu served in a buffet style to allow athletes to make individual choices of their preferred volume and type of foods. The team were motivated by the knowledge that they were being helped to fuel their bodies for maximum performance. There were fewer complaints of fatigue and gastrointestinal distress from the athletes, and performance improved.

Breakfast	Snacks on plane	Lunch	Dinner	Snacks after game
Skip breakfast at home Egg McMuffin and orange juice at the airport	4 bags peanuts 330 ml Coke Snickers bar Pretzels	Burger King double burger, fries and Coke at the airport	Steak Baked potato Sour cream and butter Garlic bread Salad with dressing Milk	Pepperoni pizza Coke

Chapter 8
Eating and drinking during exercise

Introduction

Ingestion of food and fluid during exercise has the potential to improve performance by influencing one or more of the factors that limit exercise performance. Prolonged hard exercise is associated with an increased body temperature, a decrease in body water content due to sweat loss, and a fall in the body's liver and muscle carbohydrate (CHO) stores. All of these factors can impair performance by reducing exercise capacity and, in some circumstances, by bringing about an impairment of skilled movements and of decision making. Ingestion of CHO and fluids before and during competition can improve performance, but athletes prone to gastrointestinal problems often avoid any solid or liquid intake for some hours before, and also during, competition. The demands of travel, precompetition preparation, and frequent competitions may also limit the opportunities for eating and drinking. The choice of food and fluids to be consumed during an event will be influenced by a variety of factors, including the nature and duration of the event, the climatic conditions, the pre-event nutritional status, and the physiological and biochemical characteristics of the individual.

Food and fluid consumed during competition are part of a specific short-term nutritional strategy aimed at maximizing performance at that particular time. There is no need to take account of long-term nutritional goals, except perhaps, and even then

only to a limited extent, in extreme endurance events such as the Tour de France or in multiday running events. A balanced nutrient composition is therefore not necessary and intake is targeted at minimizing the impact of those factors that are responsible for fatigue and impaired performance.

The primary considerations for food and fluid intake during exercise are to supplement the body's limited carbohydrate stores, and to provide water, and in some situations also electrolytes, to replace sweat losses. There is good evidence that CHO metabolism is central to the athlete's ability to perform well in competition. In warm environments, however, fatigue occurs while substantial CHO stores remain, and performance is limited more by thermoregulatory failure and dehydration. These observations point clearly to the nutritional strategies that the athlete should adopt to improve performance.

CHO supplementation during exercise

CHO ingested during exercise will enter the blood glucose pool at a rate that will be dictated by the rates of gastric emptying and absorption from the intestine; if this exogenous CHO can substitute for the body's limited endogenous glycogen stores, then exercise capacity should be increased in situations where liver or muscle glycogen availability limits endurance. Several studies have shown that the ingestion of even modest amounts of glucose during prolonged exercise will maintain or raise the circulating glucose concentration. Glucose can be replaced by a variety of other sugars, including sucrose, glucose polymers, and mixtures of sugars, without markedly affecting this response.

In well-trained marathoners running at racing pace, the rate of CHO oxidation can be about 3–4 $g \cdot min^{-1}$, but if this was sustained the available CHO stores would be depleted long before the finish line was reached. Certainly in cycling, and perhaps also in running, the point of fatigue in prolonged exercise carried out in cool or temperate conditions coincides closely with the depletion of glycogen in the exercising muscles. Increasing muscle glycogen stores prior to exercise can improve performance in both cycling and running, and performance is closely related to the size of the pre-exercise glycogen stores. Improvements in performance have also been reported in cycling time trials carried out in the laboratory, and in a variety of running models, including intermittent shuttle running tests. A laboratory study showed that ingestion of 1 l of a glucose polymer–sucrose ($50 \ g \cdot l^{-1}$) solution did not increase the total distance covered in a 2-h treadmill run, but subjects ran faster over the last 30 min of exercise when CHO was given compared with a placebo trial. A similar effect was seen when a CHO solution (50 g of glucose–glucose polymer, or 50 g of fructose–glucose polymer) or water was given in a 30-km treadmill time trial. The running speed decreased over the last 10 km of the water trial, but was maintained on the other two runs; there was no significant difference between the three trials in the time taken to cover the total distance. This ergogenic effect was initially attributed to a sparing of the body's limited muscle glycogen stores by the oxidation of the ingested CHO, but other studies have failed to show a glycogen-sparing effect of CHO ingested during prolonged exercise. The current consensus view seems to be that there is probably little or no sparing of muscle glycogen utilization in cycling exercise but there is good evidence for muscle glycogen sparing in running.

Tracer studies have shown that a substantial part of the CHO ingested during exercise is available for oxidation, but there appears to be an upper limit of about $1 \ g \cdot min^{-1}$ to the rate at which ingested CHO can be oxidized, even when much larger amounts are ingested. This has been used as an argument to suggest that CHO should not be ingested at rates of more than $1 \ g \cdot min^{-1}$, but these high rates of oxidation will not be achieved unless the amount ingested is in excess of this. Based on the feeding protocols used in studies that show performance enhancements, it has been suggested that carbohydrate should be ingested at a rate of about 30–60 g per hour.

Studies in field situations, or in laboratory settings simulating competition, have shown that CHO ingestion during team and racquet games sometimes, but not always, enhances measures of mental and physical skill by reducing the impairment seen with fatigue. A growing number of studies report benefits of CHO ingestion during high-intensity exercise lasting about 1 h. In these situations, the intake of a CHO drink was shown to enhance the performance of running and cycling time trials (lasting about 10 min) undertaken at the end of about 50–60 min of exercise, or cycling time trials lasting 1 h. CHO availability to the muscle is not considered to be limiting in the performance of such exercise, and further research is needed to confirm and explain these effects. It is possible that benefits to "central performance", involving the brain and nervous system, are involved.

In most sports, practical considerations dictate the timing and frequency of CHO (and fluid) intake during the event. Intake is generally much less in running than in cycling events of comparable duration, as few runners are able to tolerate solid food, even when the exercise intensity is low. Intake during competition may be limited by consideration of the time lost in stopping or slowing down to consume food or fluid, or the impact of such ingestion on gastrointestinal discomfort. In other events, such as team sports, formal and informal pauses in play provide opportunities to consume CHO or fluid. Experimentation and practice in training and in minor competitions will help to determine the best strategies for each situation. Strategies that may help to develop a competition eating plan are discussed in Chapter 13.

Effects of hyperthermia and dehydration on performance

The perception of effort is increased, and exercise capacity reduced, in hot climates. In a laboratory study, exercise capacity was greatly reduced at 31°C (55 min) compared to 11°C (93 min): exercise time was also reduced (to 81 min) at the comparatively modest temperature of 21°C. Other studies have shown similar effects and also showed that muscle glycogen was not depleted at the point of fatigue at high ambient temperature (40°C). Dehydration can compromise performance in high-intensity exercise as well as endurance activities. Although sweat losses during brief exercise are small, prior dehydration (by as much as 10% of body mass) is common in weight category sports. Prolonged exercise resulting in a loss of fluid corresponding to 2.5% of body weight was found to result in a 45% fall in the capacity to perform high-intensity exercise. Even very small fluid deficits may impair performance, but the methods used are not sufficiently sensitive to detect small changes.

The mechanisms responsible for the reduced exercise performance in the heat are not entirely clear, but it has been proposed that the high core temperature itself is involved. This proposition was based on the observation that a period of heat acclimatization was successful in delaying the point of fatigue, but that this occurred at the same core temperature. The primary effect of acclimatization was to lower the resting core temperature, and the rate of rise of temperature was the same on all trials. This observation is further supported by numerous studies which show that manipulation of the body heat content prior to exercise can alter exercise capacity: performance is extended by prior immersion in cold water and reduced by prior immersion in hot water. This, of course, immediately raises questions about the "warming up" strategies that should be adopted before exercise in hot climates.

Electrolyte loss and replacement

The sweat loss that accompanies prolonged exercise leads to a loss of electrolytes and water from the body. Sodium is the most abundant cation of the extracellular space, and is the major electrolyte lost in plasma; chloride, which is also mainly located in the extracellular space, is the major anion. The greatest fraction of fluid loss is therefore derived from the extracellular space, including the plasma. Although the composition of sweat is highly variable, sweat is always hypotonic with regard to body fluids, and the net effect of sweat loss is an increase in plasma osmolality. The plasma concentration of sodium and potassium also generally increases, suggesting that replacement of these electrolytes during exercise may not be necessary.

When the exercise duration is very prolonged and when excessively large volumes of low-sodium drinks (such as plain water or cola drinks) are taken during exercise, hyponatremia has been reported to occur. Hyperthermia and hypernatremia associated with dehydration are commonly encountered in athletes requiring medical attention at the end of long-distance races, and the symptoms usually resolve on treatment with oral rehydration solutions. A small number of individuals at the end of very prolonged events may be suffering from hyponatremia in conjunction with either hyperhydration or dehydration. Most of the cases have occurred in events lasting in excess of 8 h, and there are few reports of cases where the exercise duration is less than 4 h. Supplementation with sodium may be required where large sweat losses occur and where it is possible to consume large volumes of fluid. Most competitors, however, will be hypohydrated and hypernatremic.

Fluid replacement and exercise performance

Only a few studies have investigated the effects of plain water or of CHO-free electrolyte solutions on performance. In prolonged exercise at low intensity, water may be as effective as dilute saline solutions or nutrient–electrolyte solutions in maintaining cardiovascular and thermoregulatory function: when subjects ingested plain water (100 ml every 10 min) median exercise time was longer (93 min) than when no drink was given (81 min). Subjects also completed trials where dilute CHO–electrolyte drinks were given and these also extended exercise time compared to the no-drink trial. In a prolonged (90-min) intermittent high-intensity shuttle running test designed to simulate the demands of competitive soccer, ingestion of flavored water was found to prevent a decline in performance of a soccer-specific skilled task: when no fluid was given, performance deteriorated.

The effects of providing fluid and CHO were investigated in a study where subjects performed 50 min of exercise at about 80% of $\dot{V}_{O_{2max}}$ followed by a time trial where a set amount of work had to be completed as fast as possible. During the initial 50 min of exercise, subjects were given either a small volume (200 ml) of water, a small volume of water with added CHO (40% solution, 79 g of maltodextrin), a large volume (1330 ml) of flavored water, or a large volume of water with the same amount of CHO as in the other CHO trial (as a 6% solution). Water ingestion was found to be effective in improving performance; exercise time was 11.34 min on the placebo trial and 10.51 min on the water trial. Exercise time on the CHO trial was 10.55 min, indicating that CHO provision during exercise acted independently to improve performance, and the effects were found to be additive, with the shortest time (9.93 min) when the 6% CHO drink was given.

The results of these and other studies suggest that fluid replacement is effective in improving exercise performance in a variety of different situations, and that an additional benefit is gained by the addition of CHO, and possibly also of electrolytes, to fluids ingested during exercise. The optimum formulation of drinks for use in different exercise situations has not, however, been clearly established at the present time.

Guidelines for replacing fluid and CHO during exercise

As well as providing an energy substrate for the working muscles, CHO added to ingested drinks can promote water absorption in the small intestine. Because of the role of sugars and sodium in promoting water uptake in the small intestine, it is sometimes difficult to separate the effects of water replacement from those of substrate and electrolyte replacement when CHO–electrolyte solutions are ingested. It was shown in the study mentioned above that ingestion of CHO and water have separate and additive effects on exercise performance, and it might be concluded from this that ingestion of dilute CHO solutions would optimize performance. Most reviews of the available literature have come to the same conclusion.

The optimum concentration of CHO to be added to a sports drink will depend on individual circumstances. High CHO concentrations will delay gastric emptying, reducing the amount of fluid that is available for absorption, but will increase the rate of CHO delivery. If the concentration is high enough to result in a markedly hypertonic solution, net secretion of water into the intestine will result, and this will actually increase the danger of dehydration. Dilute glucose–electrolyte solutions may be as effective as, or even more effective than, more concentrated solutions in improving performance, and adding as little as 90 mmol·l^{-1} (about 16 g·l^{-1}) glucose may improve endurance performance. The consequences of severe dehydration and hyperthermia are serious and potentially fatal, but the symptoms of CHO depletion are usually nothing more than severe fatigue. It seems sensible to focus on fluid replacement and to favor low-CHO, high-sodium drinks when training or competing in warm weather.

CHO–electrolyte sports drinks are often referred to as isotonic drinks, as though tonicity were their most important characteristic. The osmolality of ingested fluids is important as this can influence the rates both of gastric emptying and of intestinal water flux. Both of these processes together will determine the effectiveness of rehydration fluids at delivering water for rehydration and substrate for oxidation. Ingestion of strongly hypertonic drinks will promote net secretion of water into the intestine and, although this effect is transient, it will result in a temporary exacerbation of the extent of dehydration. The composition of the drinks, and the nature of the solutes is, however, of greater importance than the osmolality itself. Most of the popular sports drinks are formulated to have as osmolality close to that of body fluids, and are promoted as isotonic drinks, but there is good evidence that hypotonic solutions are more effective when rapid rehydration is desired.

Electrolyte composition and concentration

The available evidence indicates that the only electrolyte that should be added to drinks consumed during exercise is sodium, which may be added in the form of sodium chloride or sodium citrate (the latter helps regulate the acidity of the drink). Sodium will stimulate sugar and water uptake in the small intestine and will help to maintain extracellular fluid volume. The optimum sodium concentration is unclear, and equilibration may occur so rapidly in the upper part of the small intestine that addition of high concentrations of sodium is not necessary. Most soft drinks of the cola or lemonade variety contain virtually no sodium ($1–2$ mmol·l^{-1}), but sports drinks commonly contain about $10–30$ mmol·l^{-1} sodium. A high sodium content may stimulate absorption of glucose and water in the upper part of the small intestine, but too much can make drinks unpalatable. Drinks intended for ingestion during or after exercise should have a pleasant taste in order to stimulate consumption. Specialist sports drinks are generally formulated to strike a balance between the twin aims of efficacy and palatability.

Taste

The thirst mechanism is rather insensitive and does not stimulate drinking behavior until some degree of dehydration has been incurred. This absence of a drive to drink is reflected in the rather small volumes of fluid that are typically consumed during exercise. In endurance running events, voluntary intake seldom exceeds about 0.5 L·h^{-1}, and seems to be largely unrelated to the sweating rate. Because the sweat losses normally exceed this, even in cool conditions, a fluid deficit is almost inevitable whenever prolonged exercise is performed. Anything that stimulates drinking behavior is therefore likely to be advantageous, and palatability is clearly important. Several factors will influence palatability, and the addition of a variety of flavors has been shown to increase fluid intake relative to that ingested when only plain water is available. The addition of flavorings can result in an increased consumption (by about 50%) of fluid during prolonged exercise. Athletes and coaches should

recognize that relying on the thirst mechanism to prompt drinking will not result in an adequate intake: a conscious effort is necessary to prevent dehydration.

Addition of other nutrients and ingredients

Many commercial sports drinks and energy products for athletes contain a wide range of added vitamins, minerals, and other ingredients. There is, however, no compelling evidence for a beneficial effect of any of these additives. The athlete's normal diet should supply the essential nutrients and, except in a few extremely unusual situations, food and fluid ingested during exercise will not make a significant contribution to an athlete's total energy or nutrient intake.

Gastrointestinal disturbances during exercise

Disturbances of both the upper and lower gastrointestinal tract may occur during exercise, with problems including reflux, burping, gastritis, and vomiting (upper), and cramp, irritable bowel, and diarrhea (lower). These problems not only cause distress or embarrassment to the athlete, but may exacerbate the performance and health impairments caused by dehydration or low carbohydrate availability during exercise. After all, symptoms such as vomiting and diarrhea cause the further loss of fluids and electrolytes from the body, as well as impeding the potential for replacement of fluid, electrolytes, and carbohydrate during the exercise session. Exercise can be a direct cause of gastrointestinal problems or it may simply exacerbate underlying problems in individual athletes. Factors that seem to be involved in the development of problems include high-intensity exercise, exercise involving "joggling" of the gut (e.g. running), moderate to severe levels of dehydration, and the intake of inappropriate amounts or types of foods and fluids before or during exercise. Dietary factors that can be modified include the timing and volume of food consumed before exercise, and the presence of large amounts of fiber, fat, protein, fructose, or lactose in pre-event meals. Factors that may cause problems during exercise include dehydration (i.e. waiting too long before attempting to replace fluids during the session), and the intake of fluids or foods that are too highly concentrated, or have an excessive amount of fructose or fiber. Females appear to be at greater risk of gut disturbances, and training appears to reduce the frequency of symptoms. Athletes who experience gut problems should seek the advice of a sports doctor, and be prepared to experiment with their pre-event and during-event nutrition strategies.

Summary

The intake of fluid and CHO offers benefits to the performance of most sports events and exercise activities. The effects of dehydration on performance are now well known, with the penalties ranging from subtle, but often important, decrements in performance at low levels of fluid deficit, to the severe health risks associated with substantial fluid losses during exercise in the heat. Beneficial effects of CHO intake during exercise appear to occur across a variety of activities, ranging from high-intensity sessions lasting about 1 h to more prolonged sessions of moderate-intensity, or intermittent high-intensity work. Optimal strategies for CHO and fluid intake during exercise are yet to be fine-tuned, and ultimately will be determined by practical issues such as the opportunity to eat or drink during an event, and gastrointestinal comfort.

Reading list

American College of Sports Medicine. (1996) Position stand: exercise and fluid replacement. *Medicine and Science in Sports and Exercise* **28**, i–vii.

Below, P., Mora-Rodriguez, R., Gonzalez-Alonso, J. & Coyle, E.F. (1995) Fluid and carbohydrate ingestion independently improve performance during 1 h of intense cycling. *Medicine and Science in Sports and Exercise* **27**, 200–210.

Coyle, E.F. (1997) Fuels for sport performance. In: *Perspectives in Exercise Science and Sports Medicine,* Vol. 10. *Optimizing Sport Performance* (eds D.R. Lamb & R. Murray), pp. 95–138. Benchmark Press, Carmel.

Galloway, S.D. & Maughan, R.J. (1997) Effects of ambient temperature on the capacity to perform cycle exercise in man. *Medicine and Science in Sports and Exercise* **29**, 1240–1249.

Gonzalez-Alonso, J., Teller, C., Andersen, C.L., Jensen, F.B., Hyldig, T. & Nielsen, B. (1999) Influence of body temperature on the development of fatigue during prolonged exercise in the heat. *Journal of Applied Physiology* **86**, 1032–1039.

Hubbard, R.W., Szlyk, P.C. & Armstrong, L.E. (1990) Influence of thirst and fluid palatability on fluid ingestion during exercise. In: *Perspectives in Exercise Science and Sports Medicine*, Vol. 3. *Fluid Homeostasis During Exercise* (eds C.V. Gisolfi & D.R. Lamb), pp. 39–95. Benchmark Press, Carmel.

McGregor, S.J., Nicholas, C.W., Lakomy, H.K.A. & Williams, C. (1999) The influence of intermittent high-intensity shuttle running and fluid ingestion on the performance of a soccer skill. *Journal of Sports Science* **17**, 895–903.

Maughan, R.J. (2000) Fluid and carbohydrate intake during exercise. In: *Clinical Sports Nutrition* (eds L. Burke & V. Deakin), 2nd edn, pp. 369–395. McGraw-Hill, Sydney, Australia.

Maughan, R.J. & Shirreffs, S.M. (1998) Fluid and electrolyte loss and replacement in exercise. In: *Oxford Textbook of Sports Medicine* (eds E. Harries, C. Williams, W.D. Stanish & L. Micheli), 2nd edn, pp. 97–113. Oxford University Press, New York.

Maughan, R.J., Bethell, L. & Leiper, J.B. (1996) Effects of ingested fluids on homeostasis and exercise performance in man. *Experimental Physiology* **81**, 847–859.

Nielsen, B., Kubica, R., Bonnesen, A., Rasmussen, I.B., Stoklosa, J. & Wilk, B. (1982) Physical work capacity after dehydration and hyperthermia. *Scandinavian Journal of Sports Sciences* **3**, 2–10.

Saris, W.H.M., van Erp-Baart, M.A., Brouns, F., Westerterp, K.R. & ten Hoor, F. (1989) Study on food intake and energy expenditure during extreme sustained exercise: the Tour de France. *International Journal of Sports Medicine* **10**, S26–S31.

Schedl, H.P., Maughan, R.J. & Gisolfi, C.V. (1994) Intestinal absorption during rest and exercise: implications for formulating oral rehydration beverages. *Medicine and Science in Sports and Exercise* **26**, 267–280.

Vergauwen, L., Brouns, F. & Hespel, P. (1998) Carbohydrate supplementation improves stroke performance in tennis. *Medicine and Science in Sports and Exercise* **30**, 1289–1295.

EXPERT COMMENT 1 Is there a perfect formula for a sports drink? Susan M. Shirreffs and Ronald J. Maughan

The ability to sustain a high rate of work output requires that an adequate supply of carbohydrate substrate be available to the working muscles, and fluid ingestion during exercise has the aims of providing a source of carbohydrate fuel to supplement the body's limited stores and of supplying water to replace the losses incurred by sweating. The rates at which substrate and water can be supplied during exercise are limited by the rates of gastric emptying and intestinal absorption. Although it is not clear which of these processes is limiting, it is commonly assumed that the rate of gastric emptying will determine the maximum rates of fluid and substrate availability. Increasing the carbohydrate content of drinks will increase the amount of fuel which can be supplied, but will tend to decrease the rate at which water can be made available. Even dilute glucose solutions (40 g·l^{-1} or more) will slow the rate of gastric emptying, but active absorption of glucose, which is co-transported with sodium in the small intestine, stimulates water absorption: the highest rates of oral water replacement are thus achieved with dilute solutions of glucose and sodium salts. The highest rates of glucose emptying from the stomach are observed with concentrated glucose solutions (200 g·l^{-1} or more), even though the volume emptied is small when such solutions are consumed. There is some evidence, however, that the rate of glucose absorption is already maximal at more moderate glucose concentrations.

There is clearly never going to be one perfect formula for a sports drink to meet the needs of all athletes in all situations. The ideal composition of drinks consumed during exercise is influenced by the relative importance of the need to supply fuel and water. This in turn depends on the intensity and duration of the exercise task, on the ambient temperature and humidity, and on the physiological and biochemical characteristics of the individual. Carbohydrate depletion will result in fatigue, but is not a life-threatening condition. However, disturbances in body fluid balance and temperature regulation can not only impair exercise performance but can also be potentially life threatening. Therefore, the emphasis for most people should be on proper maintenance of water and electrolyte balance.

Where provision of water is the first priority, therefore, the carbohydrate content of drinks will be low, perhaps about 30–50 g·l^{-1}, even though this restricts the rate at which substrate is provided. The substitution of other sugars for glucose may have benefits for energy provision, but the evidence is not convincing. The addition of sodium to sports drinks has been questioned on the grounds that secretion of sodium into the intestinal lumen will occur sufficiently rapidly to stimulate maximal rates of glucose–sodium cotransport. The evidence here is doubtful, but there are other good reasons for addition of sodium to rehydration fluids. Added sodium will maintain plasma sodium levels, stimulating the drive to drink and helping to ensure an adequate intake. There is little evidence to support the addition of other electrolytes, and no evidence that the addition of vitamins or other components has any benefit.

The suggestion that availability of drinks is enhanced if they are chilled before ingestion is not supported by the most recent evidence. Taste, however, is an important factor and athletes should experiment with different types of drinks to find the one that they like best.

CASE STUDY 1 Fluid intake during tennis play. Melinda M. Manore

Athlete

Steve was a 21-year-old collegiate tennis player (85 kg) on an athletic scholarship, as the number one singles player on his team. Steve attributed his achievement of this status to the increased weight training and aerobic training program that he had undertaken to complement his sport-specific practices. The increase in exercise, in addition to his normal practice time, had started to leave Steve fatigued, especially after tournaments. He now needed 2–3 days to recover after a tournament. He also complained of poor sleep patterns and headaches after practice. Steve usually worked out for an hour in the morning before breakfast, and then completed a 4-h afternoon practice. At the time of consultation, the average court temperature in the afternoon was 30–35°C (~ 85–95°F), with the expectation of further increase in the temperature over the next 2 months.

Reason for consultancy

Steve was referred to a nutritionist to help with his fatigue and to see if the headaches and poor sleeping patterns were related to his diet.

Current dietary and activity patterns

Steve was lean (10% body fat) and unconcerned about his weight. At the onset of the training program he had gained 2–3 kg, but had been relatively weight stable over the last 5 years, apart from the dramatic weight loss seen after practice. He drank large amounts of water to help replace this fluid loss. He ate out for most of his meals due to lack of time for cooking. His typical diet is outlined below.

Professional assessment

Mean daily intake from this self-reported eating plan was assessed to be ~ 20 500 kJ (4900 kcal), with adequate protein intake (1.6 g·kg^{-1}) but a relatively high intake of fat (~ 38% of energy). Food choices were often poorly made with a low intake of whole fruits and vegetables, and a lack of wholegrain cereals. He consumed snacks and drinks frequently over the day, including 2–3 cups of coffee in the morning, Coke and a candy bar before practice, and Coke or a coffee with takeaway foods as after-dinner snacks. During practice he drank lots of iced water to combat the heat and dehydration. It was possible that his headaches and poor sleeping were due to dehydration during and after practice or games and were exacerbated by a high use of caffeine.

Intervention

Steve was interested to try to improve his food selections during the day and at meals to more nutrient-dense, carbohydrate choices. However, a focused strategy for improved fluid and carbohydrate intake during training and matches was the main dietary change suggested to combat his problems. This would be supported by better postexercise recovery meals, and a reduced intake of caffeine. The changes suggested to Steve included the following advice.

1 Use a sports drink during exercise sessions to replace fluid losses and to refuel. Work at better replacing fluids lost during practice, by observing weight changes as a guide to fluid losses and continuing to replace fluids after practice and in the evening before bed.

2 Limit intake of coffee and Coke during the day. Use replacements such as sports drinks or fruit juice which also provide carbohydrate and allow caffeine intake to be reduced.

3 Switch to a higher-carbohydrate breakfast—for example, wholegrain breakfast cereal, low-fat milk, orange juice, and toast.

4 Find alternatives to chips and burgers for lunch and snacks—for example, deli sandwiches at lunchtime, and fruit and energy bars as snacks—to supply adequate energy and prevent weight loss.

5 Look for healthier dinner choices—include some wholegrain cereals and greater intakes of vegetables.

Outcome

Steve noticed an immediate effect of implementing dietary change. The headaches associated with exercise were eliminated, his sleep improved, and his fatigue was greatly reduced. He was successful with using sports drinks throughout practice or games and in the evening, and limited himself to 2–3 servings of coffee or coke per day. He still ate at Burger King, but limited his visits to two or three times per week and ate breakfast at home rather than stopping for fast food. He packed oranges or apples to snack on during the day and used a sports bar to fuel up before practice. He recognized that his vegetable intake still fell short of the suggested plan, but was working to improve this. Overall fat intake has decreased to 30% of energy intake, with a greater intake of carbohydrate.

Breakfast	Lunch	Dinner	Snacks
2 Egg McMuffin	Burger King:	Spaghetti with meat sauce	Coke
Orange juice	hamburger	Small salad with ranch dressing	Snickers bar
2% milk	large fries with tomato ketchup	Garlic bread	Beer and pizza
Coffee with cream and sugar	500 ml Coke	Ice cream	Apple or banana
	Power bar	2% milk	Popcorn
		Coffee or Coke	Chips
			Coffee

CASE STUDY 2 Gastrointestinal problems during exercise. Melinda M. Manore

Athlete

Megan was a 28-year-old physical therapist training for her first marathon (55 kg, 170 cm). She had been training with a group which usually did a long run on Saturday morning. Lately she had been so fatigued during these runs she had been forced to stop and walk home. At other times she had suffered such severe stomach pains that she could not continue. She had experimented with eating dried toast before her early morning runs, but nothing seemed to help. She felt she needed to eat to fuel up for the long run, but was afraid to eat because food might upset her stomach. The marathon was only 6 weeks away and she was now concerned about being able to complete the run.

Reason for consultancy

Megan was referred to a nutritionist by one of the physicians at her clinic who suggested that a better eating/drinking strategy would help to overcome her fatigue and her stomach problems.

Current dietary and activity patterns

Megan was lean and unconcerned about her weight. Although she had been weight stable for the previous 5 years, she had recently experienced a loss of 2.5 kg. She described herself as being conscious of the need to eat well, but found that opportunities were limited by a physically demanding job, often working until 8 PM. She did not have time to snack between meals and did not snack after dinner. She trained early in the morning, before breakfast and work, and was currently running about 60 miles (100 km) per week. Her typical diet is outlined below.

Professional assessment

Mean daily intake from this self-reported eating plan was assessed to be ~ 10 500 kJ (2300–2500 kcal), relatively low in fat (~ 20–25% of energy), and chosen from nutrient-rich foods. Although her food selection is good, the recent weight loss suggests that she is failing to consume enough energy to compensate for the increased training load. She reports that she does not like to cook and eating is more of a chore than a pleasure. The fatigue from her morning runs might be explained by inadequate CHO intake before and during the session, as well as inadequate fluid. Stomach pains may be caused by gastritis, which is irritated by coffee and other foods (e.g. orange juice and spicy foods). Although she is frightened to eat before the run, the practice of having only coffee may be exacerbating the problem.

Intervention

Megan needed to increase her intake of energy and carbohydrate by incorporating more eating events into her day. She also needed to eliminate foods that irritated her stomach and check with a physician regarding her stomach problems. Better fueling and drinking practices during and after all training sessions, particularly the long run, would help to improve her training performance and start to develop an eating/drinking plan for race day. The following dietary suggestions were made.

1 Drink a sports drink before the morning run, and become practiced at drinking it during and after the session.

2 Slowly experiment with eating a small amount of food before the long Saturday morning runs. If food continues to cause problems, try a sports drink and a carbohydrate gel to improve energy intake.

3 Find time for a mid-morning and mid-afternoon snack (fruit, energy bar, half a sandwich, yoghurt).

4 Eat a healthy dinner, even after a long day at work, and have a sports drink or carbohydrate snack in the evening before bed.

Outcome

The dietary plan worked well for Megan. She began using a sports drink on a regular basis, especially before, during, and after her runs. She altered her work schedule so she could eat more snacks during the day. She stopped skipping dinner and enjoyed a carbohydrate snack in the evening. The day of the race she felt confident to use her well-practiced tactics of pre-event gel and sports drink throughout the race, and finished the event below her planned time. Her stomach still bothers her but she found that avoiding certain drinks on an empty stomach (coffee, orange juice) helped.

Breakfast	Lunch	Dinner	Snacks
Wholegrain cereal	Turkey or tuna sandwich (wholegrain bread)	Grilled chicken/fish or a pasta meal	No snacking during the day or
Skimmed milk	Salad filling (lettuce, tomato and mustard)	Salad with reduced-fat dressing	after dinner
Orange juice	Low-fat chips	Breadsticks	
	Apple or banana	Water	
Two slices wheat	Power bar	Skips dinner if working late	
toast + margarine	Water/sports drink		
Coffee			

Chapter 9
Post-event recovery

Introduction

In the world of sport, success is often determined by the athlete's ability to recover between one exercise bout and the next. In sports such as track and field or swimming, athletes compete in a program of brief races—heats, semifinals, and finals—often performing more than once each day. In cycling stage races, and tennis or team sport tournaments, the schedule consists of one or more lengthy events each day, with the competition extending for 1–3 weeks. Even where teams compete in a weekly fixture, the athlete must train between matches or races to maintain fitness.

Perhaps even more importantly, the daily training program for many sports, even at a recreational level, involves one or more workouts, with less than 24 h separating each session. The ability to recover between training sessions and to maintain quality training without succumbing to the effects of cumulative fatigue and injury is a key characteristic of the top athletes. To meet these challenges, an athlete must practice special recovery strategies between sessions.

Recovery encompasses a complex range of nutrition-related issues including:
• restoration of muscle and liver glycogen stores;
• replacement of fluid and electrolytes lost in sweat; and
• regeneration, repair, and adaptation processes following the catabolic stress and damage caused by the exercise.

This chapter will provide an overview of the well-defined issues of postexercise refueling and rehydration. The biochemical and physiological events that make up the regeneration and repair processes remain somewhat nebulous, and involve activities ranging from the synthesis of protein (muscle cells, enzymes, etc.) to the activities of the antioxidant defense systems and the immune system (see Expert Comment 1). At present, we are unable to make definite recommendations on strategies to optimize all the recovery processes. However, it seems prudent to promote a varied intake of nutrients in postexercise eating strategies. Such variety will help to meet the needs of recovery processes that are yet to be well defined.

Postexercise refueling

There is a strong drive to restore glycogen levels in a muscle whose carbohydrate stores have been depleted by exercise, with muscle glycogen storage taking priority over the restoration of liver glycogen content. The rate of synthesis is determined by factors that regulate glucose transport into the cell (for example, glucose supply and glucose uptake) as well as glucose disposal (for example, the activity of glycogen synthase enzyme). Brief periods of high-intensity exercise resulting in high postexercise levels of lactate are associated with rapid recovery of muscle glycogen stores, even in the absence of carbohydrate intake after exercise. In the case of prolonged moderate-intensity exercise, however, muscle glycogen synthesis is largely dependent on the postexercise carbohydrate supply. In the absence of dietary intake of carbohydrate, synthesis occurs at a low rate (1–2 mmol per kg wet weight (ww) of muscle per hour), with some of the substrate being provided through gluconeogenesis (see Chapter 2). Glycogen storage follows a two-phase timescale: a very rapid synthesis during the first hour after exercise, followed by a slower restoration phase that is under the influence of factors such as insulin. When optimal amounts of carbohydrate are consumed, maximal rates of postexercise muscle glycogen storage during the first 12 h of recovery are within the range of 5–10 mmol·kg ww^{-1}·h^{-1} and gradually decline as restoration continues. In the face of substantial glycogen depletion, 20–24 h of well-fed recovery are required for the restoration of muscle glycogen stores.

Liver glycogen stores are more labile than muscle glycogen stores, and may be depleted by an overnight fast as well as a prolonged bout of exercise. Strategies to enhance the restoration of liver glycogen store have been less well studied due to practical problems in obtaining liver biopsy samples. However, it is considered that liver glycogen is restored by a single carbohydrate-rich meal.

Dietary factors that can impair or enhance the refueling of muscle glycogen stores will be reviewed in greater detail below.

Amount of carbohydrate

The most important dietary factor affecting muscle glycogen storage is the amount of carbohydrate consumed. There is a direct relationship between the quantity of dietary carbohydrate and the rate of postexercise glycogen storage, at least until the muscle storage capacity or threshold has been reached. Studies suggest that the threshold varies between individual athletes but generally occurs within the intake of 7–10 g carbohydrate per kg body mass (BM). Maximal refueling during the first 0–6 h of recovery is achieved when foods or drink providing a carbohydrate intake of about 1 g·kg^{-1} are consumed during the first hour, and repeated every 2 h until the normal meal pattern can be resumed.

These figures form the basis of carbohydrate intake guidelines for athletes who desire to optimize muscle glycogen recovery within a busy training or competition schedule. However, total carbohydrate intake recommendations or requirements may be higher in some situations. For example, athletes who undertake strenuous daily competition may need to meet the fuel requirements of their continued exercise in addition to postexercise recovery needs. For example, cyclists undertaking prolonged daily training sessions or stage races may need to consume carbohydrate intakes of more than 12 g·kg BM^{-1}. In fact, the ingestion of substantial amounts of carbohydrate during low to moderate intensity exercise has been reported to cause a net glycogen storage during the session, particularly within nonactive muscle fibers that have been previously depleted. Increased carbohydrate intake may also be useful in the case of muscle damage (e.g. following eccentric exercise or substantial contact injuries), which typically impairs the rate of postexercise glycogen resynthesis. In this case, low rates of glycogen restoration in damaged muscles may be partially overcome by increased amounts of carbohydrate intake during the first 24 h of recovery. A summary of the guidelines for carbohydrate intake for athletes is presented in Table 9.1.

Timing of carbohydrate intake

The highest sustained rates of glycogen storage occur during the first few hours after exercise. In addition to the activation of the glycogen synthase enzyme, early postexercise recovery is marked by an exercise-induced permeability of the muscle cell membrane to glucose and an increased muscle sensitivity to insulin. Carbohydrate feeding during these early stages appears to accentuate these effects by increasing blood glucose and insulin concentrations. The intake of carbohydrate immediately after prolonged exercise has been shown to result in higher rates of glycogen storage (~ 8 mmol·kg ww^{-1}·h^{-1}) during the first 2 hours of recovery, slowing thereafter to the more typical rates of storage (~ 4 mmol·kg ww^{-1}·h^{-1}). However, failure to consume carbohydrate in the immediate postexercise phase of recovery leads to very low rates of glycogen restoration (1–2 mmol·kg ww^{-1}·h^{-1}) until

Table 9.1 Summary of carbohydrate (CHO) intake guidelines for athletes (from Burke *et al.* 2001).

Situation	Recommended CHO intake
Acute/single event	
Optimal daily muscle glycogen storage (e.g. for postexercise recovery, or to fuel up or CHO load prior to an event)	$7-10 \text{ g} \cdot \text{kg BM}^{-1} \cdot \text{day}^{-1}$
Rapid postexercise recovery of muscle glycogen, where recovery between sessions is < 8 h	$1 \text{ g} \cdot \text{kg BM}^{-1}$ immediately after exercise, repeated after 2 h
Pre-event meal to increase CHO availability prior to prolonged exercise session	$1-4 \text{ g} \cdot \text{kg BM}^{-1}$ eaten 1–4 h pre-exercise
CHO intake during moderate-intensity or intermittent exercise of > 1 h	$0.5-1.0 \text{ g} \cdot \text{kg}^{-1} \cdot \text{h}^{-1}$ ($30-60 \text{ g} \cdot \text{h}^{-1}$)
Chronic or everyday situation	
Daily recovery/fuel needs for athlete with moderate exercise program (i.e. < 1 h, or exercise of low intensity)	$5-7 \text{ g} \cdot \text{kg}^{-1} \cdot \text{day}^{-1}$
Daily recovery/fuel needs for endurance athlete (i.e. 1–3 h of moderate to high-intensity exercise)	$7-10 \text{ g} \cdot \text{kg BM}^{-1} \cdot \text{day}^{-1}$
Daily recovery/fuel needs for athlete undertaking extreme exercise program (i.e. > 4–5 h of moderate to high intensity exercise such as Tour de France)	$10-12+ \text{ g} \cdot \text{kg BM}^{-1} \cdot \text{day}^{-1}$

feeding occurs. If ingestion of carbohydrate is delayed for 2 h or more, this phase of very rapid carbohydrate synthesis is missed. Thus the importance of early intake of carbohydrate following strenuous exercise is to start effective refueling by ensuring the provision of substrate to the muscle cell. This strategy is most important when there is only 4–8 h of recovery between exercise sessions, but may be of less significance when there is a longer recovery time (24 or more hours).

Overall it appears that when the interval between exercise sessions is short, the athlete should maximize the effective recovery time by beginning carbohydrate intake as soon as possible. However, when longer recovery periods are available, the athlete can choose their preferred eating schedule as long as total carbohydrate intake goals are achieved. It is not always practical or enjoyable to consume substantial meals or snacks immediately after the finish of a strenuous workout.

Whether carbohydrate is best consumed in large meals or as a series of snacks is of practical interest to athletes. One study has shown that very high rates of glycogen synthesis can be achieved during the first couple of hours after exercise when substantial amounts of carbohydrate are consumed every 15 min during recovery. However, these rates were simply compared with the values reported in other studies rather than being directly measured against a different eating schedule. This finding needs to be confirmed by other studies. In terms of long-term refueling (24 h of recovery), several studies have reported that as long as total carbohydrate is adequate, the rate of muscle glycogen synthesis appears unaffected by the frequency of intake. One benefit of small frequent meals may be in overcoming the gastric discomfort often associated with eating large amounts of bulky high-carbohydrate foods. It is also possible that when total carbohydrate intake is limited, there may be some advantage in altering the pattern of intake to promote greater blood glucose and insulin profiles at key times.

Type of carbohydrate intake

Different types of carbohydrate and carbohydrate-rich foods appear to have different effects on rates of muscle glycogen synthesis. Studies using feedings of simple sugars have found that glucose and sucrose feedings produce similar rates of muscle glycogen recovery after exercise, whereas the intake of fructose produces a lower rate of glycogen storage in the exercised muscles. However, these studies are of little practical relevance to athletes who need to eat real food to achieve their everyday nutrition goals.

Since glycogen storage is influenced by both insulin and a rapid supply of glucose substrate, it has been proposed that dietary carbohydrates designated as high glycemic index (GI) might enhance postexercise refueling. The GI system classifies carbohydrate-rich foods according to actual measurements of blood glucose levels following the intake of each food. Older studies investigating the effect of different types of carbohydrate-rich foods on glycogen storage failed to find consistent results, most probably because they used the confusing system of classifying carbohydrate foods as "simple" or "complex". However this system does not truly differentiate the effects of different carbohydrate-rich foods on glucose and insulin responses.

One study supports the benefits of refueling with high GI carbohydrate-rich foods, observing greater glycogen storage during 24 h of postexercise recovery on a diet based on high GI carbohydrate-rich foods compared to a diet based on low GI carbohydrate sources. However, the magnitude of increase in glycogen storage (~ 30%) with the high GI carbohydrate trial was far greater than the increase in 24-h blood glucose and insulin concentrations following the high GI trial. In other words, while the outcome of the study was as predicted, it could not be explained in terms of alteration of glucose and insulin responses. The cause of reduced glycogen storage with low GI carbohydrate foods is unclear, but may be in part due to the relatively poor digestibility of many of these foods. A diet or meals based on indigestible carbohydrate foods may overestimate the real amount of carbohydrate that is available for glycogen storage by the muscle. This issue needs to be further studied.

Form of carbohydrate feeding

Solid and liquid forms of carbohydrate appear to be equally effective in providing substrate for muscle glycogen synthesis. Practical issues such as compactness and appetite appeal may be important in choosing a menu that meets the athlete's total carbohydrate intake goals. Liquid forms of carbohy-

drate or carbohydrate foods with a high fluid content may be particularly appealing in hot weather or to athletes who are too fatigued to eat bulky foods.

Co-ingestion of protein

It is possible that other macronutrients present in carbohydrate-rich foods or simultaneously ingested at a meal may influence muscle glycogen storage—for example, by affecting digestion, insulin secretion, or the satiety of meals. The effect of adding protein to a carbohydrate-rich meal or snack has been the focus of attention because of the suggestion that it achieves a greater postmeal insulin response, which might in turn stimulate glycogen synthesis. Indeed, one well-quoted study reported that the 2-hourly feedings of protein (40 g) and carbohydrate (112 g) achieved a greater rate of muscle glycogen storage during 4 h of recovery than the carbohydrate alone. More recent versions of this type of study involve the comparison of concentrated carbohydrate–protein sports supplements to sports drinks.

Unfortunately, studies of this type are flawed by the failure to match the energy content of the diets—it is impossible to know whether additional glycogen storage is due to the protein per se, or the extra energy consumed by the subjects. Although it is a good marketing ploy by the manufacturers of various sports supplements, it is unfair to compare equal volumes of a concentrated (e.g. 20% carbohydrate) drink with a dilute (e.g. 6% carbohydrate) drink. In fact, in several recent studies of postexercise refueling in which carbohydrate and carbohydrate–protein mixtures of equal energy value have been compared, identical rates of glycogen storage have been seen. Nevertheless, snacks or meals providing substantial amounts of carbohydrate and protein may be useful for achieving other recovery goals—in particular, promotion of protein synthesis or retention during and after exercise (see Expert Comment 4 and see also Chapter 13 for practical suggestions for choosing suitable snacks).

In general it appears that the addition of fat and protein to carbohydrate foods and meals does not affect glycogen storage as long as targets for carbohydrate intake are met. However, it should be remembered that the presence of large amounts of protein and fat can displace carbohydrate foods within the athlete's energy requirements and gastric comfort, thereby indirectly interfering with glycogen storage by promoting inadequate carbohydrate intake.

Issues in postexercise rehydration

Ideally, an athlete should aim to fully restore fluid losses between exercise sessions so that the new event or workout can be commenced in a euhydrated state. In normal healthy people, the daily replacement of fluid losses and maintenance of fluid balance are well regulated by thirst and urine losses. However, under conditions of stress (e.g. exercise, environmental heat and cold, altitude) thirst may not be a sufficient stimulus for maintaining fluid balance. Furthermore, there may be a considerable lag of 4–24 h before body fluid levels are restored following moderate to severe hypohydration.

Studies of voluntary fluid intake patterns across a range of sports show that athletes typically replace only 30–70% of the sweat losses incurred during exercise. As a result, most athletes can expect to finish training or competition sessions with a mild to moderate level of hypohydration. After exercise, people fail to drink sufficient volumes of fluid to restore fluid balance, even when drinks are made freely available—this effect was first described in the 1940s and termed "voluntary dehydration". More recently, the name has been changed to "involuntary dehydration" to recognize that the dehydrated individual has no desire to rehydrate even when fluids and opportunity are available.

An additional challenge to postexercise rehydration is that the athlete may continue to lose fluid during this phase, partly due to continued sweat losses, but principally due to urination. The success of postexercise rehydration ultimately depends on the balance between fluid intake and ongoing fluid losses.

In summary, although hydration is generally well maintained in the long term, special attention is needed for an acute situation of a moderate to high degree of hypohydration (i.e. fluid deficit of 2–5%

BM or greater) and a recovery interval of less than 6–8 h. Optimal rehydration requires a scheduled plan of fluid intake, to overcome both physiological challenges such as inadequate thirst, and practical problems such as poor access to fluids. A number of factors affecting postexercise rehydration have been identified and will now be discussed.

Palatability of fluid

Numerous studies have reported that the palatability of a drink affects how much a person will voluntarily consume, and this probably becomes more important when very large volumes must be consumed. Flavor and temperature are two important characteristics determining the drink palatability. It should be noted that most studies of rehydration in athletes have been undertaken *during* moderate-intensity exercise rather than *after* exercise, so it is uncertain whether the findings apply directly to postexercise recovery. However, some studies show that an athlete's perception of what tastes good to drink may change according to the environmental conditions, their body temperature, and their degree of dehydration. In some situations palatability may not always determine the total intake of a rehydration fluid. For example, while a person who is hot and thirsty may regard very cold water (0°C) as the most desirable drink, it is easier to drink larger quantities of cool water (15°C).

Flavoring of drinks has also been considered to contribute to voluntary fluid intake, with studies reporting greater fluid intake during postexercise recovery with sweetened drinks than with plain water. Further research is needed to differentiate whether subjects are responding to a sweet flavor or to energy replacement. Drinks that are too sweet may reduce voluntary intake, and there is some evidence of "flavor fatigue"—that after several hours of drinking, people tire of drinking things they initially preferred.

Replacement of electrolytes

Drinking water following dehydration leads to a dilution of plasma osmolality and sodium content, which in turn causes an increased diuresis (urine production) and reduction of thirst. Therefore, water is an ineffective rehydration fluid since it is likely to inhibit fluid intake and stimulate urine losses—even while the athlete is still dehydrated. By contrast, when sodium is replaced in conjunction with fluid, there is a greater voluntary intake of fluid and a lower urine output, leading to faster restoration of plasma volume. Sodium can be replaced in the drink itself, or by simultaneously eating sodium-containing foods or meals with added salt.

Varying the sodium content of rehydration fluids has effects on both the taste of the fluids (affecting voluntary intake) and the degree of fluid retention. Sports drinks provide a source of sodium, but this is less than the amount present in the specially formulated oral rehydration solutions used in the medical treatment of dehydration (e.g. for diarrhea and gastrointestinal upsets). This lower sodium content reflects the needs for these drinks to have a well-accepted taste that will lead to wide commercial appeal. Studies show that even low sodium concentrations have a mild advantage over plain water in terms of restoration of plasma volume. However, when this effect is added to the improved palatability of the drink, it appears that sports drinks may confer some rehydration advantages over plain water. The composition of the postexercise recovery drink is discussed in greater detail in Expert Comment 2.

Volume and pattern of drinking

Since sweat and urine losses occur during recovery, an athlete must drink a volume greater than the postexercise fluid deficit to restore total fluid balance. Typically, studies show that replacement of fluid in volumes equal to the deficit results in only a 50–70% fluid restoration over 2–4 h of recovery (based on body weight restoration). However, forced rehydration with greater volumes of fluid will not achieve fluid balance unless sodium losses are simultaneously replaced. In general, a volume of fluid equal to 150% of the fluid deficit will be required to restore fluid balance in conjunction with sodium replacement.

There is little information about the preferred drinking pattern—for example comparing the effect of a large volume consumed immediately after exercise with a pattern of frequent small drinks throughout the recovery period. However issues such as gastric comfort must also be considered, especially if the athlete has to undertake another exercise session within a short period.

Caffeine and alcohol—potential diuretics

Urine losses are required to get rid of waste material. However, urine production is further stimulated by dilution of blood osmolality and by the action of pharmacological agents including caffeine and alcohol. These constituents are frequently found in beverages consumed after exercise. A study comparing the postexercise consumption of a diet cola drink containing caffeine with water and sports drink found less effective restoration of body fluid losses with the cola drink than with the other fluids. In fact, although subjects consumed volumes of fluid equal to their sweat losses in all trials, the cola drink resulted in a net restoration of only 54% of body mass. Compared to the other drinks, there were substantially greater urine losses and a small but significantly greater loss of fluid through continued sweating. The balance of evidence, however, suggests that the amount of caffeine present in cola-type drinks and in tea or coffee does not have a strong diuretic effect, especially in those who habitually consume these drinks. There are likely to be more problems from avoiding these drinks than from consuming them in moderation.

Alcohol consumption has also been shown to increase urinary losses during postexercise recovery. Subjects consuming drinks containing 4% alcohol showed slightly greater urinary losses than when drinks containing 0, 1, or 2% alcohol were consumed. Therefore drinks containing alcohol at concentrations of more than 2–3% (e.g. full-strength beer, wine, coolers, spirits) are not considered good rehydration drinks. Excessive intake of alcohol may have other detrimental effects on recovery and health (see Chapter 5).

Summary

Recovery after exercise poses an important challenge to the modern athlete. Important nutrition goals include resynthesis of glycogen stores in the muscle and liver, as well as the replacement of fluid and electrolytes lost in sweat. Effective recovery of muscle glycogen stores occurs with the intake of carbohydrate—with targets of at least 1 g·kg BM^{-1} during the first 2 h of recovery and a daily total of 7–10 g·kg BM^{-1}. Rapid refueling, beginning with the intake of carbohydrate as soon as possible after the session, may be important for the athlete who has less than 8 h between lengthy exercise sessions. As long as the athlete consumes enough carbohydrate, it appears that the frequency of intake, the form (liquid vs. solid) and the presence of other macronutrients do not appear to affect the rate of glycogen storage. Practical considerations such as the availability and appetite appeal of foods or drinks and gastrointestinal comfort may determine ideal carbohydrate choices and the pattern of intake.

Rehydration requires a special fluid intake plan since thirst and voluntary intake will not provide for full restoration of sweat losses in the acute phase (0–6 h) of recovery. Steps should be taken to ensure that a supply of palatable drinks is available after exercise. Cool sweetened drinks are generally preferred and can contribute towards achieving carbohydrate intake goals. Replacement of the sodium lost in sweat is important in maximizing the retention of ingested fluids. Beverages containing large amounts of caffeine and alcohol are not ideal rehydration fluids since they promote an increased rate of diuresis. It may be necessary to consume 150% of fluid losses to allow for complete fluid restoration.

Reading list

Burke, L. (2000) Nutrition for recovery after competition and training. In: *Clinical Sports Nutrition* (eds L. Burke & V. Deakin), 2nd edn, pp. 396–427. McGraw-Hill, Sydney, Australia.

Burke, L.M., Cox, G.R., Cummings, N. & Desbrow, B. (2001) Guidelines for daily carbohydrate intake: do athletes achieve them? *Sports Medicine* **31**, 267–279.

Costill, D.L., Sherman, W.M., Fink, W.J., Maresh, C., Witten, M. & Miller, J.M. (1981) The role of dietary carbohydrates in muscle glycogen resynthesis after strenuous running. *American Journal of Clinical Nutrition* **34**, 1831–1836.

Greenleaf, J.E. (1992) Problem: thirst, drinking behaviour, and involuntary dehydration. *Medicine and Science in Sports and Exercise* **24**, 645–656.

Ivy, J.L., Katz, A.L., Cutler, C.L., Sherman, W.M. & Coyle, E.F. (1988) Muscle glycogen synthesis after exercise: effect of time of carbohydrate ingestion. *Journal of Applied Physiology* **64**, 1480–1485.

Sherman, W.M. & Wimer, G.S. (1990) Insufficient dietary carbohydrate during training: does it impair athletic performance? *International Journal of Sport Nutrition* **1**, 28–44.

Shirreffs, S.M. (2000) Rehydration and recovery after exercise. In: *Nutrition in Sport* (ed. R.J. Maughan), pp. 256–265. Blackwell Science, Oxford.

Shirreffs, S.M., Taylor, A.J., Leiper, J.B. & Maughan, R.J. (1996) Post-exercise rehydration in man: effects of volume consumed and sodium content of ingested fluids. *Medicine and Science in Sports and Exercise* **28**, 1260–1271.

EXPERT COMMENT 1 Nutrition and immune function—can you close the "open window"? Bente Klarlund Pedersen

Our immune system is the body's defense against invading organisms that can cause illness and infection, but immune impairment is seen following intense exercise lasting more than 1 h. This impairment is quantitative as well as qualitative. Following exercise white blood cells (lymphocytes) disappear from the circulation and the cells left in the circulation do not function well. Thus, in the postexercise period lymphocytes have an impaired ability to proliferate and to mediate cytotoxic functions against virus-infected and tumor target cells. Following strenuous exercise there is also a decrease in the locally produced secretory antibodies, secretory IgA, in saliva. *In vivo* immune monitoring (the skin test) has further demonstrated impaired immune function in the recovery period after endurance exercise. This temporary impairment has been called "the open window" in the immune system, suggesting that during this window of opportunity, microorganisms may invade the body and establish as infections. The open window period lasts from 4 h to 3 days, depending on the intensity, but especially the duration, of the exercise.

If an athlete performs two or more exercise periods on the same day, the stress elicited by the second bout of exercise is much greater than that elicited by the first bout of exercise. In addition, the immune changes in response to the second bout of exercise are much greater than those observed in relation to the first bout. Athletes are therefore advised to make the recovery period between the two bouts of exercise as long as possible.

Several studies have investigated the possibility that nutritional products might protect against postexercise immune impairment. Can you eat something to close the open window? Research has concentrated on the effects of carbohydrate, glutamine, fish oil, and antioxidant vitamins.

There are now a number of studies showing that carbohydrate supplementation during exercise abolishes the exercise-induced immune changes. In line with these observations, training in a glycogen-depleted state induces more severe immune changes than training during glycogen-loaded conditions. Although the results of these studies are exciting, further research is needed to show that the improved immune status arising from better carbohydrate intake practices is clinically significant—that is, that it reduces the frequency of illness in athletes. Glutamine is an important fuel for lymphocyte growth, and since plasma glutamine levels decline during exercise, it has been suggested that glutamine is linked causally to exercise-induced immune impairment. Four randomized placebo-controlled glutamine intervention studies have shown that it is possible to feed athletes with glutamine and thereby keep the plasma glutamine concentration stable during exercise. However, this does not influence exercise-induced immune changes and glutamine supplementation is therefore not recommended.

There is some controversy regarding the effects of antioxidant vitamins on resistance to infections. While some studies show fewer infectious episodes in athletes who receive vitamin C prior to a marathon race compared to those who receive placebo, other studies do not confirm this finding. Also, conflicting results exist regarding the direct effect of antioxidant vitamins on the immune system. Lipids rich in n-3, such as fish oil, may potentially inhibit prostaglandin production during exercise and thereby protect against their inhibitory effects on the immune system. However, due to a limited number of studies it is not possible to reach any firm conclusions on the effects of different lipids on exercise-induced immune changes.

EXPERT COMMENT 2 Postexercise rehydration: is there an ideal rehydration drink? Susan M. Shirreffs

Dehydration incurred during exercise must be corrected if performance in a subsequent bout of exercise is not to be impaired. Obligatory urine losses persist even in the dehydrated state, ensuring the elimination of metabolic waste products. It is clear therefore that the total fluid intake after exercise-induced sweating must amount to a volume greater than the volume of sweat that has been lost if effective rehydration is to be achieved. Ingestion of plain water in the postexercise period results in a rapid fall in the plasma sodium concentration and in plasma osmolality. These changes have the effect of drastically reducing voluntary fluid intake and of stimulating urine output, both of which will delay the rehydration process. When the same volume of drinks with different sodium concentrations is ingested following exercise-induced hypohydration, the resultant volume of urine output is inversely related to the sodium content of the ingested fluid—that is, the greater the sodium content, the smaller the volume of urine produced.

Rapid, complete and sustained rehydration after exercise can only be achieved if both fluid and electrolyte losses are replaced. Ideally, rehydration drinks should have a moderately high sodium concentration, perhaps similar to that of sweat. The upper end of the normal range for sweat sodium concentration (80 mmol·l^{-1}) is similar to the sodium concentration of the oral rehydration solution recommended by the World Health Organization for rehydration in cases of severe diarrhea (90 mmol·l^{-1}). By contrast, the sodium concentration of most sports drinks ranges from 10 to 30 mmol·l^{-1}, and most fruit juices and carbonated soft drinks contain virtually no sodium.

It has been speculated that inclusion of potassium, the major cation in the intracellular space, would enhance the replacement of intracellular water after exercise and thus promote rehydration. Potassium is usually included in sports drinks in concentrations similar to that in sweat. However, there is no conclusive information on the requirement of K$^+$ for postexercise rehydration at present. Similarly, the importance of the inclusion of magnesium in sports drinks has been the subject of much discussion. Magnesium is lost in sweat and many believe that this causes a reduction in plasma magnesium levels, which have been implicated in exercise-induced muscle cramp. Even though there can be a decline in plasma magnesium concentration during exercise it is most likely to be due to redistribution of sodium between compartments rather than sweat loss. On this basis, there does not seem to be any good reason for including magnesium in postexercise rehydration and recovery sports drinks.

While there are clear guidelines as to how to optimize postexercise rehydration, there is never going to be one ideal drink to meet the needs of all athletes. There are two steps that should be taken by an athlete to ensure postexercise rehydration is as ideal as possible. First, they should ensure a palatable drink is available in order that a large enough volume can be consumed to provide for elimination of metabolic waste products and body water restoration. Second, they should ensure that the drink, or snacks and meals that accompany this drink, contain sodium, thus avoiding an inappropriate stimulation of urine production before body water balance is restored.

EXPERT COMMENT 3 Carbohydrate in the recovery period: how much and when? Clyde Williams

In order to train hard and recover quickly it is essential that the carbohydrate stores in the liver and skeletal muscles are restocked as quickly as possible after each training session or competition. The most rapid rate of glycogen resynthesis occurs during the first few hours after exercise when glucose transport proteins are mobilized and the glycogen synthase enzyme complex is active. In order to capitalize on these conditions and so improve the rate of glycogen resynthesis carbohydrate should be ingested immediately after exercise and at frequent intervals until the next meal. Recovering between daily training sessions or competition demands careful attention to nutrition and hydration, especially if the aim is to restore or improve performance. Under these conditions carbohydrate should be ingested immediately after exercise, and this may be most convenient as a carbohydrate–electrolyte solution, in an amount that is equivalent to about 1 g of carbohydrate per kg body mass every 2 h. The first meal of the recovery period should contain mainly high glycemic index carbohydrates, such as potatoes and white rice. The total carbohydrate intake for the whole recovery period should amount to approximately 9–10 g·kg body mass^{-1}. In order to cope with this large intake of carbohydrate, concentrated glucose drinks can be used to supplement the high carbohydrate meals. Ad libitum eating will probably not achieve the carbohydrate intake

necessary to achieve glycogen resynthesis in the time available. Therefore, when recovery in 24 h must be achieved then the amount of food in general, and the quantity of carbohydrate in particular, should be prescribed for each individual.

When only a few hours are available for recovery between exercise sessions then drinking a well-formulated carbohydrate–electrolyte solution is of more benefit to subsequent exercise performance than ingesting only water or fruit juice. The effective amount is about 1 g por kg body mass, again at 2-h intervals during the recovery period. Paradoxically, doubling the amount of carbohydrate ingested does not improve subsequent exercise capacity more than the recommended amount. The reason for the lack of a dose–response between carbohydrate ingestion and exercise capacity is not entirely clear. However, a reasonable suggestion is that the increased carbohydrate intake reduces fat metabolism during exercise such that the deficit is covered by an increase in the metabolism of the ingested carbohydrate but with no apparent gain in endurance capacity. Finally in translating these principles from nutritional science into practice the key word is "practice", i.e. the strategies should be rehearsed and refined in training in order to ensure that prescribed amounts of carbohydrate can be ingested at rates that are tolerable and effective.

EXPERT COMMENT 4 Does protein intake immediately after exercise promote recovery and enhance adaptation? Peter W.R. Lemon

As the increased dietary protein needs for regular exercisers have become recognized, scientific interest has shifted toward attempts to understand the underlying reasons responsible. One possibility involves providing exercise fuel, but this is not likely to be important as protein provides little energy for exercise, especially when sufficient carbohydrate is available. Other possibilities include providing the stimulus and the materials necessary to enhance muscle recovery and repair following exercise. The latter might include adaptations induced by training (i.e. increases in contractile or functional protein). Specifically, exercise has dramatic effects on protein metabolism both during and following the session. For example, there appears to be a period of time following exercise where protein synthesis is greatly enhanced relative to baseline. Consequently, providing adequate raw materials (i.e. amino acids and energy) during this time period might enhance exercise recovery, resulting in improved readiness for subsequent exercise. Unfortunately, the time course of this increased protein synthetic response has not been well characterized, as yet, so specific recommendations regarding how much protein or amino acids and when to ingest them would be premature. There are data indicating that the first few hours after exercise may be critical, but other results suggest the period of enhanced synthesis extends much longer. Some amino acids (i.e. the branched-chain amino acids) or other nutrients may be particularly important as controllers. Consequently, if the necessary amino acids are available in the

muscle free pool and energy stores are sufficient, very small amounts of a few specific nutrients might be sufficient to stimulate this enhanced recovery rate. On the other hand, following strenuous exercise, and especially when it is prolonged, it is quite likely that gram (or perhaps hundreds of gram) quantities will be needed to maximize muscle recovery. It appears that a mixture of carbohydrate (high glycemic index) and protein is best, due to the insulin-stimulated amino acid uptake by muscle. Because hunger may be suppressed immediately following strenuous exercise, liquid formulations or compact food choices are recommended. There is a large variability between individuals in their tolerance of solid and liquid meals, so experimentation outside of competition would be wise. Although several protein types are available (whey, casein, soy, etc.) few data suggest one is superior to another in terms of speeding exercise recovery. There is some evidence that whey protein enters the bloodstream at a faster rate than casein protein. Until further study clarifies this issue, it recommended that during the immediate postexercise period (30 min) a mixture of proteins be consumed in combination with high glycemic index carbohydrate. Choices that are easy to prepare or consume (e.g. drinks such as liquid meal supplements, fruit smoothies) are valuable when it is impractical to eat whole foods or meals. Finally, this strategy should be repeated hourly for the first few hours after intense exercise because the exact time course of elevated protein synthesis is unclear.

CASE STUDY 1 Eating to recover after training. Linda Houtkooper

Athlete

JJ was a 19-year-old male collegiate Division I American football quarterback competing to be the team's number one pick for starting quarterback in the upcoming season. JJ was 188 cm in height and weighed 89 kg at the end of the previous football season. In preparation for the new season JJ undertook a program of 1½ h per day weight training five times a week, an additional 1½ h running and skill development six times a week, and about 1 h playing a game of pick-up basketball most days of the week.

Reason for consultancy

Within the first month of spring training JJ had lost 3 kg despite reporting eating "lots and lots." He was fatigued and starving by the end of workouts and was frustrated with his weight loss. He felt that lack of recovery between training sessions was preventing him from making the desired weight and performance gains.

Existing dietary patterns

JJ ate the bulk of his energy in the afternoon and evening. He grabbed a sports bar and Gatorade in the morning before weight training around 10.30 AM and typically went without breakfast during the week. He ate his lunch out every day, usually a burrito or sub sandwich. JJ avoided soda but drank lemonade with meals, and water before and after practice. Sometimes between afternoon practice and pick-up basketball JJ grabbed another sports bar, but his main energy intake came at dinnertime. On the drive home he would stop and get a medium pizza with sausage and lemonade. Before bed, he always had a protein shake made with 1% milk. A typical training day of food intake is outlined below.

Professional assessment

Mean daily intake from this self-reported eating plan was ~ 14 650 kJ (3500 kcal); 498 g carbohydrate (5.8 g·kg body mass^{-1}); 145 g protein (1.7 g·kg body mass^{-1}); 106 g fat (27% of kJ). JJ reported a low energy intake, ~ 4200 kJ (1000 kcal) below the estimated requirements for his activity level. His daily menu was low in fiber intake (18 g vs. recommended 20–30 g), and failed to provide the recommended number of servings for fruit and vegetables. Estimated intake of protein was adequate and his intake of calcium was at the upper recommended intake of calcium (~ 2500 mg·day^{-1}). Sodium intake was very high (~ 6000 mg·day^{-1}), and although sodium replacement is part of postexercise recovery, his intake was well above the required levels. His carbohydrate intake was estimated to be in the lower end of the recommended range of intake, but more importantly was not well timed to promote effective refueling after training sessions. For example, little of the carbohydrate intake was achieved during the morning after his first training session, and he often waited a couple of hours after the afternoon session before eating dinner.

Intervention

Goals were set to increase JJ's daily energy and carbohydrate intake, obtain the recommended fiber and fruit and vegetable intake, and moderate his sodium intake. To achieve these changes the following recommendations were made.

1 Start the day off with a wholewheat bagel, peanut butter, and banana before morning weight-training session.

2 Eat a high carbohydrate snack with a high glycemic index providing at least 1–5 g of carbohydrate per kg BM within 30 min after all training sessions: fruit, bagel or sports bar, and Gatorade.

3 Replace high-fat dinner choices with a meal that is higher in carbohydrate, has adequate protein, and is low in fat. For example, replace whole sausage pizza with half a medium thin crust vegetarian pizza with plain breadsticks, a garden salad, and orange juice.

4 Replace Mexican rice with a large vegetable salad to help reduce sodium intake and increase intake of vegetables.

5 Replace sports bar with whole foods such as wholewheat bagel, and add a piece of fruit in the afternoon, or wholegrain breakfast cereal and milk.

6 Encourage fluid intake throughout the day and during training sessions, especially sports drinks.

7 Switch to 2% milk in protein shake to increase energy content.

Outcome

JJ managed to start eating a high carbohydrate snack immediately after his workouts and found that his body recovered more completely from intense training. Though hesitant to eat breakfast, JJ did so on the days he weight trained in the morning and noticed increased energy during weight-training sessions as well as a 2-kg gain in muscle. JJ's fruit and vegetable consumption increased and his carbohydrate and fiber intakes both reached recommended levels: 622 g of carbohydrate (7.2 g·kg body mass^{-1}) and 37 g of fiber. Cutting out sodium-packed Mexican rice and reducing his serving size of pizza reduced his overall sodium intake and moderating his serving of cheese on the pizza helped reduce calcium intake to less than the recommended upper limit level of 2500 mg. JJ's coach noticed his improvements and recommended him for the top pick for quarterback during the opening game.

Morning snack	Lunch	Afternoon snack	Dinner	Evening snack
Sports bar Gatorade	Large chicken burrito Mexican rice Lemonade	Sports bar Water	Medium sausage pizza Lemonade	16 oz (460 ml) 1% milk and a scoop of protein powder

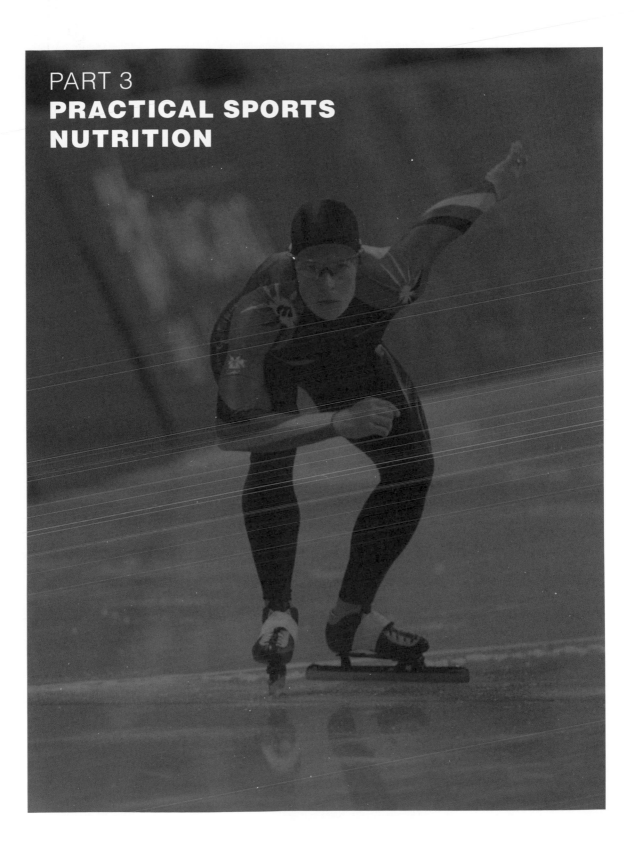

PART 3
**PRACTICAL SPORTS
NUTRITION**

Chapter 10
Assessing nutritional status and needs

Introduction

Athletes often expect precise information and feedback to guide them in their sporting pursuits. After all, they are used to following a strict training prescription and to receiving detailed information about their training and competition performances, and they are generally more impressed if measurements are made to several decimal places. It is understandable that an athlete might want clear guidelines about when and what to eat, and from time to time, a precise assessment of how well they are meeting their dietary goals. In this chapter, issues related to setting and assessing the achievement of nutritional goals will be addressed.

Assessment of nutritional status

Although alternative practitioners often advertise that they can do a complete nutritional and medical assessment via a single technique such as hair analysis or iridology (examining the eyes), in fact, the assessment of nutritional status is complex and often inexact. No single technique or piece of information can tell the full story. Instead, an assessment is made by piecing together information from a variety of sources. Many serious athletes undertake a complete screening that includes a variety of medical, physiological, and psychological measures at critical times of their competitive year—for example, at the beginning of a new season, and perhaps around competition peaks (to gain a picture of measurements that are consistent with optimal performance). Some of these assessments might be usefully repeated to distinguish the causes of suboptimal health or performance if they occur.

Components of a complete screening include a medical check-up, a musculoskeletal screening by a physiotherapist, physiological testing in the laboratory, and a psychological assessment. A complete nutritional screening should include a dietary evaluation (an overview of what the athlete is eating), biochemical and hematological testing of blood and perhaps urine, anthropometric testing to assess body composition, and a clinical assessment of the athlete's appearance and well-being. In previous chapters we discussed that many parameters cannot be assessed as optimal or suboptimal in isolation. Occasionally a reading is found to be clearly suboptimal, but the usual situation is that readings need to be compared to information previously collected from the same athlete and interpreted in conjunction with other data. For example, in Chapter 4 we saw that a diagnosis of iron deficiency required an examination for clinical signs of fatigue and pallor, indications of suboptimal intake of dietary iron, and a clear reduction in biochemical and hematological measures of iron status. Since an evaluation of the dietary patterns of the athlete provides a key piece of the puzzle, it is important to understand what is involved and how the information should be used in light of the limitations of the various methods of evaluation.

Assessment of dietary intake

A complete evaluation of an athlete's dietary patterns is time-consuming and requires special expertise. Throughout this book, case histories of different athletes have been included to illustrate various nutritional challenges and issues arising in sport. Each has included a brief summary of key findings in the nutritional assessment of the athlete or athletes involved, without the opportunity to discuss how the information was collected or interpreted. In fact, there are a number of methods that can be used to monitor dietary intake; each has specific advantages and disadvantages and each adds a typical bias to the information collected. The dietary survey method chosen to monitor the intake of an individual athlete or group of athletes will depend on the type of information that is sought, and the resources and opportunities available. When assessing the intake of an individual athlete, most sports dietitians use several techniques in combination, using one method to cross-check the results of another technique. For example, the results of an athlete's food diary may be compared with the information collected using a dietary history protocol.

It is important to underpin all the information provided by dietary recalls or records with an appreciation of the athlete's lifestyle and commitments, and their interest in and understanding of nutrition. After all, issues such as motivation, finances, food availability, nutrition beliefs, domestic skills, and time will influence the athlete's present dietary patterns and their ability to make changes. Therefore, the primary contact with the athlete should include a thorough interview to collect information such as where they live, who cooks their meals, how often they travel, how and why they have chosen their present eating patterns, what supplements they take, and how their time is spent in a typical day. Against this background, the athlete's eating patterns can then be monitored and assessed. The following techniques for monitoring dietary intake collect information about the athlete's typical consumption of food and drinks. Sometimes, this information is compared directly against dietary benchmarks, while on other occasions an assess-ment is made of the typical nutrient intake provided by these foods and fluids.

Techniques for monitoring dietary intake fall into two major categories: "retrospective" or "recall" techniques that monitor behavior in the past or immediate past, and "prospective" techniques that monitor ongoing behavior. Popular retrospective techniques include dietary history, diet recall, and food frequency questionnaires (FFQs).

Retrospective or recall techniques

The technique that is generally called a dietary history (and is actually a shorter modified version of the original technique) asks the athlete to describe their food intake during a typical day over recent times. A skilled interviewer, using prompts and probing questions, ascertains the athlete's whereabouts and activities over each section of the day, and the food and drink that is usually consumed. Ideally, the athlete will be assisted to build up a composite of their usual eating patterns, including descriptions of serving sizes of various items as well as a summary of how different options might be chosen weekly, monthly, or seasonally. Aids such as food models may help the athlete to accurately describe their usual portion sizes. The dietary history is usually cross-checked against a brief FFQ (see below).

The advantages of the dietary history are that it focuses on usual intake, is relatively quick, and places relatively little burden on the athlete. On the other hand, it requires a skilled interviewer and assumes that the athlete can provide an accurate (and truthful) recall of their intake. An athlete who has a chaotic lifestyle and erratic eating habits, or a poor memory or insight into their eating patterns, will not necessarily be able to provide an objective account of a typical day.

The dietary recall technique involves questioning about actual intake of foods and fluids on a previous occasion, usually the last 24 h. Again, a skilled interviewer is needed and should use prompts and aids to stimulate the athlete to provide accurate information about the type and amounts of foods and drinks consumed. Although most subjects will find it easier to remember what they ate yesterday, rather than create an overview of what is typically eaten, a major disadvantage of this technique is that it does not provide a picture of usual intake. After all, we eat differently from day to day, and the athlete may have followed a totally unrepresentative eating plan the day before their interview. The 24-h recall is often used in dietary surveys of large groups where a number of accounts of a day's eating can build up a picture of the typical eating habits of a population. Alternatively, it may be undertaken on a number of separate occasions in the same individual to build up a picture of the daily or weekly changes in their intake.

A food frequency questionnaire (FFQ) takes the form of a checklist of commonly eaten foods and drinks, with each item requiring one response denoting the size of the serving that the athlete typically consumes, and another response listing the frequency of consumption of this item. This list is often supplemented with questions on other foods eaten by the respondent but not on the list, and questions about food preparation, supplement use, and other food-related behaviors. FFQs can be undertaken by interview, or as a self-administered questionnaire. In its early form, the FFQ was designed as a qualitative method, seeking information on the frequency of consumption of specific food items without specification of the actual serving or portion sizes usually consumed. More recent versions of FFQs focus on portion sizes so that a quantitative determination of food and nutrient intake can be achieved. The accuracy of FFQs is dependent on how well the checklist has been prepared to include the foods and drinks consumed by the athlete, and how well and accurately the athlete can summarize his or her usual intake. Many FFQs are developed to focus on the intake of a specific nutrient (e.g. carbohydrate or calcium), and are validated against the results achieved by other dietary survey techniques. A particular advantage of the FFQ is that it is relatively quick and easy for both the athlete and the interviewer.

In general, all recall or retrospective techniques are limited by the athlete's memory, insight, and cooperation. Research shows that young and adolescent subjects have limited insight into their food intake, and that a "typical" day is difficult to picture in an erratic and chaotic lifestyle. Furthermore, people deliberately or unconsciously "rewrite" their usual food intake to downplay the foods they see as undesirable (e.g. snacks and sweets) and increase their stated intake of foods seen as desirable (e.g. fruit). Many athletes give biased responses either in fear of revealing inappropriate dietary behavior to a coach or investigator, or to impress the investigator. Many studies have shown that people have poor skills in recalling portion sizes of foods and fluids. In general, retrospective methods of assessing food and nutrient intake tend to overestimate true intake, although they may underestimate the true intake of large eaters.

Prospective monitoring techniques

The duplicate portion method is an old technique that was sometimes used to monitor the ongoing dietary intake of an individual in the era before extensive food composition tables were available. To undertake this technique, the athlete would collect a duplicate sample of all food and drinks consumed over a specified period of time; this collection would then be thoroughly homogenized and a chemical analysis of the energy and nutrient content would be undertaken. Clearly, such a method is time-consuming and expensive and is very rarely used in modern times.

The most popular method of dietary survey work is the food diary or food record, in which a completed account of all food and fluid intake is kept over a specified period of time, either by the subject, or in special cases (such as the monitoring of children or athletes in extreme competition such as a cycling tour) by the designated food handler. As in all dietary survey methods, accuracy in describing the type and amount of food and fluid intake is critical. In some food record protocols, the athlete is required to use scales to weigh all food and drinks, whereas other techniques ask the athlete to estimate portion sizes using a combinations of household measures and grids. The weighed food record is sometimes considered the "gold standard" of dietary survey techniques, but although this protocol improves the accuracy of the quantification of the athlete's intake, it may be a source of other errors if increased demands on the athlete lead to reduced compliance or distortion of their true intake.

In general, all dietary surveys are hampered by errors of validity (how well they measure the subject's actual intake), and reliability (how closely the period of monitoring reflects the athlete's usual intake). Prospective techniques carry a disadvantage in that athletes may deliberately or subconsciously alter their eating habits during the period of recording so that it no longer reflects their usual intake. This may happen, as in the case of recall techniques, because the athlete is embarrassed about their true intake and wants to appear to "eat better" than they usually do. On the other hand, the requirement to record all intake is intrusive and time-consuming, and the athlete may subconsciously try to simplify the demands by choosing to eat foods that are easier to record, or by omitting to eat or record the consumption of meals or snacks altogether if it is inconvenient.

Extensive study of the accuracy of food diaries in the general population shows a bias towards widespread and significant under-reporting of true intake; comparison of energy intakes estimated from food diaries and other techniques such as doubly labeled water show that records typically underestimate intake by about 20% (see Chapter 1). However, not all subjects under-report, and studies have identified that some individuals under-report to an even greater extent. This latter population includes those who are overfat and those who are dissatisfied with their body mass and body image. Under-reporting errors can be divided into under-eating (reducing food intake during the period of recording), and under-recording (failing to record all food consumed during the observation period), but few studies have tried to measure the relative contribution of each aspect to the total error. Several sophisticated energy balance studies have also been carried out on athletes and most, but not all, have found discrepancies between reported energy intakes and energy requirements, particularly among female athletes and those in weight-conscious sports. It is not known whether the under-reporting of all nutrients mirrors the under-reporting of energy intake.

Typically, food records are kept for periods of 1–7 days, although there have been rare studies which have monitored food intake over several years. The duration of the food diary is important both for the reliability of the estimate of energy or nutrient intake (a longer period of recording reduces the variability in estimation of daily intakes) and for the compliance of the subject (longer periods reduce the attention and compliance of the subject). In the general population, a 3–4-day record is considered a reasonable compromise, although it is limited in being able to accurately estimate typical intakes of only the stable dietary components such as energy and carbohydrate. Other more variable nutrients such as vitamin A and cholesterol may require up to 3–4 weeks of recording to accurately estimate the daily intake of an individual to within 95% of true intake. In athletic populations, where individuals are highly motivated and familiar with regimented assessment of other aspects of their preparation, many researchers and clinicians like to use a 7-day food diary, since this usually represents a complete microcycle in the athlete's training program. An alternative method to increase the reliability of monitoring is to have the athlete complete a number of food diaries over shorter periods (e.g. 4-day food diaries completed two or three times over a period of training). If 3–4-day food diaries are used, they should be undertaken over a period that is representative of the different influences on food intake (for example, 1 weekend day and 3 weekdays, or 3 heavy training days and 1 light day or rest day).

In summary, although food records offer advantages as a dietary survey tool, these must be balanced against the disadvantages such as an increased burden on the subject, and the time involved (initial interview to train the athlete about recording, the daily recording commitment, and the processing of the completed diary). Most athletes are likely to under-report or underconsume their usual intakes when undertaking dietary records, and those who are weight or physique conscious or dissatisfied with their body image are at highest risk of significant underestimation errors. Reporting errors can be minimized where athletes are motivated to receive a true dietary assessment, and where training to enhance record-keeping skills has been undertaken. Nevertheless, researchers and practitioners should be cautious in their interpretation of the results of self-reported assessments of dietary intake.

Problems in converting information about food intake into nutrient intake

Dietary surveys collect information about the food intake of athletes, which is often then analysed quantitatively, in terms of intake of energy and nutrients. The conversion of food into nutrients is a major source of error in dietary surveys and is a reflection of the skills and knowledge of the researcher, the method of data collection, and the available food composition database. Errors arise from the lack of specificity in the description of food or quantities consumed, insufficient knowledge about common preparation methods, differences in handling situations which are not instantly matched by the food composition database, and simple mistakes in coding and data entry. Food composition databases do not contain all of the large number of different foods consumed, so appropriate food substitutes, omission of foods, and guesswork must be used. The importance of defining a standard protocol for coding and entering data, and for handling food substitutions is crucial for minimizing error when analysing food record data. When interpreting nutrient data derived from food composition tables, the following limitations should be recognized. Food composition data are only estimates of the average nutrient composition of foods, are specific to the country of origin, and suffer from incomplete information on many nutrients and on many commonly eaten foods. The common portions of foods documented in software programs are not necessarily the serving sizes consumed by people, especially athletes who have extremes in energy requirements.

Benchmarks for assessing or setting dietary intake

There are various sources of information against which dietary intake can be monitored or a new dietary plan can be developed. These vary from qualitative messages about food use to quantitative benchmarks for nutrient intake. Most are aimed at the nutrition of the general population, although some guidelines have been prepared especially for athletes.

Nutritional guidelines for athletes and physically active people

Over the past two decades, recognition of the specialized nutritional needs of athletes and the importance of nutrition in determining sports performance has led to the release by expert bodies of position stands on sports nutrition. These have attempted to provide a state of the art summary of current thinking, either over the broad spectrum of nutrition and exercise performance, or on a special issue such as alcohol and exercise, creatine supplementation, or acute techniques of weight loss by athletes. Expert bodies that have issued position stands, either individually or as joint commentaries, include professional organizations representing sports medicine and science or nutrition and dietetics as well as the international governing bodies of sport. The evolution in knowledge of sports nutrition has meant that new position stands often have to be issued to update, or even contradict, the recommendations made in previous statements (see Expert Comment 1). However, in general, these position stands can provide a valuable reference for athletes.

Guidelines can be found for principles of meeting the nutritional goals of training and competition, ranging from recommendations guiding the selection of the type and timing of meals and snacks, to guidelines for nutrient intakes especially adapted for athletes undertaking a heavy exercise program. Even though the expert bodies in most countries have failed to take the special needs of exercise into account in formulating official daily reference intakes, in the case of some nutrients (e.g. protein and carbohydrate), there is sufficient evidence to provide reasonably precise guidance to athletes at various levels of performance and training commitment.

Qualitative benchmarks: dietary guidelines and food guides

The nutrition and health experts in many countries have developed a series of dietary guidelines which provide a set of qualitative recommendations for ways in which the typical dietary patterns of the population should be modified to fit the model of healthy eating. The goals of such eating are to achieve nutrient requirements in the short term, as well as to minimize eating behaviors associated with risks for the development of long-term health problems. In some countries such as Australia, separate dietary guidelines have been prepared for adults, children and adolescents, and the aged. The education messages contained in dietary guidelines are generally similar across countries—for example, eat more cereals, fruits, and vegetables, or reduce the intake of fats, particularly saturated fats. However, the ways in which these guidelines are expressed can differ between countries. For example, while the dietary guidelines for Australia and America encourage people to "eat a variety of nutritious foods", the Japanese dietary guidelines are more specific in recommending that "30 or more different foods" should be eaten each day. These messages are appropriate for nutrition education of athletes and are used by sports dietitians in combination with other qualitative guides to assess and advise athletes about food choice (see Expert Comment 2). Other qualitative education tools include "food pyramids", "food plates", and "rainbows" that provide a pictorial representation of the proportion in which foods should be chosen to make up meals and diets.

Food guides are nutrition education tools to assist children and adults to plan and select nutritionally desirable diets consistent with the dietary guidelines. Most countries have devised food selection guides specific to the food supply, nutrient recommendations, and cultural needs of their population. These food guides translate dietary standards and recommendations into suggested servings of foods from groups that can be easily understood and used by people who have little formal training in nutrition. Examples of food guides include "The Core Food Group" and "CSIRO 12345+ Food and Nutrition Plan" (Australia), "Four Food Groups Guide" (USA), and "Food Guide for Healthy Eating" (Canada). Food guides categorize food into groups that are usually based on similar nutrient content, and make recommendations about the number of servings from each group that should be consumed

daily so that requirements for key nutrients are probably achieved. In many countries, specific recommendations are given according to gender, age, or special nutritional need (e.g. pregnancy and breastfeeding). A quick way of assessing nutrient intakes is to check if the recommended number of foods from each group is represented in a day's dietary intake. Such an achievement is by no means a foolproof or precise assessment of dietary adequacy, and will not meet the energy requirements for most people, especially athletes. Athletes need to increase the number of servings to meet their energy and nutrient requirements. Nevertheless, food guides can provide a baseline tool for assessing dietary intake.

Recommended nutrient intakes

All major countries have a set of recommended intakes for energy, protein, and micronutrients for use in their populations. These recommendations vary in name from country to country, and include recommended nutrient intakes (RNIs) (UK), recommended dietary intakes (RDIs) (Australia) and the recommended dietary allowances (RDAs), which are in the process of evolving into the dietary reference intakes (DRIs) (USA). The original use of these recommendations (hereafter, simply referred to as RNIs) was to set a standard for an adequate diet for different groups of the population. Their use has spread so that they have become the basic unit of nutrition education, a benchmark for planning therapeutic diets and food programs, and a benchmark for food enrichment and food labeling programs. Their use as a tool for assessing the dietary intakes of individuals has also become widespread, although this is a purpose for which they were not designed.

In each country, expert committees in nutrition and health set RNIs from a mathematical treatment of information about requirements for individual nutrients. These requirements are generally derived from studies that have identified the lowest levels of intake that are consistent with the absence of evidence of a nutrient deficiency or with maintenance of the body pool. RNIs are extrapolated and interpolated from these data, taking into account the distribution of values around the mean value for the minimum requirement (i.e. adding $2 \times SD$ to the mean value so that it theoretically encompasses the needs of 99% of a population). The special needs of different groups within the population, and factors of dietary quality or nutrient absorption are also taken into account. The final RNI value is meant to represent the intake of a nutrient that should meet the requirements of nearly all members of a community. The DRIs that are currently being issued in the USA are broader in scope and application than RNIs, encompassing a family of markers for nutrient intakes ranging from estimated average requirements to an upper limit that takes into account problems of excessive intake or toxicity. It is interesting to note that values for RNIs differ between countries, based on the way that their expert committees have interpreted the available data on nutrient requirements and the priority that is given to simply avoiding symptoms of deficiency vs. consuming an intake that might promote optimal health.

The use of RNIs to assess the adequacy of the dietary intake of an individual is problematic, since these standards are recommendations for the average daily amounts of nutrients that population groups should consume over a period of time, rather than requirements for a specific individual. Differences in the nutrient requirements of individuals are unknown, and by definition the RNI values overestimate the real nutrient needs of most of the population. RNIs should be considered a general assessment tool that assesses the likelihood that an individual is meeting his or her requirements for various nutrients. By convention, nutrient intakes that are below two-thirds of the RDI are considered to be at high risk of being inadequate. However, the accuracy of the assessment of nutrient intake must also be taken into account when comparing such values to RNIs.

Although very few countries have included special RNIs for athletes, or contemplated any changes to nutrient requirements arising from a heavy exercise program, the RNIs are generally considered suitable for use with athletic populations. In the case of some micronutrients, there is recognition that requirements are related to energy requirements, so that an athlete with a high turnover of energy would also have an increased requirement for those micronutrients (e.g. some of the B group vitamins). Nevertheless, some elite athletes may not fit within the range of these "average" population values on which nutrient standards are based. Evidence for a slightly higher requirement for protein and carbohydrate than the general population is well documented in some groups of athletes (see Chapters 3 & 9). Recent evidence supports a slight increase in micronutrient needs in physically active people to compensate for losses in sweat, urine, and perhaps feces, and for an increase in free radical formation. However, this evidence is based on biochemical and physiological indices of micronutrients, which are highly variable among athletes and difficult to interpret (Chapter 4). More research is needed on large groups of athletes participating in different sports to allow micronutrient recommendations to be quantified; however, for the present time, RNIs are considered to be satisfactory for use by the majority of athletes.

Summary

The collection of nutritional status measures in sports people is critical to our understanding of the association between nutrition, health, and sports performance, and is information that is often requested by the athlete or coach. A complete nutritional screening should include a dietary evaluation, biochemical and hematological testing of blood and perhaps urine, anthropometric testing to assess body composition, and a clinical assessment of the athlete's appearance and well-being. Many of these parameters cannot be assessed as optimal or suboptimal in isolation. Occasionally a reading is found to be clearly suboptimal, but the usual situation is that readings need to be compared to information previously collected from the same athlete and interpreted in conjunction with other data. Collection of information about the dietary intakes of athletes requires highly trained people who are familiar with limitations and bias in collecting and interpreting these data. Despite measures to improve the accuracy and reliability of information collected in dietary surveys, misreporting, particularly under-reporting true intake, is a major problem in all methods. Population reference standards and guidelines for interpreting dietary intakes and biochemical indices can be applied to athletes with caution. Because of the extensive research on carbohydrate and protein intakes in athletes, specific values for daily intakes of these nutrients as well as other recommendations for sports nutrition practice are available in position stands prepared for athletes and people who are active.

Reading list

American College of Sports Medicine. (1975) Position statement of the American College of Sports Medicine: prevention of heat injuries during distance running. *Medicine and Science in Sports and Exercise* **7**, vii–ix.

American College of Sports Medicine. (1987) Position stand of the American College of Sports Medicine: the prevention of thermal injuries during distance running. *Medicine and Science in Sports and Exercise* **19**, 529–533.

American College of Sports Medicine. (1996) Weight loss in wrestlers. *Medicine and Science in Sports and Exercise* **28**, ix–xii.

American College of Sports Medicine. (1996) Position stand: exercise and fluid replacement. *Medicine and Science in Sports and Exercise* **28**, i–vii.

American College of Sports Medicine, American Dietetic Association, and Dietitians of Canada. (2000) Nutrition and athletic performance. *Medicine and Science in Sports and Exercise* **32**, 2130–2145.

American College of Sports Medicine. (2000) Roundtable: The physiological and health effects of oral creatine supplementation. *Medicine and Science in Sports and Exercise* **32**, 706–717.

Deakin, V. (2000) Measuring nutritional status of athletes: clinical and research perspectives. In: *Clinical Sports Nutrition* (eds L. Burke & V. Deakin), 2nd edn, pp. 30–68. McGraw-Hill, Sydney, Australia.

Institute of Medicine, Food and Nutrition Board. (1998) *Dietary Reference Intakes for Thiamine, Riboflavin, Niacin, Vitamin B-6, Folate, Vitamin B-12, Pantothenic Acid, Biotin, and Choline.* National Academy Press, Washington, DC.

National Health and Medical Research Council. (1992) *Dietary Guidelines for Australians.* Australian Government Publishing Service, Canberra.

National Health and Medical Research Council. (1991) *Recommended Dietary Intakes for use in Australia.* Australian Government Publishing Service, Canberra.

National Research Council. (1989) *Recommended Dietary Allowances*, 10th edn. National Academy Press, Washington, DC.

EXPERT COMMENT 1 Changes in dietary recommendations for athletes. Louise M. Burke

The science of sports nutrition has evolved over the past 40 years and continues to evolve with new studies and new techniques. Position statements or position stands, even when made by experts, can only make guidelines based on the knowledge of the day. We generally recognize that expert statements are prepared by consensus, and, as such, generally represent a conservative view that is well supported by research. Therefore, guidelines may be considered "state of the art" at the time of their release, but may need to be altered over time in view of new information or the recognition that a more practical education message is needed. A good example of the way that knowledge has evolved and changed with time can be seen in the guidelines for fluid and carbohydrate intake during prolonged exercise. Excerpts from position stands from the American College of Sports Medicine over the last two decades are presented below.

"Rules prohibiting the administration of fluids during the first 10 kilometers of a marathon race should be amended to permit fluid ingestion at frequent intervals along the race course. . . . It is the responsibility of the race sponsors to provide fluids which contain small amounts of sugar (less than 2.5%) and electrolytes. . . . The addition of even small amounts of sugar can drastically impair the rate of gastric emptying. During exercise in the heat, carbohydrate supplementation is of secondary importance and the sugar content of oral feedings should be minimized."
American College of Sports Medicine: 1985 position statement on prevention of heat injuries during distance running.

"An adequate supply of water should be available before the race and every 2–3 km during the race . . . Aid stations should be stocked with enough fluid (cool water is the optimum) for each runner to have 300–360 ml at each aid station."
American College of Sports Medicine: 1987 position statement on prevention of thermal injuries during distance running.

"During intense exercise lasting longer than 1 h, it is recommended that carbohydrates be ingested at a rate of 30–60 g per hour to maintain oxidation of carbohydrates and delay fatigue. This rate of carbohydrate intake can be achieved without compromising fluid delivery by drinking 600–1200 ml/hr of solutions containing 4–8% carbohydrates."
American College of Sports Medicine: 1996 position stand on exercise and fluid replacement.

These excerpts show that the focus of statements in the early 1980s was to promote rehydration by athletes during endurance events. In fact, the first guidelines targeted the rules of the International Amateur Athletic Federation, which had previously prevented race organizers from providing fluids during the first 10 km of distance races, and either directly prevented or discouraged competitors from drinking adequate amounts of fluids during competition. During the 1970s most studies of fluid intake during exercise were based on techniques that emphasized the inhibitory effect of solutes in fluid on gastric emptying. Therefore, recommendations for fluids to be consumed during exercise promoted drinks with a low solute content (water or dilute solutions of carbohydrate). These guidelines can now be seen as proactive in terms of hydration messages, but conservative in view of the accumulating data from studies showing the benefits of consuming carbohydrate during prolonged exercise.

When the guidelines were rewritten a couple of years later, the focus on hydration over refueling remained, despite even greater amounts of evidence supporting performance enhancement with carbohydrate intake. Again the emphasis was on combating dehydration by promoting fluid intake during distance events, and it was considered helpful to provide athletes with guidelines in terms of volumes of fluid that should be consumed during a race.

In addition to expanding its focus to a range of sports and exercise activities instead of distance running, the most recent position stand on exercise and fluid replacement has been updated in two important ways. First, it now recognizes that carbohydrate and fluid can be simultaneously replaced during exercise without compromising hydration status, and that refueling provides a performance benefit across a range of exercise activities. This change in thinking is supported by newer studies of gastric emptying and fluid replacement during exercise, as well as studies of carbohydrate intake and exercise performance. However, the other change is that the position stand goes on to recognize that blanket recommendations for fluid intake during exercise do not take into account the myriad factors that govern fluid needs and fluid intake practices across sports. The new guidelines recognize that each athlete needs to consider issues in their sport such as individual sweat rates, access to fluid, opportunities to drink, and risk of gastrointestinal discomfort when organizing a plan of fluid intake. Therefore, it provides advice that helps athletes to assess the needs and opportunities for fluid and carbohydrate intake in their sport and to devise their own plan.

The goals of sports nutrition include issues of health as well as performance, and issues that have an immediate effect on performance as well as those of long-term importance. Clearly athletes need to have a central dietary pattern, to which specialized needs can be added. It is of interest to nutritionists to see whether the dietary guidelines prepared for the general population can address the basic needs of athletes. This would have a twofold advantage. Not only might they form a backbone for sports nutrition guidelines, but they might also provide a strong advertisement for the benefits of healthy nutrition to the community. Since athletes are admired and often presented as role models in our society, they can provide a strong positive message about the importance of healthy eating.

An examination of the Australian dietary guidelines for the general population shows that they are generally consistent with the nutritional needs of the athlete.

1 *Enjoy a wide variety of nutritious foods*

Eating nutrient-rich foods to meet additional energy requirements will ensure that the athlete can also meet their increased requirements for a number of important nutrients. Many athletes need to learn that being motivated and focused on nutrition does not equate to being extreme and restrictive with food choices. Dietary restriction and fad diets are a common cause of suboptimal intake of key nutrients.

2 *Eat plenty of breads and cereals (preferably wholegrain), vegetables (including legumes), and fruits*

Carbohydrate is a critical fuel for training and competition activities, and the athlete's diet must supply adequate carbohydrate to meet the fuel needs of exercise and recovery. Choosing nutrient-rich carbohydrate foods to meet fuel needs will help to supply other nutrient needs as well.

3 *Eat a diet low in fat, and in particular, low in saturated fat*

Moderation with fat intake ensures that the athlete can concentrate on carbohydrate fuel needs. Reducing fat intake is an effective way for an athlete to reduce energy intake to achieve and maintain optimal weight or body fat levels.

4 *Maintain a healthy body weight by balancing activity and food intake*

Body weight and body fatness play a role in the performance of most sports. Athletes should seek to achieve levels that are consistent with good health as well as good performance. It may be necessary to alter food and exercise patterns to achieve such goals.

5 *If you drink alcohol, limit your intake*

Alcohol use and sport are closely linked through sports sponsorship and social drinking customs. Athletes must also practice moderation with alcohol intake, especially so that it does not interfere with nutrition goals during postexercise recovery.

6 *Eat only a moderate amount of sugars and foods containing added sugars*

Moderation of sugar intake is regarded as desirable in the general population where excessive weight gain is a common problem. However, sugars and energy-dense carbohydrate-rich foods and drinks may be particularly useful for athletes who have increased requirements for carbohydrate before, during, and after exercise, and can help them to meet fuel needs in a practical way. Good dental practices, including brushing teeth after meals and snacks, are important for athletes as well as sedentary people. All carbohydrate-containing foods pose a risk for dental health if they are consumed in a grazing pattern without an opportunity to rinse the mouth and teeth.

7 *Choose low-salt foods and use salt sparingly*

Advice about moderating salt intake is aimed at the general population because of the possible association of a high sodium intake with the later development of hypertension in susceptible individuals. For most athletes, sodium needs are adequately met through the sodium content of processed foods. However, for athletes who lose large amounts of sweat over repeated days of training or competition in hot conditions, additional sodium through the salting of meals or consumption of sodium-containing fluids may be desirable to ensure adequate body sodium and to assist with rehydration following sweat loss.

8 *Encourage and support breastfeeding*

Many top athletes become mothers! Many mothers maintain their fitness before and after the birth of their children. By successfully breastfeeding, an active mother looks after the nutritional needs of her child, and provides a role model for the community.

Guidelines on specific nutrients

9 *Eat foods containing calcium. This is especially important for girls and women*

Some female athletes are at particular risk of reduced bone density due to hormonal disturbances related to menstrual dysfunction. Such problems should be referred for early intervention and management. All athletes should meet their calcium needs, so that in combination with the beneficial effects of weight-bearing exercise, they can achieve healthy bones.

10 *Eat foods containing iron. This applies particularly to girls, women, vegetarians, and athletes*

Reduced iron status impairs sports performance, and some athletes, particularly females, are at risk of developing inadequate iron status.

EXPERT COMMENT 3 How much do coaches and athletes know about food and nutrition? Mikael Fogelholm

The use of nutritional supplements in athletes seems to increase year after year. Since the available scientific data only rarely support the ergogenic benefits of most supplements, does this indicate that the nutritional knowledge of athletes and coaches is not adequate? Could the use of supplements be decreased by better education?

The answers to the above questions are not straightforward. Many studies on dietary intake among athletes indicate adequate intakes of protein and most micronutrients, but too low an intake of carbohydrates. Many components of a diet, hence, seem to be in balance, although many athletes could improve their eating patterns. The problem seems to be that the nutritional "knowledge" of athletes and their coaches is focused too much on single nutrients and the need for supplements, whereas the composition of food intake in a balanced diet awakes less interest. This leads to a high use of some single food items and supplements, but less attention on general dietary guidelines, such as "eat at least five servings of fruit or vegetables each day".

It is not easy to educate athletes about nutrition, because of the many channels of persuasive nutrition "information" they already receive. All athletes' magazines, particularly those that are meant for body builders and strength athletes, contain advertisements with all kinds of claims related to the benefits of supplements. Moreover, some magazines are owned by companies that make or distribute supplements—this may bias the articles written in the magazines. Athletes also observe other athletes and especially those who win the highest medals in international events. Because many, if not most, of the successful athletes use supplements or claim to follow unusual dietary practices or popular diets, other athletes regard this as evidence for ergogenic benefits.

A more revealing question than "how much do athletes and coaches know about nutrition?" is "how much of their nutrition knowledge can be put into practice?" The answer here is that coaches and athletes often know many facts correctly, but are unable to integrate the various pieces of information into a single eating plan, or translate facts into practice. Sometimes they are also distracted by false information. Separating facts from fiction is apparently difficult, because of multiple and discrepant information available for athletes. Moreover, many athletes and coaches seem to have abandoned their interest in basic training, rest, and dietary patterns. Background eating patterns that support everyday needs for health, training, and recovery are often regarded as dull and "out of date". Instead, athletes and coaches are drawn to glamorous-sounding supplements, or single nutrients and food items that promise a direct performance enhancement. New diets that are in direct contrast to the principles of healthy eating also seem to capture the imagination of sportspeople, since challenging the status quo always seems to sound "state of the art". It is becoming increasingly difficult for the evidence-based nutrition educator to overcome the false claims from the marketing hype surrounding fad diets and supplements, because these now form an ever larger base of the athletes' and coaches' "knowledge".

Chapter 11
Changing size and body composition

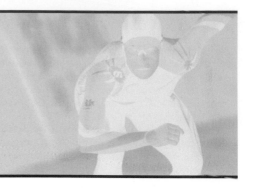

Introduction

Many athletes want to know what their ideal body size and composition is, so that they can work towards achieving this. This is particularly common in sports where the athlete's body weight, muscle mass, or body fat level have an effect on performance. However, other athletes are motivated to lose body fat or gain muscle mass for their appearance or for health reasons. Optimum body weight and body fat levels vary from sport to sport, and even with team positions or specific events within the same sport. In some sports, athletes commonly set their body weight and body fat goals below a level that is "natural" or "healthy" for many of the individuals concerned. There is some evidence that this is most likely to involve female athletes. This chapter will discuss issues in deciding on body weight and body composition goals, and eating strategies that underpin changes in body fat or lean body mass.

Measurement of lean body mass and body fat levels in athletes

Athletes come in a range of sizes and shapes—from the 40-kg gymnast to the 200-kg sumo wrestler. Contributions of lean body mass and body fat to the athlete's total body mass also vary widely. Although body mass (weight) does not distinguish between muscle mass or body fatness, many athletes, like sedentary people, rely on regular measurements of body weight to judge the suitability of their size and body composition. This is often a source of misinformation and frustration. Changes in body weight over the long term (a week or more) can sometimes be used to monitor energy balance (see Chapter 1), but changes in body mass are often difficult to interpret. Instead, the most valuable use of weighing scales is to determine acute body weight changes during a training or competition session, and thus estimate the sweat losses that must be replaced (see Chapter 8).

Assessment of body composition, particularly muscularity and fatness, is valuable for monitoring the characteristics that promote good performance in certain sports. Often these measurements are made on elite athletes, and it is assumed that mean values, or the values of the best athletes, provide a template that all aspiring athletes should attempt to achieve. However, it should be realized that even at the elite level there is some variety in size and shape, and there are too many exceptions to make all but the broadest generalizations about what is desirable. In fact, the most valuable use of body composition assessments is to sequentially monitor the same athlete, looking for changes that occur with growth and maturation, training or dietary manipulations, and stages of the competition season. Over a period of time, this information can be used to determine the athlete's body weight and body fat goals, and their success in achieving them. "Ideal" body mass and composition (i.e. body fatness, muscle mass) should only be determined for the individual athlete after consideration of the factors that are consistent with good performance and good health in the long term. The picture is further complicated by the wide variety of different methods used to assess body composition. Not all will give the same answers for an individual, even though the average values for a group may be the same, so athletes and those who advise them must be aware of the need for selection of an appropriate method.

Criteria for choosing a technique for measuring body composition in athletes include validity and reliability of the technique and the ease of access within the athlete's lifestyle. Techniques such as underwater weighing (hydrodensitometry) or dual-energy X-ray absorptiometry (DEXA) are generally considered to be the "gold standard" protocols for assessing body composition. However, these techniques are relatively expensive and are not available to many athletes, especially for use in the field or for sequential monitoring. Other methods which may be more portable or less expensive such as TOBEC (total body electrical conductivity), bioelectrical impedance analysis, and infrared spectrophotometry all need to be validated on athletic populations before absolute accuracy can be guaranteed. In surveys of large populations, the body mass index (BMI) may be used to give an estimate of fatness. This is calculated as the body mass (in kg) divided by the height (in m) squared. This measure is reasonable for the general population but should not be used with athletes as it will be misleading when the muscle mass is high.

In the field, the measurement of anthropometric data, such as girths, circumferences, and subcutaneous fat levels (via skinfold calipers) remains the most practical, simple, and inexpensive technique for the estimation of body fatness and muscularity of athletes.

Measurements of skinfold fat thickness, often together with other anthropometric data, can be used to estimate percentage body fat levels and lean body mass by means of prediction equations. However, these equations are only considered accurate and reliable when they have been derived from the specific group of athletes on which they will then be applied. Therefore, many sports scientists use anthropometric data as a direct measure on which

feedback can be provided. For example a "sum of skinfolds" (the sum of measurements of subcutaneous fat from a number of standard sites) can be used as an absolute indication of body fat levels, and the athlete can be counseled about desirable levels or desirable changes in levels based on comparisons to previous determinations of this measure. Regardless of which anthropometric information is collected for the sequential monitoring of individual athletes, it is important that technical errors in collecting data are minimized. Strategies include the expert training of anthropometrists, the use of the same anthropometrist in sequential monitoring, consistency in following a set protocol and well-defined landmarks for choosing sites, and the use of standard equipment.

Effect of body mass and body fat levels on sports performance

An athlete's muscle mass and body fat levels are determined by both genetics and the changes achieved through the conditioning effect of high-level training and diet. These characteristics exert a range of effects on performance, and different values will be more likely to bring success in different sports. As a result, successful sportspeople tend to fall into some predictable patterns of body weight and body fat levels according to the demands of their sport.

In sports that are essentially based on skill (e.g. golf, archery, bowling), performance is largely independent of body size and fatness. Since the level of physical activity in these sports, however lengthy, is low to moderate in terms of energy expenditure, participation does not contribute significantly to energy balance. Both selection and conditioning factors tend to allow higher body fat levels to occur in these sports—in some cases, elite athletes may have body fat levels that are considered obese by normal community standards. Often, strategies to reduce body fat are undertaken for improvements in health, general fitness, and appearance, rather than as a direct benefit to performance.

By contrast, low body mass, and in particular, low body fat levels, are considered important for performance across a number of sports. A small body size decreases the energy cost of activity, and allows the athlete to achieve tight movements like turns and twists in a restricted space (e.g. diving, gymnastics). The advantages of low body fat levels include physical and mechanical gains, for example, an increased "power to weight" ratio or simply a reduced amount of "dead weight" that must be moved by the athlete. This is a particular advantage in sports such as distance running, triathlon, and road cycling where the athlete transports his or her body mass over long distances, and in hill cycling and jumping for height or distance, where the athlete must move vertically against greater gravity effects. However, low body fat levels are often also important for reasons of aesthetics and appearance in sports such as gymnastics, diving, figure skating, and bodybuilding.

In other sports, competition takes place in specific weight divisions that are intended to match opponents of similar size and strength and therefore promote fair competition. Such sports include weightlifting, boxing, amateur wrestling, lightweight rowing, and horse racing. However, in these sports, most competitors attempt to compete in a weight division that is below their typical training weight, trying to gain an advantage over a smaller, lighter opponent. Athletes in these sports often show large and frequent fluctuations in body weight, and pursue weight loss even when they are already very lean.

Finally, in sports in which power and momentum are important, athletes are interested to increase body mass, primarily though an increase in muscle mass. In some of these sports (e.g. throwing events and heavyweight division lifting events), athletes are not necessarily penalized by also having high levels of body fat. However, in the case of athletes who must also possess speed and agility (e.g. track sprinters and mobile players in rugby and the various codes of football), low levels of body fat are typical.

Although some athletes easily achieve a body weight and composition suited to their sport, others may need to manipulate characteristics such as muscle mass or body fatness through changes in diet or training. It is important that the athlete can identify suitable and realistic goals, take appropriate measures to achieve them, and have a suitable means of monitoring progress. The optimal body fat level for an athlete should be obtained from their individual history and should meet the following criteria:

1 be associated with (consistent) good performances;
2 promote good health in the athlete—including the absence of evidence of "underweight" or over-training; and
3 allow the athlete to consume a diet providing adequate energy and nutrients to meet all nutritional goals and to remain reasonably free of food-related stress.

Strategies to reduce body fat in sport

Although most sedentary people may find it hard to imagine, many athletes consider themselves to be overfat. In fact, a desire to lose body fat is one of the most common reasons for an athlete to seek dietary advice from a sports doctor or dietitian. Weight loss counseling for athletes shares many features with counseling for the general community. Athletes have the same misconceptions about body composition, and about safe and long-term methods of reducing body fat. However, they may need specialized help to identify and achieve their individual ideal body weight and body fat levels. Sports-specific knowledge and empathy are important to combat the misconceptions and unsafe weight loss practices that become entrenched within many sports.

There are common situations, at both elite and recreational levels of sports participation, in which energy mismatches have caused the athlete to become overfat. Athletes in skill-based sports that have low energy expenditure may be considered essentially sedentary, especially if their sporting commitments prevent them from having other active hobbies or pursuits. A rapid gain of body fat is a common experience for highly active athletes who suddenly reduce or cease their training or competition activities. Athletes who are injured or are in the off season of their sport, are often unable or unwilling to regulate their energy intake to their lower energy needs. As a result they resume their sports activities with substantially increased body fat levels. Other lifestyle issues associated with some sports interfere with the achievement of optimum nutritional goals. Athletes with irregular lifestyles (e.g. travel commitments) and without a settled domestic routine (e.g. living outside a family environment) may have erratic eating patterns and rely on high-fat food choices from restaurants and fast food outlets. Young athletes pursuing a sports career are often required to move away from home before they have accumulated adequate nutrition knowledge or food preparation skills. Financial constraints may also limit food choices. Practical nutrition advice will be important in weight loss counseling for these athletes.

Athletes with "aesthetic" requirements for a low body fat level often find their goals and energy expenditure mismatched. Although typical training commitments for elite performers may be in the order of 20–40 h per week, these activities generally involve strength, skill, and flexibility exercises, with only short bursts of high-intensity work. Therefore, training activities do not assist the athlete to achieve the energy deficit required to reduce body fat easily. While athletes in high energy expenditure sports may be assisted by both selection and conditioning to achieve low levels of body fatness, many individuals still consider themselves overfat and wish to further reduce body fat levels. At present it is fashionable among some athletic groups to try to achieve the lowest possible body fat levels. However, statistical evidence that reduced body fat correlates with improved performance cannot always be applied to individual cases. There are many examples of athletes who achieve world-class performance with atypical body physiques, including body fat levels that are at the high end of (or even above) the typical range for that sport. There are also many case histories to show that short-term improvements in performance following substantial loss of body fat are soon compromised by long-term health and injury problems.

Problems of setting goals for very low body fat levels

Many athletes set unrealistic weight loss goals—either seeking to reach an unnecessarily and harm-fully low body fat level, or to achieve body fat loss in an unacceptably short timescale. The pressure to set these goals may come from a number of sources. Athletes—at least most of the successful ones—are, by nature, compulsive and focused. The same traits that encourage good sports performance in many athletes—perfectionism, dedication, ability to work hard and withstand discomfort—may lead to false expectations and preoccupation with body fat levels. Parents, trainers, coaches, and other athletes are often guilty of providing pressure and misguided expectations. Many people do not understand that "natural" or "healthy" standards of weight and body fat are an individual characteristic. Instead they focus on the lowest possible body fat levels, or the very low body fat levels of another successful competitor. The situation appears worse for female athletes, perhaps reflecting the general dissatisfaction of females in the community with their body shape and the biological predisposition for female athletes to have higher levels of body fat than their male counterparts, despite undertaking similar training.

Surveys of athletes involved in sports in which body fat levels are considered important, and female athletes in general, often report problems with eating disorders and disordered eating behaviors and body perceptions. Pathogenic weight control techniques include fasting or very low energy diets, dehydration techniques (saunas, diuretics, exercise in the heat), excessive training, self-induced vomiting, and the use of appetite suppressants or laxatives. These strategies may have detrimental effects on health and well-being as well as on exercise performance. Such problems appear to occur at a higher rate than seen in the general community or in sports in which weight or fatness is not an issue. The extent of eating disorders among athletes remains unknown, but should be seen as a continuum that includes clinical cases of anorexia and bulimia nervosa at one end, to food-related stress and unhealthy eating practices at the other. Eating disorders also occur among male athletes, although at a lower rate, and require special consideration and treatment.

It should be noted that many of the athletes reporting the use of abnormal eating and training practices do not appear to have classical eating disorders. Some athletes use these techniques simply as a method of achieving their weight and body fat goals, and are supported by the similar practices and beliefs of their peers. Indeed, we applaud other examples of extreme behavior in the athlete's lifestyle (e.g. rising very early in the morning to train, minimizing normal social and leisure activities to concentrate on sports goals). Some studies have reported that unhealthy weight control behaviors and preoccupation with weight and body fat levels do not persist in the off season in the majority of these athletes.

However, even in these groups, the potential problems associated with extreme dieting and achieving unnaturally low body fat levels should be recognized. Very low energy diets and specific low-carbohydrate diets will result in low muscle (and perhaps liver) glycogen stores in athletes, and are likely to cause fatigue and poor performance in athletes undertaking strenuous daily training. Rapid weight loss may also lead to loss of muscle mass, which will also adversely affect sports performance. In the longer term, frequent periods of dieting may place the athlete at risk of an inadequate intake of protein and micronutrients. There is speculation that hormonal and metabolic function may be compromised, including impairment of growth and development in young athletes. Psychological distress, including anxiety, isolation and depression, is also common.

The disadvantages of very low body fat levels *per se* include loss of body insulation and cushioning, but these effects are hard to separate from the indirect consequences of the techniques used to achieve them. Some racial groups and some individuals appear to have naturally low levels of body fat, or at least to be better able to tolerate low body fat levels. However, there is accumulating evidence that individuals who chronically restrict energy availability to reduce body fat below the natural level that their body wishes to defend may induce complex metabolic and hormonal changes. This work remains speculative, and offers no real cure for affected athletes other than to encourage them to reassess their body fat goals. The present emphasis on the prevention of this problem may be best achieved by safe and conservative methods of body fat loss.

The special case of "making weight"

The tradition of "making weight" to meet a competition division in weight category sports has been well described among jockeys, lightweight rowers, wrestlers, and weightlifters. Body builders are also known to "cut up" immediately prior to competition, although their intention is not directly related to body weight. Instead they claim to increase muscle definition by minimizing the subcutaneous fat cover or dehydrating themselves in the hope of making skin tissue "paper thin". Rapid and short-term weight loss is typically achieved over the days leading up to an event using techniques such as dehydration, food restriction, self-induced vomiting, and the use of diuretics and laxatives. Competition may occur in these sports from once or more a week (e.g. lightweight rowers, wrestlers, and jockeys), to once or twice a year (body builders, professional boxers). Weight loss and gain will cycle between these periods. The interval between weigh-in and competition varies from 1 to 12 h, and generally leaves little time to overturn the effects of rapid weight loss strategies.

Techniques of "making weight" can threaten health as well as athletic performance. The seriousness of the effects will be greatest in athletes who are required to lose the greatest amounts of weight and in sports where this is repeated most often. The acute and chronic effects of restricted eating have already been discussed. The effect of dehydration will vary according to the degree of fluid deficit, the method by which it was induced (e.g. thermal stress, exercise, or diuretics) and the type of exercise that is performed. Nevertheless, the outcome may vary from reduced performance to severe health risks, including death from hyperthermia or renal failure.

"Making weight" practices exist in most weight category sports in spite of the continued attention of medical, educational, and research bodies. It appears that the traditions, however negative, have become part of the culture of these sports and are resistant to change. Coaches and athletes are also convinced that performance benefits result from competing in the lowest possible weight category, in spite of the acknowledged performance decrement that results from the procedures that are used to make this possible. It is unlikely that sound nutrition and weight loss education will be embraced by athletes in weight category sports without additional reinforcement from the governing bodies in these sports. In some sports considerable discussion has led to proposals for rule modifications that might discourage weight cutting. These include certification of athletes at a weight division at the beginning of a season, measuring the level of hydration in competitors before an event, redistributing weight divisions to better match the normal weight distribution in the sports population, and making weigh-in closer to the event to prevent the reliance on post-weigh-in recovery.

Education programs for athletes and coaches should target the need for the athlete to make informed decisions about the weight category in which they compete. The core advice should be to achieve any desired weight loss through safe and realistic changes to body fat levels well in advance of competition. Minor adjustment of body mass (e.g. loss of 1–2 kg) in the week leading up to the event might be achieved by light dehydration and a low-residue diet to reduce gastrointestinal contents.

The female athlete triad: disordered eating, menstrual dysfunction, and reduced bone density

Disturbed menstrual function, including amenorrhea (absence of periods), is commonly reported in athletic groups, particularly in sports where body weight and body fat levels are considered important. Although low body fat levels *per se* have not been implicated as the cause of impaired menstrual function, there is evidence that restrained or disordered eating practices present a risk factor in some individuals. Studies have shown that practices which reduce energy availability below a critical threshold cause metabolic and hormonal adaptations. These changes may be mediated, at least in part, by the hormone leptin.

Whatever the underlying cause, menstrual dysfunction presents a concern for the bone health of young women and adolescents. In contrast to the protective effects of weight-bearing exercise on bone health, menstrual dysfunction is associated with reduced bone mass, perhaps as a result of low levels of the sex hormone, estrogen. Bone health is influenced by a complex array of factors, and athletes with menstrual disturbances seem at risk of suffering a reduction in bone mass or a failure to gain optimal bone mass during their early adult years. This may increase the risks of developing stress fractures in the short term, as well as an earlier onset of osteoporosis in later life. Of course, for the athlete who is concerned about their sporting career, the problem of chronic injury is the most immediate concern. The interrelationship and frequent coexistence of disordered eating, menstrual dysfunction, and poor bone health including stress fractures have led to the identification of the "female triad" syndrome. This is discussed in more detail in Chapter 4, with consideration of calcium intake as another issue in bone health.

Awareness of the female triad and associated problems may help to alert athletes to the need to avoid dangerous eating/training practices and to seek assistance as soon as problems do occur. It may also help sports medicine to develop early identification and treatment programs. However, it is important to remember that each of these problems can occur independently, and the athletes with problems should receive comprehensive and individualized attention, rather than expecting a simple cure. The treatment should attend to symptoms, but must also address the underlying causes. Intensive therapy from a team involving the athlete's coach, family, doctor, psychologist or psychiatrist, dietitian, and other members is typically required. The athlete may need to address her training load, eating practices, and body fat goals.

Guidelines for safe and effective weight (fat) loss by athletes

Few studies have systematically investigated the effects of various body fat levels, or the safety and effectiveness of weight loss techniques, on sports performance. Therefore we are left to develop general guidelines for weight loss in athletes based on common sense rather than rigorous scientific research. Guidelines and practical strategies to achieve these goals are summarized in Chapter 13.

A clear role for the sports dietitian or sports nutrition expert exists at all levels of this plan. Services provided by these professionals may include:

1 monitoring and counseling of individual athletes;
2 screening of athletes at high risk of developing disordered eating and eating disorders;
3 developing programs to incorporate sound nutrition practices into the plans of sports groups, clubs, or teams;
4 developing nutrition education resources based on safe and effective strategies for management of weight and body fat in specific sports; and
5 providing input into the programs underpinning the management and development of each specific sport (e.g. development of the coaching syllabus, rule changes to discourage unsafe weight loss practices such as "making weight").

Guidelines for effective weight (muscle) gain by athletes

At the other end of the spectrum are athletes who are interested in gaining muscle mass and strength. Size and power are key factors in the successful performance of many sports such as sprinting, lifting and throwing events, bodybuilding, rowing, and many team games, particularly the various codes of football. The core components for increasing muscle size and strength are genetic predisposition, a suitable resistance training program and adequate energy intake. Goals for gain of muscle mass and strength should be tailored to the athlete's individual potential and the type and volume of training that can be managed. However, athletes often focus their interest on protein intake and special supplements that claim to enhance the gain of lean body mass. These factors are covered in more detail in Chapter 12. Adequate energy intake is an important dietary factor that underpins the results of a resistance training program. In addition, there is some evidence that the timing of carbohydrate and protein intake may also be important in providing fuel for a resistance work-out, and optimizing protein balance during the recovery phase. It is often difficult for the athlete to achieve adequate or additional energy intake to support effective gain of muscle mass, or to organize meals and snacks to optimize recovery and adaptation to training. Guidelines and practical strategies to achieve an appropriate eating strategy to support these goals are summarized in Chapter 13.

Summary

Athletes require access to simple and inexpensive techniques to identify body fat and body weight goals and to monitor changes that occur with training, growth, and maturation. The physique characteristics of elite athletes might be used to provide general guidelines for the range of body fat levels that are consistent with good performance in a sport. However, they should not be used to provide rigid body fat prescriptions for individual athletes. The optimal weight and body fat level for an athlete should be obtained from their individual history and should consider a range of goals including good performance and good health over the long term. Athletes in sports in which low body fat levels are deemed necessary for optimal performance, and in particular, female athletes in these sports, should be considered at high risk for the development of disordered eating. These sports may benefit from education programs promoting safe and effective weight loss strategies, and from screening techniques to identify athletes in the early stages of developing disordered eating and body image problems.

Reading list

Brownell, K.D., Steen, S.N. & Wilmore, J.H. (1987) Weight regulation practices in athletes: analysis of metabolic and health effects. *Medicine and Science in Sports and Exercise* **19**, 546–555.

Brownell, K.D., Rodin, J. & Wilmore, J.H. (eds) (1992) *Eating, Body Weight and Performance in Athletes: Disorders of Modern Society*. Lea & Febiger, Philadelphia.

Houtkooper, L. (2000) Eating disorders and disordered eating in athletes. In: *Clinical Sports Nutrition* (eds

L. Burke & V. Deakin), 2nd edn, pp. 210–240. McGraw-Hill, Sydney, Australia.

Kerr, D. (2000) Kinanthropometry: physique assessment of the athlete. In: *Clinical Sports Nutrition* (eds L. Burke & V. Deakin), 2nd edn, pp. 69–89. McGraw-Hill, Sydney, Australia.

O'Connor, H., Sullivan, T. & Caterson, I. (2000) Weight loss and the athlete. In: *Clinical Sports Nutrition* (eds L. Burke & V. Deakin), 2nd edn, pp. 146–184. McGraw-Hill, Sydney, Australia.

Steen, S.N. & Brownell, K.D. (1990) Patterns of weight loss and regain in wrestlers: has the tradition changed? *Medicine and Science in Sports and Exercise* 22, 762–768.

Walberg-Rankin, J. (2000) Making weight in sports. In:

Clinical Sports Nutrition (eds L. Burke & V. Deakin), 2nd edn, pp. 185–209. McGraw-Hill, Sydney, Australia.

Withers, R.T., Craig, N.P., Bourdon, P.C. & Norton, K.I. (1987) Relative body fat and anthropometric prediction of body density of male athletes. *European Journal of Applied Physiology* 56, 191–200.

Withers, R.T., Whittingham, N.O., Norton, K.I., Ellis, M.W. & Cricket, A. (1987) Relative body fat and anthropometric prediction of body density of female athletes. *European Journal of Applied Physiology* 56, 169–180.

Wilmore, J.H. (1991) Eating and weight disorders in the female athlete. *International Journal of Sport Nutrition* 1, 104–117.

EXPERT COMMENT 1 What is the best (practical) way to assess body fat in athletes? Mikael Fogelholm

The human body may be divided into compartments by several approaches, but the molecular model forms the basis of most body composition assessment methods used today. According to the molecular model, the body is composed of molecules—that is, lipids, proteins, water, glycogen, and bone mineral molecules. Athletes and coaches are most often interested in fat mass of the body (FM = total lipids), or in the fat-free mass (FFM = body weight – FM).

There are no direct measures of body composition. Instead, the assessment techniques are based on measurements of one or more properties that have a known (or assumed) relationship with body composition. The result of the measurement is then placed in an equation to derive an estimation of body fat and fat-free mass. Two kinds of techniques exist.

1 Mechanistic methods, also considered to be laboratory methods. These methods, which include underwater weighing (UWW) and dual-energy X-ray absorptiometry (DEXA), use regression equations based on physical–anatomical assumptions to derive estimates of body composition.

2 Descriptive methods, also known as field methods, which include measurements of subcutaneous (skinfold) fat and bioimpedance (BIA). Since the regression equations used to estimate body composition in these methods have been derived by comparison against a mechanistic method (usually UWW), these techniques can be considered doubly indirect.

Assessment of body composition is characterized by two types of errors (biases). A systematic bias shifts the mean value of a population, but does not affect the population distribution. There are systematic biases in all methods and even between different equations used within the same method. Therefore, the result is affected by the method used or the equations employed in this method. Moreover, different outcomes will result from the use of

different protocols or equipment in undertaking a certain technique. Unreliable measurement techniques and random errors of the assumptions or regression equations increase the distribution of results (scattering the results around the mean value). Random errors are about twice as large in descriptive methods, compared with mechanistic methods.

All body composition methods identify obese subjects as obese, and lean subjects as lean. However, the accuracy of the methods is not good enough to reliably identify a relatively small (less than 5%) difference between two individuals. Therefore, use of any body composition method (and especially any of the descriptive methods) in a cross sectional setting, e.g. to identify "ideal body composition", is not warranted. Any single cut-off point may be misleading, especially because the relationship between small differences in body composition and physical performance is not straightforward.

Measurements of body composition are more valuable when they are used for sequential monitoring of the same athlete over a period of their training and development. The most practical and accessible method used in the field is monitoring of skinfold fat levels. This is considered a reliable technique when it is undertaken by a trained technician using a standardized protocol. By comparison, mechanistic methods are expensive and rarely in use, and another commonly available descriptive method, BIA, may be too much affected by water balance to be useful for monitoring of athletes. Particular care should be undertaken with body composition assessments of pubertal girls, because a careless use and interpretation of body composition assessment might increase the risk for restricted or disordered eating in this vulnerable group. The measurement and interpretation of body composition characteristics of athletes can be open to abuse, and should only be done with care and sensitivity.

CASE STUDY 1   Weight loss in a weight-sensitive sport. Melinda M. Manore

Athlete

Molly was in her first year of collegiate gymnastics, living in the college dorm with another gymnast. She was training well, but was anxious to lose 5 kg from her present body mass of 54 kg. Her body fat level had been assessed at 23%, and her coach wanted her to achieve a level of 20%.

Reason for consultancy

Molly wanted to lose weight but needed expert advice on how to achieve this. She admitted that her eating habits were often poor, especially when sharing meals with her room-mate, another gymnast who didn't need to watch her weight. She did not eat in the dorm cafeteria and had no access to cooking facilities. Therefore, all meals were eaten out.

Current dietary and activity patterns

Molly didn't have much time to eat during the day. She ate a good breakfast but skipped lunch, apart from a sports bar, to fit in extra classes before going to gymnastics practice. Practice, from 1 to 5 PM, was followed by an hour of physical therapy. She was starving by the time she ate dinner at a fast food restaurant, and continued to snack during the evening while she studied or watched TV. She didn't consume anything during practice and didn't take any supplements. Menstrual status was reported to be normal. Molly's typical dietary patterns are outlined below.

Professional assessment

Mean daily intake from Molly's self-reported eating plan was estimated to be ~ 10 460 kJ (2500 kcal) providing an adequate intake of protein (1.3 g kg^{-1}). Molly failed to meet the general guidelines for daily intake of fruits and vegetables, and dairy products. Her low fiber intake was also explained by her carbohydrate choices coming only from processed grains (white bread, rice, or pasta) and sweets. Her intake of many micronutrients (including iron, calcium, and folate) failed to meet the recommended daily intakes. Molly did not do any other physical activity besides gymnastics.

Intervention

Molly needed a meal plan that would accommodate her daily schedule and living situation. To achieve weight loss, Molly needed to decrease energy intake by 800–1200 kJ·day^{-1} (200–300 kcal·day^{-1}) and add an aerobic activity component to her overall training plan. Molly was encouraged to spend three nights a week at the gym doing aerobic activity on the treadmill (30–40 min) instead of watching TV. The following dietary suggestions were made to Molly.

1 Continue to choose a good breakfast, but have a skimmed milk coffee or hot chocolate instead of coffee with cream to increase calcium intake.

2 Buy a sandwich (wholewheat bread, low-fat meat, cheese and salad) and a piece of fruit on the way to classes each morning. Eat lunch between or during class, but before practice.

3 Bring a piece of fruit or half an energy bar to eat immediately after practice while working with the physical therapist. This will curb hunger and reduce overeating at dinner. Use a sports drink during exercise.

4 Decide on three separate eating plans for dinner at various "healthier" restaurants near campus. Select specific menu items and set an appropriate amount to be consumed, then stick to the plan.

5 Allow a snack of yogurt and fruit or pretzels at night.

6 Use a multivitamin/mineral supplement while energy intake is restricted.

7 Review her dietary plan and exercise goals with her gymnastics coach.

Outcome

After 8 weeks, Molly reported feeling in charge of her eating patterns and happy with her aerobic exercise plan. She had lost 1.5 kg and was feeling better about herself. At the end of the year she planned to move out of the dorm, and get an apartment so she could begin to cook some of her own meals.

Breakfast	Lunch	Dinner	Snacks during the evening
Bowl instant oatmeal with skimmed milk Orange juice Coffee with cream	Power Bar	Dinner at a fast food restaurant (sub sandwich; soup and salad; chicken, rice and vegetable; pizza; hamburger and fries)	Popcorn, fat-free chocolate cookies, pretzels, ice cream, diet pop, cheese, brownies

CASE STUDY 2 Loss of body fat. Patricia Thompson

Athlete

Maria was a 17-year-old swimmer who held many local and regional records including the national record for 100-m backstroke. She had been swimming at national team level for 4 years, and at the age of 15 had just failed to qualify for the 1996 Olympics. Although her typical training commitment was at least nine sessions a week, in recent times her weekly training load had been reduced to four or five sessions.

Reason for consultancy

Maria was referred by her coach for assistance to lose body fat. Following the Olympic trials, Maria had reduced her training significantly and had gained weight—from a pretrial level of 72 kg to her current weight of 81 kg. Although she had always been stocky, she was now definitely overfat. She complained of feeling weak and out of breath. Her best time in the 100-m backstroke was 1.06.51 but she was now struggling to achieve 1.10.00. Her coach felt she was capable of better performance, even with her curtailed program.

Current dietary patterns

Prior to the consultation, Maria had never paid much attention to her eating habits. On training days, her eating pattern consisted of two meals and two snacks. On race day, she skipped breakfast, and ate a big lunch and maybe a snack at night. Fluid replacement was not given high priority, although during competition she made an effort to drink more water. During competition periods she also tried to increase her carbohydrate intake by increasing her intake of vegetables and fruit. A sample daily intake is shown below.

Professional assessment

Maria's body fat was assessed to be 28%. Mean daily intake from her self-reported eating plan was estimated to be ~ 8400 kJ (2000 kcal) of which 36% of the energy was supplied from fat, 54% from carbohydrate (270 g or 3.3 $g \cdot kg^{-1}$) and 10% from protein (50 g). Her post-training recovery snack was the smallest meal of the day, and dinner following evening training was based

on fried food choices. Her meal plan was assessed to be low in both protein and carbohydrate, compared with the guidelines for training nutrition. Her intake of some micronutrients, for example calcium, was also assessed to be below recommended dietary allowances.

Intervention

The energy deficit needed to produce a loss of body fat was achieved primarily via an increase in training level rather than a reduction in energy intake. A reorganization of macronutrient intake was desired—primarily to increase protein and carbohydrate, while moderating fat intake. Suggestions to improve nutrient intake from a similar energy intake included the following strategies.

1 Adjustment of the timing and volume of meals so that eating would coincide more appropriately with the training schedule. In particular, the size of the breakfast snack was increased to promote recovery after the morning training session.

2 A reduction in fat intake, particularly fats added in cooking and food preparation. This energy was replaced by increasing the consumption of staple foods such as bread and rice.

3 Replacement of some salads with steamed vegetables, so that oily dressings could be replaced.

4 Increased intake of protein, and simultaneous improvement of calcium intake by adding reduced-fat dairy foods to meals and snacks.

5 Increased intake of fresh fruit.

Outcome

Maria's energy level increased and her training improved. Loss of body fat occurred as a result of her increased training level, rather than a drastic restriction of energy intake. Within 2 months, her weight showed a substantial decrease, and her body fat measurement was reassessed at 25% (a fat loss of 2.5 kg). Importantly, her times gradually improved so that she was able to secure a swimming scholarship to college within the year. Within one semester, she had achieved her best race times and qualified for the national championships.

Post-training snack	Lunch	Snack (3.00 PM)	Dinner
One slice pineapple Half large bread roll	Salad with lots of dressing Baked chicken thigh Orange drink	One glass juice	Fried rice, fried plantain, fried fish 1 cup pineapple juice

CASE STUDY 3　Loss of body fat. Patricia Thompson

Athlete

Sharon was the national female table tennis champion, but at 32 years of age her game had started to slip. Three years previously she had gained an enormous amount of weight (from 65 kg to 85 kg) during a failed pregnancy. After this she had adopted a sedentary lifestyle and had stopped a regular playing routine.

Reason for consultancy

Sharon was referred by her coach, who wanted her to compete in a forthcoming tournament. At the time of the referral, she weighed 88 kg and was sluggish and demotivated. She had tried "crash dieting" towards her goal weight of 67 kg, but the effort had only made her weak. She had resumed training with a 3-hour session of table tennis practice each day at 5 PM.

Current dietary pattern

Sharon's breakfast consisted of a small snack of bread and coffee for breakfast, while lunch and dinner were eaten as large fully cooked meals. She loved peanuts, but was conscious of trying to reduce her intake of such tempting snack foods. Fruit was not generally available so she snacked mainly on cheese and cream biscuits. A typical daily meal plan, excluding snacks, is shown below.

Professional assessment

Sharon's body fat was assessed to be 37%. Mean daily intake from her self-reported eating plan was assessed to be ~ 9240 kJ (2200 kcal) which was equivalent to her daily energy requirement. Because she required a relatively rapid weight loss, it was decided to trial a 5 MJ (1200 kcal) eating plan, aiming to provide maximum nutrient intake from this minimum energy allowance.

Intervention

Three main meals were planned, providing 55% calories from carbohydrate (173 g), 30% from fat (45 g), and 15% from protein (50 g). Features of this plan included the following.

1 Fruits were recommended for snacks, and a plan was worked out to ensure that these were purchased and made accessible.
2 Excess fat was removed from soup, and bread was consumed without fatty spreads.
3 A protein-rich food was included at breakfast.
4 A mid-afternoon snack was included to provide fuel for training.
5 The size of dinner was reduced, with an adjustment to increase carbohydrate intake at lunch, thus better fueling the afternoon training session.
6 Following initial weight loss, further changes were made to increase carbohydrate intake and to eliminate oil in cooking and in gravy.

Outcome

After 6 weeks, a loss of 5 kg had been recorded, and after 11 weeks, the total loss had reached 10 kg. Sharon was able to increase her training level and work on her skills, while weight loss continued at a steady rate of ~ 1 kg a week. Eventually she reached a plateau of 72 kg and a percentage body fat of 29%. This was sufficient encouragement for her to enter the championship, and to regain the title! After retiring, she took up coaching younger players.

Morning	Lunch (noon)	Dinner (8–9 PM)
1 cup coffee with full cream milk One or two slices hard-dough bread with butter spread thin	1 bowl soup—fish, beef or chicken with noodles, vegetables, peas, margarine, flour dumplings Cocoa	Rice Beef or chicken (breast and wing) with gravy Vegetables

Chapter 12
Dietary supplements and ergogenic aids

Introduction

The sports world is filled with products that claim to prolong endurance, enhance recovery, reduce body fat, increase muscle mass, minimize the risk of illness, or achieve other characteristics that enhance sports performance. Athletes are major consumers of supplements, and an important target group for the multibillion dollar supplement industry. The distinction between a supplement and a sports food is sometimes arbitrary. If the distinction is based on the form of the product, we might consider supplements to exist in the form of pills, potions, capsules, or powders, whereas sports foods would take a more traditional form of energy-containing bars, drinks, and other edible products. However, the definitions differ between countries according to the way that food and pharmaceutical products are regulated. This distinction can have important practical implications for the way that these products are manufactured and marketed. This chapter will review the range of products that are currently available, noting items that have true value as part of the athlete's nutrition program and compounds that have been proven by rigorous scientific testing to be ergogenic (work enhancing).

Issues that should be considered in contemplating the use of a supplement include, first, the effectiveness of the product; the amount and timing of supplementation and the specific exercise conditions under which its effects may be optimized must be considered. A second concern relates to whether there is a possibility of contravening the antidoping code imposed by the governing bodies of sport, as this might lead to suspension from competition. Thirdly, and perhaps most importantly of all, the question of safety of supplementation must be considered. This should perhaps be the primary concern, but the use by athletes of pharmaceuticals with well-recognized harmful side-effects shows that this is often not the case.

As a general principle, it is safe to assume that most supplements that offer a direct performance-enhancing effect are against the rules of sport: this category includes drugs and hormones. Most substances that are not banned are not effective: this includes most of the vitamin and mineral supplements as well as the herbal products sold in health food shops. There are, however, some exceptions to these generalizations: substances in this category might include creatine, bicarbonate as well as antioxidant nutrients. There are also grey areas, sometimes referred to as "nutraceuticals", and including compounds such as caffeine, that may be classified as foods but which are consumed for their pharmacological action. Of course, we will also see that many sports foods are effective when used by the athlete to meet a special nutritional goal for training or competition.

Supplements

Supplement use is widespread in sport. Reviews of the published literature suggest that the use of supplements is more prevalent in athletes (about 50%) than in the general population (35–40%), while among elite athletes almost 60% report supplement use. All these surveys find that the overall prevalence and the types of supplements used vary with the nature of the sport, the sex of the athletes, and the level of competition. In some surveys, 100% of bodybuilding and strength-training athletes use some form of nutritional supplementation.

It is not possible to review all of the nutritional supplements used by athletes, nor to consider in any detail the evidence relating to more than a few. However, consideration of some specific examples will illustrate the general principles that determine usage, and the evaluation that ought to be applied to these supplements.

Creatine

Creatine supplementation has been practiced by many successful athletes, particularly in track and field athletics, but also now in many, if not most, other sports. Some indication of the extent of its use is gained from the fact that the estimated sales of creatine to athletes in the US alone in 1997 amounted to over 300 000 kg. This represents a remarkable growth, as its use first became popular in sport after the 1992 Olympic Games in Barcelona. What distinguishes creatine from most other ergogenic aids is that it seems to be effective in improving performance. More significantly, perhaps, its use is not prohibited by the governing bodies of sport, and there appear to be no harmful side-effects even when very large doses are taken, at least in the quantities that are necessary to produce an ergogenic effect. Issues relating to the use of creatine will be considered in some depth as these highlight the questions that relate to all supplement use.

Creatine metabolism

Creatine phosphate (CP) itself is present in resting muscle in a concentration approximately 3–4 times that of ATP, the immediate energy source for muscle contraction. The amount of ATP in muscle cells is small, and only a fraction of this can be viewed as an energy store: when the cellular ATP concentration falls too far, fatigue ensues. Muscle ATP content rarely falls by more than about 25–30% at the point of fatigue in high-intensity exercise.

Regeneration of ATP at a rate close to that of ATP hydrolysis is essential if fatigue is to be delayed. Transfer of the phosphate group from CP to ADP is catalysed by the enzyme creatine kinase, resulting in the restoration of ATP and the release of free creatine (C). The situation during intense muscle contraction can be represented as follows:

$$ATP \rightarrow ADP + P_i$$

$$CP + ADP \rightarrow ATP + C.$$

The rate of ATP hydrolysis is set by the power output of the muscle, and can exceed 10 mmol·kg dry muscle^{-1} in maximum efforts. The resting ATP content of muscle is about 24 mmol·kg^{-1}, but this cannot fall by more than about 30%, so the need for rephosphorylation of the ADP formed during contraction is obvious. This reaction is extremely rapid, and since the muscle CP concentration can fall to almost zero, it can make a significant contribution to the energy supply necessary for brief bursts of very high intensity exercise. The CP store is also limited, however, and increasing the CP content of muscle ought to allow a greater amount of work to be done using this energy source.

During the recovery process after exercise, the creatine kinase reaction is reversed, using energy made available by oxidative metabolism that occurs within the mitochondria:

$$C + ATP \rightarrow CP + ADP$$

$$ADP + P_i + metabolism \rightarrow ATP.$$

In high-intensity exercise, glycolysis will result in the formation of pyruvate at a rate higher than that at which it can be removed by oxidative metabolism, leading to an accumulation of lactate within the muscle. The hydrogen ions associated with anaerobic glycolysis cause muscle pH to fall, and this increasing acidity is a factor in the fatigue process. A number of buffers within the cell resist changes in pH, and the breakdown of CP is such a mechanism. The creatine kinase reaction can be rewritten to take account of the charges involved:

$$CP^{2-} + ADP^{3-} + H^+ \rightarrow ATP^{4-} + C.$$

An increased availability of CP for breakdown has the potential to increase the intramuscular buffering capacity, delaying the point at which pH reaches a critically low level.

CP has been reported to play another role within the muscle cell, which is to transfer ATP equivalents from within the mitochondria, where ATP is generated by oxidative phosphorylation, to the cytoplasm where it is required. There is, however, no evidence from studies of human skeletal muscle that this process is limited by the availability of creatine. The apparent failure of creatine supplementation to influence the metabolic response to exercise of moderate intensities or performance in this type of exercise also argues against an important—or at least limiting—role for this shuttle.

Creatine supplementation and muscle CP concentration

Creatine is an amino acid (methylguanidine-acetic acid) which occurs naturally in the diet, being present in meat: 1 kg of fresh steak contains about 5 g of creatine. The normal daily intake is less than 1 g, but the estimated daily requirement for the average individual is about 2 g. The body has a limited capacity to synthesize creatine in the liver, kidney, pancreas, and other tissues, but the primary site of synthesis in humans is the kidney. This supplies the amount required in excess of the dietary intake, and is also the only way in which vegetarians can meet their requirement. Synthesis occurs from amino acid precursors (methionine, arginine, and glycine), but the synthetic pathway is suppressed when the dietary creatine intake is high.

Studies of resting human skeletal muscle have shown the CP concentration to be about 75 mmol·kg dry weight^{-1} and the free creatine concentration to be about 50 mmol·kg^{-1}. There is, however, quite a large range of values reported in the literature, and it seems clear that there is considerable interindividual variability. The first studies of creatine supplementation in the 1990s showed that taking creatine (5 g four times per day) over a period of 4–5

days resulted in a marked increase in the total creatine content of the quadriceps femoris muscle. An increase in muscle creatine content was apparent within 2 days of starting this regimen, and the increase was greatest in those with a low initial level: in some cases an increase of 50% was observed. Approximately 20% of the increase in total muscle creatine content was accounted for by creatine phosphate. More recent studies show that creatine supplementation of ~ 3 g·day^{-1} will result in similarly increased muscle creatine concentrations, but it may take 3 weeks to reach the creatine storage threshold. Once creatine loading has been achieved, a continued daily intake of 1–2 g of creatine will maintain the increased muscle creatine content, whereas cessation of all supplemental intake will cause muscle creatine concentrations to gradually return to presupplementation levels over 3–4 weeks. Since coingestion of creatine with carbohydrate (75–100 g) enhances the uptake of creatine into the muscle cell, many sports scientists recommend that creatine supplements be taken with a meal or substantial carbohydrate-rich snack.

Effects of creatine supplementation on exercise performance

Muscle creatine content will remain elevated for several weeks following creatine supplementation. If athletes are used as subjects, the increased training loads that seem to be possible after creatine supplementation make it difficult to interpret results of crossover studies where placebo is administered as the second treatment. For these reasons, most of the reported studies have used matched groups of subjects. The past decade has seen the publication of a large number of studies that have investigated the effects of creatine supplementation on the performance of a variety of modes and types of exercise. This literature shows that there appears to be no significant benefit to the peak power output that can be achieved in a single high-intensity exercise bout, but the balance of the available evidence suggests that performance is improved in tasks involving repeated high-intensity exercise with short recovery intervals. In fact, some very recent studies have shown that these benefits are seen in well-trained subjects undertaking field tests or laboratory protocols that simulate competitive events such as team sports. On this basis, creatine supplementation may be a useful adjunct to the training programs of athletes that involve interval or resistance training and to the competition performance of field and court sports involving intermittent high-intensity bursts of play.

There is little information on the effects of creatine supplementation on the performance of more prolonged exercise. In an incremental treadmill running test there was no effect of creatine supplementation on the cardiorespiratory or metabolic response to submaximal exercise, but exercise performance was not measured in this study. However, another study has reported no beneficial effect of creatine supplementation on performance in an endurance running test. In fact, the performance was impaired, perhaps as a result of the small weight gain (~ 1 kg) that is usually associated with acute supplementation with creatine.

The mechanism by which creatine supplementation might improve performance is not entirely clear, although it seems clear that this effect is related to the increased muscle CP content. Recent results indicate that the rate of CP resynthesis after intense exercise is enhanced after high-dose creatine supplementation. This allows faster recovery after sprints as well as allowing more work to be done during each subsequent high-intensity effort.

Creatine and muscle strength

Although there have been numerous investigations into the effects of creatine supplementation on the ability to generate high levels of muscle power, few studies have looked for possible effects on muscle strength. This seems surprising in view of the importance of a high force-generating capacity for the development of power. In an early study, subjects were required to perform five sets of 30 maximal voluntary isokinetic contractions before and after supplementation with creatine or placebo. No effect was seen in the placebo group, and an increase in muscle peak torque production was seen in the creatine group only in the later stages of some of the sets. No effect of creatine supplementation on peak torque was seen, but this experimental model might not allow subjects to generate max-

imum forces because of the large number of contractions to be performed.

More recently, it has been shown that 5 days of creatine supplementation was effective in increasing maximum voluntary isometric strength of the knee extensor muscles in individuals engaged in a strength training program. This gain was maintained in a subsequent test after a period during which a placebo was administered. In a second group of subjects, the treatment order was reversed: no gain in strength was seen after the first period of placebo administration, but an increase was observed in the third test, after the creatine supplementation period. Isometric endurance capacity at various fractions of maximal voluntary contraction was also increased after creatine supplementation but was not affected by the placebo treatment. Other studies have also shown bigger improvements in strength gains in naïve subjects embarking on a strength training program.

Creatine and body mass

Many studies and anecdotal reports support the suggestion that acute supplementation with creatine is associated with a prompt gain in body mass. This typically seems to amount to about 1–2 kg over a supplementation period of 4–5 days, but may be more than this. Because of the rapid increases in body mass, it must be assumed that this is mostly accounted for by water retention. Increasing the creatine content of muscle by 80–100 mmol·kg^{-1} will increase intracellular osmolality, leading to water retention. There is some preliminary evidence for a stimulation of protein synthesis—perhaps secondary to this osmotically induced swelling of the cells—in response to creatine supplementation, but further experimentation is required. It seems unlikely that major effects on muscle protein content can be achieved within 4–5 days. It must be conceded, however, that the reported gains in muscle strength within the same timescale are difficult to explain.

Health concerns of creatine supplementation

Many concerns have been raised that the effects of long-term use of large doses of creatine are unknown and that its use may pose a health risk. Concerns seem to focus primarily on the possible effects on renal function, in particular in individuals with impaired renal capacity. Studies on the response to long-term creatine use are in progress at this time, but results are not yet available. There have, however, been no reports of adverse effects in any of the studies published in the literature, and the few reports of medical problems that have received attention in medical journals have concerned a few individuals who have had pre-existing renal problems prior to taking creatine. One study that specifically examined renal function in individuals supplementing with creatine found no reason to believe that renal complications were likely. Anecdotal reports of an increased prevalence of muscle cramps in athletes taking creatine supplements have been circulating for some time, but there seems to be no substance to any of these stories. It seems likely that any injury suffered by an athlete will be ascribed to an easily identifiable change in habit, such as the introduction of a new supplement.

Uninformed comment blamed the deaths of three American collegiate wrestlers on creatine use, but this was not substantiated at the formal inquiries conducted. Given the increase in body mass that often accompanies supplementation, it does seem possible that athletes who must acutely reduce body mass to qualify for a particular weight category might face problems. It is not unusual in some sports for body mass to be reduced by as much as 10% in the few days before competition: if the mass loss necessary to make the qualifying weight is 1–2 kg more than anticipated due to the weight gain associated with creatine use, the measures required to achieve the target mass will be unusually severe and may provoke problems related to dehydration and hyperthermia.

The concern over possible adverse effects is entirely justified. It is usually recommended that athletes take 20 g of creatine per day for 4–5 days (a loading dose) followed by 1–2 g per day (maintenance dose). Many athletes, however, work on the principle that more is better and may greatly exceed these amounts. Even with very large doses, however, the possibility of adverse effects seems remote. Creatine is a small water-soluble molecule easily cleared by the kidney, and the additional nitrogen load resulting from supplementation is small. The same concerns over renal damage have been raised in the context of protein supplementation among strength athletes and body builders. These athletes may consume up to 400 g of protein per day over very long periods, but there is no evidence that the theoretical problems of clearance of the extra solute load are real.

Carnitine

Depletion of the intramuscular glycogen stores is recognized as one of the primary factors involved in the fatigue that accompanies prolonged exercise. The importance of carbohydrate as a fuel for the working muscles is confirmed by the close relationship between the pre-exercise glycogen concentration and the time for which exercise can be sustained. Further evidence comes from studies that show that increasing the combustion of fat during prolonged exercise, and thus sparing the limited carbohydrate stores, can improve endurance capacity. Increasing fatty acid mobilization by heparin administration has been shown to be effective in improving performance, even though this method is not practical for competitive sport.

Although the supply of plasma free fatty acids to the exercising muscle is an important factor in determining the relative contributions of fat and carbohydrate to oxidative metabolism, a number of other steps are recognized as being involved in fat oxidation. Fatty acid uptake into the cell and translocation across the mitochondrial membrane are also key steps and carnitine is involved in this process, allowing fatty acids to enter the mitochondrion. Within the mitochondrion, carnitine also functions to regulate the acetyl-CoA concentration and the concentration of free CoA. It has been proposed that an increased availability of carnitine within the mitochondrion might allow the cell to maintain a higher free CoA concentration, resulting in a stimulatory effect on oxidative metabolism.

Because of the key role of carnitine in the oxidation of both fat and carbohydrate, it has been proposed that carnitine supplementation may improve exercise performance and also that it may help promote loss of body fat. On the basis of this logic, carnitine is widely sold in sports shops as a supplement for endurance athletes and for those seeking to lose weight. There is, however, no good evidence that carnitine deficiency occurs in the general population or in athletes. Carnitine is present in the diet in red meat and dairy products, so it might be thought that individuals who follow a vegan lifestyle might be at increased risk of deficiency, but it can also be synthesized from lysine and methionine in liver and kidney. Studies have failed to find clear evidence that carnitine supplementation enhances exercise performance. Surprisingly, only a few studies have examined the effect of carnitine on fat oxidation or on success in reducing body fat levels. However, studies of carnitine supplementation have failed to find evidence that it causes an increase in muscle carnitine levels; this would be a necessary starting point for expecting a change in muscle function in response to the supplementation.

It must be concluded from the studies published in the scientific literature that, although there is a theoretical basis for an ergogenic effect of carnitine on performance of both high-intensity and prolonged exercise, this is not supported by the experimental evidence. Supplementation of the diet with carnitine is unlikely to be beneficial for athletes.

Bicarbonate

In exercise that causes fatigue within a few minutes, anaerobic glycolysis makes a major contribution to energy metabolism. Although glycolysis allows higher rates of ATP resynthesis than can be achieved by aerobic metabolism, the capacity of the system is limited, and fatigue is inevitable when high rates of anaerobic glycolysis occur. The metabolic acidosis that accompanies glycolysis has been implicated in the fatigue process, either by inhibition of key glycolytic enzymes, by interfering with calcium transport and binding, or by a direct effect on the actin–myosin interaction. Because of these effects of acidosis on the muscle, it is intuitively attractive to believe that induction of alkalosis prior to exercise, an increase in the muscle buffering capacity, or an increased rate of efflux of hydrogen ions from the active muscles will all have the potential to delay fatigue and improve exercise performance.

Several investigators have reported a decrease in perceived exertion or an increase in performance during high-intensity exercise after bicarbonate administration. Others, however, have shown no benefit of an induced metabolic alkalosis on perceived exertion or performance. In one study designed to simulate athletic competition, trained non-elite (best 800 m time about 2 min 5 s) middle-distance runners were used as subjects and the exercise consisted of a simulated 800-m race: in the alkalotic condition, subjects ran almost 3 s faster than in the placebo or control trials. A more recent report has indicated similar improvements (3–4 s) over a distance of 1500 m in runners who completed simulated races in about 4 min 15 s. Although these effects on performance might seem small, they are of considerable significance to the athlete: an improvement of even a fraction of a second in these events is considered to be a major achievement. The reason for the conflicting effects reported in the published literature is not altogether clear, but some at least is probably due in part to variations in the intensity and duration of the exercise tests used, in the nature of the exercise task, in the dosage of sodium bicarbonate administered, and in the time delay between bicarbonate administration and the beginning of the exercise test (i.e. in the degree of metabolic alkalosis induced).

There are, of course, potential problems associated with the use of increased doses of bicarbonate. Vomiting and diarrhea are not infrequently reported as a result of ingestion of even relatively small doses of bicarbonate, and this may limit any attempt to improve athletic performance by this method, certainly among those individuals susceptible to gastrointestinal problems. There have been reports of athletes using this intervention, which is not prohibited by the rules of sport, being unable to compete because of the severity of these symptoms. Although unpleasant and to some extent debilitating, these effects are not serious and there are no long-term adverse consequences of occasional use. Sodium citrate administration, which also results in an alkaline shift in the extracellular fluid, has also been reported to improve peak power and total work output in a 60-s exercise test, but without any adverse gastrointestinal symptoms.

Where an increase in performance after bicarbonate ingestion has been observed, it has been ascribed to an increased rate of hydrogen ion efflux from the exercising muscles, reducing the rate of fall of intracellular pH, and relieving the pH-mediated inhibition of phosphofructokinase. The higher blood lactate levels after exercise associated with metabolic alkalosis, even when the exercise duration is the same, may therefore be indicative not only of a higher rate of lactate efflux, but also of an increased contribution of anaerobic glycolysis to energy production. There is also a loss of adenine nucleotides from muscle when the exercise intensity is very high, and this loss may be reduced by ingestion of bicarbonate before exercise. Whatever the mechanism, however, it seems reasonable to suggest that bicarbonate administration prior to high-intensity exercise will only enhance performance when the intensity and duration of the exercise are sufficient to result in significant muscle acidosis and adenine nucleotide loss.

Caffeine

Caffeine is a drug that, because of its longstanding and widespread use, is considered socially acceptable. Caffeine and the related compounds theophylline and theobromine are naturally occurring food components (Table 12.1). For many people, these substances are part of the normal daily diet and caffeine is probably the most widely used stimulant drug in the world. Caffeine is included among the list of prohibited (banned) stimulants in the Olympic Movement Anti-Doping Code (1 September 2001), with the comment that "the definition of a positive test is a concentration in urine greater than 12 µg/ml". This wording is ambiguous since it can be interpreted to mean that either:

1 caffeine intake is banned at all times, with the reporting level being 12 $\mu g \cdot ml^{-1}$; or
2 caffeine intake is permitted up to the level that causes a urinary concentration above 12 $\mu g \cdot ml^{-1}$.

Actions of caffeine

Caffeine achieves a complex array of effects within the body, including stimulation of the central nervous system, cardiac muscle and epinephrine release and activity. Caffeine has several effects on skeletal muscle involving calcium handling, sodium–potassium pump activity, elevation of cyclic AMP, and direct action on enzymes such as glycogen phosphorylase. Increased catecholamine action, and the direct effect of caffeine on cyclic AMP, may both act to increase lipolysis in adipose and muscle tissue, causing an increase in plasma free fatty acid concentrations and increased availability of intramuscular triglyceride.

It has been proposed that an increased potential for fat oxidation during moderate-intensity exercise promotes glycogen "sparing"; indeed the early studies of caffeine ingestion and endurance performance identified this as the most likely mechanism to explain the beneficial outcomes. However, more recent studies have provided considerable evidence that the ergogenic benefits of caffeine on exercise

Table 12.1 Caffeine content of various foodstuffs. Values for tea and coffee vary widely, depending on the source and the method of preparation.

Food or drink	Serving	Caffeine content (mg)
Instant coffee	250-ml cup	40–160
Brewed coffee	250-ml cup	40–200
Tea	250-ml cup	10–60
Hot chocolate	250-ml cup	5–10
Chocolate bar—milk	60 g	5–15
Chocolate bar—dark	60 g	10–50
Caffeinated chocolate bar (e.g. Viking bar)	60 g	58
Coca Cola	375-ml can	49
Pepsi Cola	375-ml can	40
Jolt soft drink	375-ml can	72
Energy drinks	250-ml can	50–80
Caffeinated sports gel	30–40-g sachet	20–25

performance are not limited to, or always explained by, the so-called "metabolic theory". Several studies have reported an enhancement of performance following caffeine intake in the absence of any change to substrate oxidation, or have found that glycogen sparing is limited to the first 15–20 min of exercise. Others have found individual variability in the metabolic response to caffeine: half of a group of subjects was shown to "spare" glycogen during the first 15 min of exercise following caffeine intake compared with a placebo treatment, while glycogen utilization was unaffected in the other half of the group following caffeine treatment.

Other popular explanations for performance enhancement with caffeine ingestion include effects on the central nervous system (CNS) or a direct effect of caffeine on skeletal muscle. Caffeine ingestion has been shown to elicit greater motor unit recruitment and alter neurotransmitter function in the muscle. It also affects the CNS in ways that cause it to override fatigue signals during exercise. Breakdown products of caffeine such as paraxanthine and theophylline may also have actions within the body. Caffeine supplementation is complex to investigate due to the difficulty in isolating individual effects of caffeine and the potential for variability between subjects.

Effects of caffeine on performance

There are a number of studies showing beneficial effects of caffeine ingestion in a variety of laboratory tests, and a smaller number showing improvements in field tests. Caffeine is unusual in that it appears to provide ergogenic effects across a range of exercise protocols, from shorter efforts of high-intensity exercise to prolonged submaximal exercise. Different mechanisms may be involved to explain the observed performance outcomes. Early studies focused on the effects of caffeine intake on the performance of endurance exercise protocols, with subjects ingesting caffeine doses of 6 mg·kg body mass^{-1}, 1 h before the start of exercise. An increased time to exhaustion was observed in a number of these studies, but performance in simulated race situations, where a fixed amount of work has to be done in the shortest possible time, is also improved.

More recent studies have focused on exercise of shorter duration, and a number of studies have shown beneficial effects on the performance of higher-intensity exercise lasting 4–6 min (e.g. track cycling events, 1500-m running) or 20–60 min (e.g. 1500-m swimming, 40-km cycling). There is little information on performance in sprint tasks, and what is reported is conflicting. There appears to be considerable individual variability in the response to caffeine, for reasons that are unclear, but, surprisingly, seem unrelated to habitual caffeine use.

Whereas the traditional protocol for caffeine ingestion was a 5–6 mg·kg^{-1} dose, consumed 1 h prior to the start of exercise, recent studies have shown performance benefits when caffeine is consumed throughout the exercise bout, or even just towards the end of the protocol. Furthermore, performance enhancement is seen with lower doses of caffeine (i.e. 1–3 mg·kg^{-1}). There does not seem to be a dose related effect of caffeine intake; when benefits are seen with a low dose, there are no further improvements with consumption of larger amounts of caffeine.

There is some variability in urinary caffeine excretion between individuals, but in general a caffeine intake of < 6 mg·kg^{-1} is unlikely to cause the urinary caffeine concentration to exceed 12 µg·ml^{-1}. Indeed, such concentrations are typically not reached until caffeine intakes reach 9 mg·kg^{-1} or more. It is therefore clear that positive effects of caffeine can be obtained in a variety of exercise situations with caffeine doses that are far below those necessary to produce a "reportable" sign of caffeine usage. Although some people feel that caffeine is technically a drug that enhances performance and is therefore against the ethics of sport, others feel that the widespread intake of caffeine-containing foods and drinks prevents a meaningful ban from being practical. It is also important for athletes to remember that caffeine is not tested for in out-of-competition samples. Clarification of the present status of caffeine in relation to doping is needed.

Other effects of caffeine

Caffeine has a number of unwanted side-effects that may limit its use in some sports or by sensitive individuals: these effects include insomnia, headache, gastrointestinal irritation and bleeding, and a stimu-lation of diuresis. There are also some suggestions that high levels of caffeine intake may be a risk factor for bladder cancer. This is unlikely to be modified by occasional use of modest doses prior to competition, but the athlete who may contemplate using high doses of caffeine prior to training on a daily basis should consider this. In the very high doses that were sometimes used by athletes, notice-able muscle tremor and impairment of coordina-tion have been noted.

The diuretic action of caffeine is often stressed, particularly in situations where dehydration is a major issue. This affects particularly competitions held in hot, humid climates where the risk of dehy-dration is high, and is more important for all athletes whose performance might be negatively affected by dehydration. Athletes competing in these conditions are advised to increase their intake of fluid, but are usually also advised to avoid tea and coffee because of their diuretic effect. It seems likely, however, that this effect is small for those habituated to caffeine use and the negative effects caused by the symptoms of caffeine withdrawal may be more damaging.

Protein and amino acid supplements

Chapter 3 provided a summary of protein metabol-ism and requirements for training and competition. This chapter concluded that protein supplements are expensive and are unnecessary for achieving an increase in muscle mass or strength. However, as we will discuss in the following section in this chapter on sports foods, products like liquid meal supple-ments, which provide a compact source of carbohy-drate, protein, and micronutrients, are often useful in helping athletes to meet their sports nutrition goals. Typical scenarios include meeting the high-energy needs involved in heavy training, a growth spurt, or a muscle hypertrophy program, or provid-ing a postexercise recovery meal which can simulta-neously promote a positive protein balance and glycogen restoration. In both situations a liquid meal supplement might provide a practical altern-ative or adjunct to everyday foods. The cost of this sports food is usually considerably less than high-protein, or all-protein supplements, but is typically

higher than that of normal foods. Nevertheless, this expense may be justified when convenience is an important issue in achieving nutrient intake goals.

Several individual amino acids, or amino acid groups, have been singled out for special attention in sports nutrition. During the 1980s, preparations of individual amino acids were the most success-fully marketed "designer" supplement, despite a lack of evidence that "free-form" preparations of amino acids were superior in digestion or absorp-tion to amino acids found in intact proteins (i.e. in everyday foods). Today it is possible to purchase a range of tablets or powders containing individual amino acids as the sole ingredients, as well as gen-eral sports supplements (sports drinks, liquid meal powders, bars) fortified with additional amino acids. Many of these specialized products provide amino acid intakes that can easily be consumed from everyday foods, but at highly elevated prices. There is currently no good evidence that amino acid supplements enhance sports performance. Special commentaries have been provided in this chapter to address the case for branched-chain amino acids (BCAAs) and glutamine.

Chromium picolinate

Chromium is an essential trace element that has a number of functions in the body, and it has been reported to potentiate the effects of insulin. Because of the anabolic effects of insulin, it might be expected that amino acid incorporation into muscle protein would be stimulated, enhancing the adaptive response to training. There is also some evidence to suggest an increased urinary chromium loss after exercise, further supporting the idea that athletes in training may have higher requirements than sedentary individuals. Chromium is widely used as a supplement by strength athletes, and is usually sold as a conjugate of picolinic acid: this form is reported to enhance chromium uptake.

Supplementation of the diet with chromium picolinate was reported to enhance the adaptive response to a strength training program, with an increase in lean body mass. No direct measures of muscle mass were made in this study, however, and the results must be viewed with caution. A number of subsequent studies, mostly using more appropriate methodology, have failed to reproduce these results, with no effect on lean tissue accretion or on muscle performance being seen. Nonetheless, chromium supplementation remains popular.

Coenzyme Q10

Coenzyme Q10, also known as ubiquinone, is a non-essential lipid-soluble nutrient found predominantly in animal foods and in low levels in plant foods. In the body it is located primarily in the mitochondria, especially in skeletal and cardiac muscle. One of its well-known functions is as a link in the electron transport chain within the mitochondria, thus playing a role in the final production of ATP. It is also believed to have an antioxidant function, mopping up free oxygen radicals in the mitochondrial antioxidant defense system and preventing damage to DNA and cell membranes. It has been suggested that some cardiac and neuromuscular dysfunction is due to coenzyme Q10 deficiency; indeed patients with ischemic heart disease have been shown to have lower plasma Q10 concentrations. Some studies have shown that these patients respond to coenzyme Q10 supplementation with increased exercise capacity. Coenzyme Q10 supplements have recently emerged as new products marketed in the general community to promote vigor. For athletes, they are claimed to enhance energy production through the electron transport chain, and to reduce the oxidative damage of exercise. However, a summary of studies which have examined the effects of coenzyme Q10 supplementation on exercise metabolism and performance and on oxidative damage caused by exercise, has failed to find convincing evidence of positive effects. In fact, there are a number of studies that show that coenzyme Q10 has an ergolytic (negative) effect on high-intensity performance and training adaptations. A series of studies undertaken at the Karolinska Institute in Sweden has produced consistent evidence that Q10 supplementation *increases* the oxidative damage and reduces the training re-sponse in previously untrained subjects who undertake a high-intensity exercise program. Clearly, further work is required to investigate the effects of coenzyme Q10 supplementation on exercise performance and training. However, at present there is little to recommend Q10 supplementation to athletes undertaking high-intensity training, and we are reminded that the issue of antioxidant supplementation is complex and as yet unsolved (see Chapter 4).

Beta-hydroxy beta-methyl butyrate (HMB)

Beta-hydroxy beta-methyl butyrate (HMB) is a metabolite of the amino acid leucine, and is currently one of the most popular dietary supplements. It is claimed to enhance gains in strength and body mass associated with resistance training, to enhance loss of body fat, and to enhance recovery from exercise. These effects are said to occur because of its role as an anticatabolic agent, minimizing protein breakdown and the cellular damage that occurs with high-intensity exercise. Leucine administration is known to influence protein metabolism, specifically to reduce protein degradation during periods of stress or trauma that are associated with elevated protein catabolism. It has been proposed that it is the increase in leucine metabolites such as HMB that mediates this effect. To date, only a few studies of HMB supplementation in humans have appeared in the peer-reviewed literature.

In one study involving healthy but untrained males, daily HMB supplementation was found to reduce urinary 3-methyl histidine excretion (a marker of muscle protein degradation) and plasma creatine kinase concentrations (a crude indicator of cellular damage) when a training program was undertaken. HMB supplementation was associated with a dose-responsive increase in weight lifted during training (particularly in lower body strength), and there was a trend for increased gain in lean body mass with the increase in HMB dose. A second investigation of HMB supplementation (3 mg·day^{-1}) and resistance training in previously trained subjects reported trends for greater increases in fat-free mass (assessed by total body electrical conductivity) in the HMB group and increases in muscle strength measurements that were greater for some (upper body) but not all (lower body) lifts.

Although these results support the possibility of benefits from HMB supplementation, there are several methodological concerns with these investigations such as the lack of dietary control and the failure to equally match groups for their baseline values.

It is possible to explain the increased gains in the HMB group as the outcome of lower initial levels and a greater potential for change with training. Two other studies of HMB supplementation in trained individuals have failed to find any difference in gains in body mass, strength, and markers of muscle damage when undertaking a matched training program. Therefore, until further studies of HMB supplementation are conducted and reported in full, it is impossible to make a decision on the potential of this supplement, particularly when it is used in well-trained subjects.

Other compounds

Athletes use a wide range of nutritional supplements in their quest for improved performance. Even a cursory inspection of sports shops and magazines reveals the scale and diversity of supplement use. Most of the exotic supplements make extravagant claims and are sold at inflated prices. The market, however, is largely unregulated and few of the claims made for these products are supported by any evidence; instead, they rely on endorsement by top athletes (who are paid handsomely for doing so) and on the gullibility of the consumer.

Sales figures for exotic supplements such as ginseng, inosine, colostrum, bee pollen, royal jelly, and pangamic acid, together with a wide range of vitamins and minerals (including boron, vanadium, zinc, magnesium, and manganese), demonstrate that many athletes remain convinced of their effectiveness. In spite of the limited and conflicting evidence, however, the balance of the available information suggests that there is no benefit from these substances for healthy individuals consuming a normal diet. Some supplements are potentially harmful in large doses and their use should be actively discouraged. Many studies that purport to show beneficial effects are poorly designed, often with inadequate subject numbers and no control group, and few are published in reputable journals. The power of the placebo effect is well recognized, and athletes seem to be particularly susceptible.

Athletes should consider several factors before deciding to use a supplement. The likely benefits should be considered carefully, and weighed against the cost of a supplement program and the risk of negative outcomes. Supplement use, even when it provides a performance advantage, is an expense that athletes must acknowledge and prioritize appropriately within their total budget.

The other disadvantages of supplement use include the potential for side-effects and the possibility of an inadvertent doping outcome. There has been much recent publicity about doping infringements by leading athletes involving alleged use of nandrolone (an anabolic steroid) that has been attributed to their inadvertent intake of prohormones from the use of dietary supplements. Although these prohormones (e.g. 19-norandrostenedione, DHEA, androstenedione, and others) are also banned by antidoping codes, they are often found in dietary supplements both as stated ingredients and as an undeclared ingredient or contaminant. Other supplements may contain banned stimulants including ephedrine and large amounts of caffeine. Antidoping education messages warn athletes to carefully read the labels of supplements and avoid using products that contain ingredients that are banned in sport. However, several recent reports from independent analyses of dietary supplements have found that a large percentage of products contain banned substances without declaring their presence on labels. Reports from the IOC accredited laboratories in Cologne and Vienna suggest that up to 25% of supplements may contain low levels of unlisted steroids. Therefore, the use of dietary supplements carries a small but real risk of causing high-level athletes who compete in competitions governed by anti-doping codes to infringe these rules. Strict liability means that the governing bodies of sport will not accept ignorance as a valid excuse in the case of the athlete who inadvertently consumes a prohibited substance. The cost may be a ban from sport, and the loss of money and prestige.

Sports foods

Sports nutrition is a practice as much as it is a science, and many sports nutrition experts have commented that athletes fail to make appropriate food choices and eating plans. Sometimes this is due to a lack of nutrition knowledge that prevents the athlete from achieving their nutrient intake targets. At other times it can be due to practical reasons that make it difficult to obtain or consume normal foods in an exercise-related situation. Special food products targeted for use by athletes or people undertaking sports and exercise activities may provide a useful niche market for the food industry as well as a benefit for this specialized audience. In some countries there are special provisions for sports foods within their food standards codes, which provide guidelines for products of this type.

Characteristics of potential sports foods

Specialized products targeted at the exercising population might have one or more characteristics that would make them suitable for an athlete with special nutritional needs. Some characteristics may relate to helping the athlete achieve a certain nutrient intake goal—for example, the sports food may deliver a precise "dose" of nutrients for a specialized situation in sports nutrition, or provide a good source of nutrients that are "at risk" in the diets of athletes or subgroups of athletes. Sometimes the packaging or information supporting the sports food may be important in communicating an education message related to sports nutrition goals, or making the athlete take a professional and organized approach to their nutrition. At other times, practical aspects of the sports food make it easy for the athlete to take or consume in a sporting setting: for example, the product may have simple preparation or storage needs, low perishability, good portability, and convenient packaging. It may be easily consumed and provide a more compact source of nutrients compared to everyday foods. Or, finally, it may contain special ergogenic compounds claimed to enhance sports performance.

It is apparent from the array of new sports foods that hit the market, that this last characteristic—the inclusion of special ingredients claimed to enhance sports performance—is becoming the most tempting issue to sports foods manufacturers.

Notwithstanding the lucrative potential from producing and marketing products that sound alluring to athletes, it is important to consider the real need, and indeed the ethics, for such a line of sports foods. In this chapter we have already seen that few of these purported ergogenic substances have evidence to support the claims made about their amazing benefits. Expert Comment 1 in this chapter explains that some companies are prepared to try for quick profits on hot compounds regardless of their lack of true efficacy, while other companies take a more long-term and responsible view with regard to developing and marketing products.

The major categories of sports foods that are genuinely useful to athletes are presented in Table 12.2, along with a summary of the typical composition of these products, and the special goals of sports nutrition that they address. The best products in each category are those that provide detailed and specific information about their intended use, and support/provide additional education about optimal sports nutrition practices. Often the manufacturers of these products make substantial contributions to exercise science research or education activities, building an environment of credibility for the company and the products. Although most of these products have specialized uses in sport, some have crossed successfully into the general population market (e.g. sports drinks). It should be remembered that the need for these products relates to the existence of a physiological requirement or challenge, rather than the caliber or talent of the person who is involved. In other words, replacement of fluid and carbohydrate during exercise is as much a priority for a weekend warrior or recreational athlete who wants to perform at their best as it is for an elite or professional sportsperson. In fact, most of the investigations of the special needs of sport or the effects of nutritional strategies on the performance of exercise have been undertaken on recreational to well-trained individuals, rather than world-class performers. Therefore we can be confident that products such as sports drinks are of benefit to the

Table 12.2 Sports foods and their uses by athletes (adapted from Burke *et al.* 2000).

Supplement	Form	Composition	Sports-related use
Sports drink	Powder or Liquid	5–7% carbohydrate 10–25 mmol·l⁻¹ sodium	Optimum delivery of fluid and carbohydrate during exercise Postexercise rehydration Postexercise refueling
Sports gel	Gel 30–40-g sachets or larger tubes	60–70% carbohydrate (~ 25 g per sachet) Some contain medium-chain triglycerides or caffeine	Supplement high-carbohydrate training diet Carbohydrate loading Postexercise recovery—provides carbohydrate Carbohydrate source during exercise, especially when carbohydrate needs exceed fluid requirements
High-CHO supplement	Powder or Liquid	10–25% carbohydrate (+ some B vitamins)	Supplement high-CHO training diet Carbohydrate loading Postexercise CHO recovery—provides carbohydrate May be used during exercise when carbohydrate needs exceed fluid requirements
Liquid meal supplement	Powder (mix with water or milk) or Liquid	1–1.5 kcal·ml⁻¹ 15–20% protein 50–70% carbohydrate Low–moderate fat Vitamins/minerals: 500–1000 ml supplies RDIs	Supplement high-energy/carbohydrate/nutrient diet (especially during heavy training/competition or weight gain) Low-bulk meal replacement (especially pre-event meal) Postexercise recovery—provides carbohydrate, protein and micronutrients Portable nutrition for traveling athlete
Sports bar	Bar (50–60 g)	40–50 g carbohydrate 5–10 g protein Usually low in fat Vitamins/minerals: often contain 50–100% of RDIs May contain specialized ingredients such as creatine, amino acids	Carbohydrate source during exercise Postexercise recovery—provides carbohydrate, protein, and micronutrients Supplement high energy/carbohydrate/nutrient diet Portable nutrition for the traveling athlete

performance and enjoyment of sport by its much larger population of non-elite participants.

Summary

Athletes are forever searching for nutritional supplements that will give them a significant advantage over their competitors. This accounts in part for the reports of widespread use of illegal drugs in sport. The difficulty lies in finding something that is effective in improving performance but is not against the rules. It is also important that any chemical substance to be used in this way should not have harmful side-effects. All essential dietary components, including protein, essential fatty acids, vitamins, and minerals, might be considered to come into the category of ergogenic aids, since they indirectly assist performance by maintaining normal health and physiological function. However, supplementation above the level required for maintenance of health is not likely to improve exercise performance. While research supports direct benefits from compounds such as creatine, bicarbonate, and caffeine, the majority of the compounds and products targeted to athletes have not been shown to provide performance enhancements. A promise of instant and dramatic results is alluring to all athletes, regardless of their level of achievement, and the supplement industry that provides these ingredients in pills and powder (non-food form) is a multibillion dollar concern. Many athletes do not understand that the claims made for many supplements and their individual ingredients result from lack of regulation rather than the results of rigorous research. As a result, athletes can be drawn to products that are insubstantial and faddish rather than strategies that provide a worthwhile and lasting contribution to sports performance.

Sports foods that address real nutritional needs of athletes can provide a valuable, although often more expensive, way for the athlete to meet their sports nutrition goals. The most obvious examples of valuable sports foods are liquid meal supplements and sports drinks. However, if the manufacture of these products becomes driven by the inclusion of unsupported "ergogenic" compounds rather than addressing true goals of sports nutrition, there is a risk that these products will become of less value to the athlete. The use of all sports foods and supplements needs to be balanced against expense, the risk of side-effects from some ingredients, and the possibility of an inadvertent doping outcome.

Reading list

American College of Sports Medicine. (2000) Roundtable: The physiological and health effects of oral creatine supplementation. *Medicine and Science in Sports and Exercise* **32**, 706–717.

Burke, L.M. & Hawley, J.A. Short-term fat adaptation and metabolism and performance of prolonged exercise. *Medicine and Science in Sports and Exercise* (in press).

Burke, L., Desbrow, B. & Minehan, M. (2000) Dietary supplements and nutritional ergogenic aids in sport. In: *Clinical Sports Nutrition* (eds L. Burke & V. Deakin), pp. 455–553. McGraw-Hill, Sydney, Australia.

Graham, T.E. (2001) Caffeine and exercise: metabolism, endurance and performance. *Sports Medicine* **31**, 765–807.

Greenhaff, P.L. (2000) Creatine. In: *Nutrition in Sport* (ed. R.J. Maughan), pp. 367–378. Blackwell Science, Oxford.

McNaughton, L.R. (2000) Bicarbonate and citrate. In: *Nutrition in Sport* (ed. R.J. Maughan), pp. 393–404. Blackwell Science, Oxford.

Slater, G.J. & Jenkins, D. (2000) B-hydroxy B-methylbutyrate (HMB) supplementation and the promotion of muscle growth and strength. *Sports Medicine* **30**, 105–116.

Spriet, L.L. & Howlett, R.A. (2000) Caffeine. In: *Nutrition in Sport* (ed. R.J. Maughan), pp. 379–392. Blackwell Science, Oxford.

Wagenmakers, A.J.M. (2000) Amino acid metabolism in exercise. In: *Nutrition in Sport* (ed. R.J. Maughan), pp. 119–132. Blackwell Science, Oxford.

Williams, M.H. & Leutholtz, B.C. (2000) Nutritional ergogenic aids. In: *Nutrition in Sport* (ed. R.J. Maughan), pp. 356–366. Blackwell Science, Oxford.

EXPERT COMMENT 1 Commercial issues in producing products for athletes. Robert Murray

Nutrition plays a critical role in sustaining the large training volumes and high training intensities required of competitive athletes, and in helping stimulate rapid and complete recovery. Athletes generally have a difficult time selecting and consuming a well-balanced diet with adequate energy content, so there is certainly a justification for efficacious sports nutrition products.

Sports nutrition products represent a large market for manufacturers. In 1999, sales of sports nutrition products in the US topped $5 billion. Sports drinks constituted about 40% of those sales, with energy bars at 22%, and the remainder split among weight gain products, "fat burners", protein and amino acid supplements, and a variety of other products. The sports nutrition industry is characterized by a constant flux of companies entering and leaving the marketplace. Very few manufacturers have more than 5 years' tenure, a reflection not only of the competitive nature of the category but also of the difficulty of formulating and producing good-tasting, nutritious, affordable products with proven benefits.

Nonetheless, there is a plethora of sports nutrition products from which to choose, each accompanied by one or more tantalizing claims about product benefits. When it comes to benefits, separating fact from fiction is a daunting task even for scientists, and near impossible for consumers. A primary challenge for manufacturers is to overcome that hurdle by developing a strong base of consumer belief and trust in the efficacy of their products. Supporting and communicating the research behind the products is a key component of developing consumer loyalty, but many sports nutrition companies have neither the finances nor the corporate commitment to do so, relying instead on cobbled-together support from the scientific literature or, all too frequently, no support at all.

Formulating an efficacious, nutritious, and good-tasting sports nutrition product requires an in-depth understanding of the demands of sport and of the physiological and metabolic responses to nutrient ingestion before, during, and after exercise, and comprehensive knowledge of the interactions among the physicochemical properties of the product, its package, the process by which the product is made, storage conditions, and shelf-life considerations. As a rule of thumb, well-established companies produce products that have high quality control in terms of their composition and safety; such companies have too much to lose to tolerate sloppy manufacturing processes. Unfortunately, small start-up companies, looking to establish a quick profit margin, often do not follow the highest manufacturing and quality control standards. As a result, ingredient levels may not conform to label declarations and bioactive contaminants may be found in the products. Well-documented examples can be found for sports nutrition products that are grossly mislabeled or contain contaminants that produce positive results for banned substances.

EXPERT COMMENT 2 Can athletes improve their performance by fat loading? John A. Hawley

The consumption of a high-fat (> 60% of energy), low-carbohydrate (< 15% of energy) diet for 1–3 days significantly reduces resting muscle glycogen content, and is typically associated with impaired exercise tolerance at submaximal intensities. Longer periods of exposure to high-fat diets appear to induce adaptive responses that increase fat oxidation during exercise and largely compensate for the low muscle glycogen stores. While popular diet books and supplement programs suggest that such "fat loading" strategies will enhance the performance of endurance and ultraendurance athletes by making them better able to "tap into body fat stores", in fact, the few studies of this practice in well-trained athletes show that at best it maintains, rather than enhances, exercise capacity and performance. There is also evidence that long-term periods of high-fat diets (> 4 weeks) might interfere with training adaptations. However, recent studies also show that the adaptations to a high-fat diet can be achieved in well-trained subjects in as little as 5 days.

A variation on the theme of "fat loading" is for the athlete to train most of the year on a high-carbohydrate diet, adapt to a high-fat diet for several days prior to a major event, then carbohydrate load in the final 1–2 days immediately prior to competition. Such "nutritional periodization" would permit the greatest training impulse (volume × intensity × frequency) throughout the year, maximize muscle carbohydrate stores before competition, and optimize the capacity for fat oxidation during an endurance or ultraendurance race. Furthermore, a short (3–5-day) period of exposure to a high-fat diet represents a more practical period for extreme dietary change while minimizing any potential health risks.

We have recently undertaken several studies to test this model on endurance (2–3 h) and ultraendurance (5 h) exercise protocols. In each study, well-trained athletes consumed a high-fat, low-carbohydrate diet for 5 days while undertaking high-volume intense training, followed by 1 day of high carbohydrate eating and rest. In some studies, additional carbohydrate was eaten before the event and during the exercise in keeping with sports nutrition guidelines. Compared to the control treatment (high-carbohydrate diet throughout), the fat loading, carbohydrate restoration treatment increased the rate of fat oxidation and spared muscle glycogen during submaximal, constant-load cycling. In the endurance cycling protocols, despite muscle glycogen sparing, there was no improvement to a 30-min time trial undertaken at the completion of the 2-h ride. We interpreted the lack of a clear benefit to performance after fat adaptation in these investigations to mean that increased fat oxidation is of little advantage to exercise capacity if the work bout is of insufficient duration to deplete muscle glycogen stores. However, even in our ultraendurance study where a 60-min time trial was undertaken after 4 h of steady-state cycling, there was no clear-cut performance advantage following our dietary periodization strategy. It is possible that fat adaptation strategies only confer performance advantages for "responders". Further work is needed to clarify this and identify markers of those who are likely to respond.

A number of extreme diets (e.g. the Zone diet or 40/30/30 diet) have been recommended by zealous best-selling authors for optimal athletic performance. Such diets are low in total energy and restrict carbohydrate intake to levels that could never sustain prolonged, intense athletic training. The rationale for such low energy and in particular, low carbohydrate intake in the Zone diet is the belief that such a nutritional profile will promote fat oxidation during exercise. However, there are no scientific studies that have used these specific dietary recommendations to support such claims. Finally, the Zone diet is very similar to diets utilized in two well-controlled studies that reported impaired endurance capacity when subjects consumed a carbohydrate-restricted diet. A study comparing the use of Zone (40/30/30) bars during exercise to the consumption of a sports drink, found that the sports drink was more effective in assisting performance of an ultraendurance cycling protocol.

In summary, there is still no clear evidence to support the use of fat loading strategies or high-fat carbohydrate-restricted diets. Even if fat adaptation strategies can be shown to enhance exercise performance, it is likely that they are of benefit to a small group of highly trained endurance or ultraendurance athletes. Even if such a dietary regimen was shown to enhance performance, high-fat diets are associated with increased risk of a number of diseases, and although regular physical activity attenuates these risks, individuals should limit their long-term exposure to high-fat diets.

EXPERT COMMENT 3 Does BCAA supplementation enhance endurance performance? Anton J.M. Wagenmakers

Clear evidence has been presented that the main sources of fatigue in endurance exercise can be attributed to events which lead to a loss of contractility in the muscle. However, the point in time at which the athlete has to reduce running speed during a marathon or decides to give up competition for the gold medal is also influenced by central factors, such as motivation, mood, and stamina. In 1986, Dr Eric Newsholme launched a novel hypothesis about a mechanism that links changes in blood metabolites to these central factors. During prolonged exercise there is a marked increase in the blood free fatty acid (FFA) concentration. FFAs and the amino acid tryptophan both bind to albumin, a protein carrier in the blood, competing for the same binding sites. As a consequence tryptophan is displaced from binding to albumin by the increasing FFAs and, therefore, the free (unbound) tryptophan concentration in the blood rises. During prolonged exercise there also is a decrease in blood branched-chain amino acids (BCAAs) due to increases in BCAA oxidation in skeletal muscle. As a consequence there is a marked increase in the free tryptophan : BCAA ratio in the blood. The increase in this ratio will lead to increased tryptophan transport across the blood–brain barrier, as BCAA and tryptophan compete for carrier-mediated entry into the central nervous system by the large neutral amino acid transporter. Once taken up in the brain, conversion of tryptophan to serotonin will occur and lead to a local increase of this neurotransmitter. The increase in serotoninergic activity subsequently will lead to the development of "central fatigue" and the need to reduce the intensity of exercise, e.g. running speed. One of the implications of this hypothesis is that the ingestion of BCAAs should reduce brain tryptophan uptake and would improve performance.

The effect of oral BCAA ingestion on endurance performance has been investigated in many studies using several exercise and treatment designs. Only a few studies have compared the ingestion of a solution containing BCAAs in comparison with a flavored water placebo. Some of these studies, but not all, reported a positive effect on endurance performance in line with the above hypothesis. However, the most important established nutritional intervention to improve endurance performance is the ingestion of carbohydrate solutions. Therefore, to be applicable as an ergogenic supplement in endurance sports, BCAAs should have an additional benefit when added to carbohydrate solutions. Such comparisons have been made in many studies over the last 10 years, and in none of these studies was an additional benefit of the BCAAs observed.

Another implication of the "central fatigue" hypothesis is that the ingestion of tryptophan during exercise should reduce time to exhaustion. This hypothesis has also been tested in several studies and even when high doses were used, massively increasing the blood tryptophan : BCAA ratio, there was no effect on performance. Together these performance studies lead to the following conclusions: either the manipulation of the tryptophan supply to the brain by the ingestion of BCAAs or tryptophan in drinks containing carbohydrates does not change serotoninergic activity in the brain; or a change in serotoninergic activity during prolonged exercise contributes little to the development of fatigue.

The role of serotonin in fatigue development has not been underpinned with hard evidence. In neurobiology it has been established that serotonin has a role in the onset of sleep and is a determinant of mood and aggression. Evidence has been presented in rats only that there are local increases in serotonin concentration during exercise; however, this does not prove its role in fatigue development. Furthermore, exercise is associated with changes in the concentration of other neurotransmitters and metabolites, which could also have an impact on performance. The best evidence that local accumulation of serotonin may play a role in fatigue development comes from human studies using drugs that are known to influence serotonin metabolism. The use, for instance, of serotonin reuptake inhibitors has been shown to cause premature fatigue in several laboratories. However, it is well known that these drugs are not specific, so further evidence is required.

In summary, the hypothesis of Dr Newsholme is attractive and has initiated innovative research into the molecular basis of central fatigue and its contribution to endurance performance. However, the "central fatigue hypothesis" does not seem to have practical consequences for athletes during competition as the addition of BCAAs to carbohydrate supplements provides no additional benefit over ingestion of carbohydrate alone.

EXPERT COMMENT 4 Does glutamine supplementation promote recovery and immune function? Anton J.M. Wagenmakers

Glutamine is the main end-product of muscle amino acid metabolism, both in the overnight fasted state and during feeding. It is the most rapidly synthesized amino acid in the human body, and is the most abundant amino acid both in human plasma and in the muscle free amino acid pool. Glutamine produced by the muscle, among other sources, supplies glutamine to immune system cells and to the mucosal cells of the intestine. In both cell types, glutamine is an important fuel and the presence of glutamine is also needed to maintain high rates of cell division. Low muscle and plasma glutamine concentrations are observed in patients with sepsis, trauma, and burns. These conditions are also attended by mucosal atrophy, loss of the gut barrier function (bacterial translocation), a rapid net breakdown of muscle proteins, and a weakened immune response. It has been hypothesized that a reduced glutamine concentration is a cause of these functional losses. A limited number of clinical studies have reported that glutamine supplementation in these conditions may lead to small but significant improvements in nitrogen balance, and in markers of gut function and immune function. The rationale for using glutamine in clinical nutrition has been extrapolated to exercise and has led to the use of glutamine in sports nutrition.

Claims are made in the popular sport nutrition literature that oral supplementation with glutamine in the period following exercise would: (i) prevent the downregulation of the immune system following intense exercise; (ii) improve the balance between protein synthesis and protein degradation; and (iii) increase muscle glycogen resynthesis.

During exercise plasma glutamine concentrations may increase, decrease, or remain unchanged depending on the type, duration, and intensity of exercise. However, reductions of 10–50% in plasma glutamine concentration are generally seen for a period of several hours following demanding endurance exercise. In the same period there is a decline in the number of circulating lymphocytes, and in several markers of immune system activity measured in cells isolated from the blood. Suggestions have been made in the literature that the temporary decrease in glutamine is the cause of this downregulation of the immune system and that it creates an "open window" which makes athletes more susceptible to catching a common cold or infection.

However, subsequent glutamine supplementation studies have shown convincingly that normalization of the plasma glutamine concentrations following exercise has no effect on the decline in the number of circulating lymphocytes and on the indicated markers of immune system activity. Although there are some claims that glutamine supplementation decreased infection rates in athletic populations following intense exercise, such findings are not based on objective biological measurements, but on questionnaires that among others included enquiries on the presence of a sore throat. This cannot be regarded as hard scientific evidence. At the present time, the available data imply that the link between glutamine metabolism and the immune system in athletes is not nearly as strong as in critically ill or burn patients.

In vitro studies with incubated and perfused rat muscles have shown that addition of glutamine to the medium increases muscle protein synthesis and reduces protein degradation. This effect is not unique for glutamine. Other individual amino acids and balanced amino acid mixtures are at least as effective. The *in vitro* effect of glutamine has not been shown to exist in healthy human beings *in vivo* and has not been investigated in the postexercise situation.

Only one study reported that intravenous infusion of glutamine increased glycogen resynthesis rates in humans in comparison with a saline control. However, glycogen resynthesis was measured in the absence of ingested glucose and, therefore, at rates that were only about 20% of maximal. The primary stimulus of the glycogen resynthesis rate following exercise is the rate of carbohydrate ingestion. Several studies in the meantime have shown that addition of glutamine (10–60 g) to carbohydrate supplements ingested orally has no benefit on glycogen resynthesis over ingestion of carbohydrate alone.

In summary, the scientific evidence that postexercise supplementation with glutamine promotes recovery and supports the immune function of athletes is weak and circumstantial.

Chapter 13
Practical strategies to meet nutrition goals

Introduction

The previous chapters in this book have summarized the principles of sports nutrition, emphasizing the importance of underpinning these goals with rigorous science. Despite the apparent sophistication of the knowledge available to guide athletes towards sensible food choices, the evidence from studies of the dietary practices of sportspeople and from the observations of sports nutritionists is that many athletes follow nutrition practices that may prevent them from reaching their goal of optimal performance. Many factors contribute to the unsound nutrition practices of some athletes. These include a reliance on myths and misconceptions rather than expert advice, and a lack of practical nutrition knowledge and skills (e.g. knowledge of food composition; domestic skills such as food purchasing, preparation, and cooking). Many athletes face an overcommitted lifestyle, with inadequate time and opportunities to obtain or consume appropriate foods due to the heavy workload of sport, work, school, and family. There are also the challenges of inadequate finances for up and coming athletes, and the disruption of frequent travel.

This chapter will provide strategies to help athletes achieve their sports nutrition goals. Each section will explore the typical food choices and eating patterns, or manipulations of common dietary practices, which help the athlete address a specific issue or challenge in sports nutrition. It is important to be able to integrate several goals in choosing meals and

snacks, so there will be some overlap between the strategies that are useful for each goal. It is, however, impossible to cover the myriad food uses, cultural eating patterns, or individual food likes and dislikes of all athletes, or their individual nutritional needs. These specific issues are best addressed by consulting a sports dietitian or nutrition expert for individual advice. Nevertheless, there are a number of ideas that may be useful for all athletes.

Strategies to ensure that goals for carbohydrate intake are met

• The athlete should be aware that the typical eating patterns in most countries or regions are not likely to achieve a high-carbohydrate diet. To achieve the fuel needs of their training and competition, athletes may need to try new foods or to change the ratio of foods at meals to promote carbohydrate-rich sources while reducing the intake of other foods.
• Meals and snacks should be based around nutrient-dense carbohydrate-rich foods, with ideas for low-fat choices helping to promote fuel intake rather than a high fat intake. The following foods should take up at least half of the room on the plate or meal plan:
  • wholegrain breads and breakfast cereals;
  • rice, pasta, noodles, and other grain foods;
  • fresh fruit, juices, dried fruit, stewed or canned fruit;
  • starchy vegetables, e.g. potatoes, corn, kumera;

Table 13.1 Ideas for pre-event meal—high-carbohydrate, low-fat eating.

1 Breakfast cereal* with milk or yoghurt.
2 Cereal bars or breakfast bars with juice or sports drink.
3 Pancakes with syrup.
4 Toast* or English muffins* with jam.
5 Crumpets* with honey.
6 Rice cakes or bread rolls* with sliced banana.
7 Fresh fruit or fruit salad.
8 Pasta* with tomato-based or other low-fat sauces.
9 Steamed rice* or noodles* with low-fat sauce.
10 Baked potato with low-fat sauce or filling.
11 Toast* with canned spaghetti or baked beans.
12 Fruit smoothie made with milk, yoghurt, and fruit.
13 Creamed rice or rice cream.
14 Commercial liquid meal supplement.
15 Sports bars.

*For low-fiber meals choose "white" types of cereal food.

• legumes (lentils, beans, soy-based products); and
• sweetened dairy products (e.g. fruit-flavored yoghurt, milkshakes, fruit smoothies).
• Sugar and sugary foods (e.g. jam, honey, confectionery, syrups) should be considered as a compact carbohydrate source. These may be particularly useful in a high-energy diet, or when carbohydrate is needed before, during, and after exercise.
• Carbohydrate-rich drinks (e.g. fruit juices, soft drinks, fruit/milk smoothies) also provide a compact fuel source for special situations or diets very high in carbohydrate. This category includes many of the supplements specially made for athletes, e.g. sports drinks, sports gels, and liquid meal supplements.
• When energy and carbohydrate needs are high, athletes should increase the number of meals and snacks they eat, rather than the size of meals. This will mean being organized to have snacks on hand in a busy day.
• Lower fiber choices of carbohydrate-rich foods are useful when energy needs are high, or for pre-event meals.
• Carbohydrate consumed before, during, and after workouts and competition adds to the day's fuel intake, as well as addressing the acute needs of the exercise session. Tables 13.1 and 13.2 provide ideas for pre-event and postevent eating.

• Information for planning or assessing carbohydrate intake can be found in ready-reckoners of carbohydrate-rich foods or from nutrient information on food labels. This information can help the athlete keep track when carbohydrate needs are very high.

Strategies to promote adequate intake of protein, vitamins, and minerals

• Athletes should be prepared to try new foods and new recipes to keep expanding their dietary range. Including a variety of foods in the day-to-day menu greatly reduces the risk of an inadequate intake of any individual micronutrient. Explore all the varieties of foods within a group and experiment with different food forms. It is good to take advantage of foods that are in season to introduce variety into menus.
• The athlete should avoid popular diets that advise against "food combining", since these are unsound. Meals are usually improved nutritionally, and enhanced in flavor and appeal, when a number of ingredients or foods are integrated into the menu. This can be done by adding individual food items together on the plate, or by cooking recipes that already involve a mixture (e.g. stir-fries, casseroles, main meal salads).
• Most foods provide some nutrient value, even if some features are not in line with other dietary principles. Banishing a food or food group from the diet can lead to the loss of important nutrients and to dietary boredom. There are often ways to reduce or modify the intake of particular food items rather than discarding the food totally. A sports dietitian can help an athlete to explore and maximize food variety—especially when there are sound reasons for restricting food choices (e.g. food allergies or intolerances, moral or religious sanctions).
• Meals will generally be well chosen if they follow the principle of "mixing and matching" so that protein-rich foods and fruits/vegetables are added to a high-carbohydrate base. It is useful to spread protein intake over the day rather than concentrate intake to one meal each day. Obvious protein-rich foods include meats, fish, eggs, and dairy foods, but

Table 13.2 Ideas for carbohydrate-rich recovery snacks.

The following foods and drinks provide 75 g carbohydrate:

    1000–1200 ml sports drink
    two sports gels + 250–300 ml sports drink
    750 ml fruit juice or soft drink
    300–500 ml carbohydrate loader drink
    one Mars bar or chocolate bar (65 g) + 375 ml soft drink
    100–120-g packet of jelly confectionery
    three slices toast or bread with jam or honey + large banana
    three cereal bars or breakfast bars
    cup of thick vegetable soup + large bread roll + one apple
    ~ 1.5 sports bars (60 g per bar)
    100 g (one large or two small) American muffin, fruit bun or scones + 400 ml fruit juice
    375-g can creamed rice + piece of fruit
    250-g (large) baked potato with salsa filling + 250 ml soft drink
    150 g pancakes (stack of two or three) + 50 g syrup.

Postexercise carbohydrate-rich recovery snacks
The following foods and drinks provide 75 g carbohydrate, and a valuable source of protein (> 10 g) and micronutrients:

    350–500 ml liquid meal supplement
    350–500 ml milkshake or fruit smoothie
    1.5 sports bars (60-g bar)
    80 g (large bowl) breakfast cereal with milk + 200-g carton fruit-flavored yoghurt
    350 g baked beans on three slices of toast
    large bread roll with cheese/meat filling, plus large banana
    2 cups of fruit salad with 300 g fruit-flavored yoghurt or frozen yoghurt
    two crumpets or English muffins with thick spread of peanut butter + 300 ml flavored milk
    250-g (large) baked potato + cottage/grated cheese filling + two granola bars
    300 g (half medium) thick crust pizza with chicken/meat and vegetables.

grains, nuts, and seeds also add valuable amounts of protein to mixed meals.

• Since the heme form of iron found in many animal foods (e.g. red meats, shellfish, liver) is readily absorbed, it should be included regularly in meals —at least three to five times per week. These foods can be added as a partner to a high-carbohydrate meal (e.g. meat sauce on a pasta dish, liver pâté in a sandwich).

• The absorption of non-heme iron (found in wholegrains, cereal foods, eggs, leafy green vegetables, etc.) is increased by including a vitamin C food at the same meal (e.g. a glass of orange juice consumed with breakfast cereal). The absorption is also enhanced by combining with a "meat" food (e.g. legumes and meat in a chilli con carne).

• Athletes who are at high risk of iron deficiency should be aware that some food factors (e.g. excess bran, strongly brewed tea) interfere with iron absorption from non-heme iron foods. These items should be avoided, or separated from meals.

• Iron supplements should be taken only on the advice of a sports dietitian or doctor. They may be useful in the supervised treatment and prevention of iron deficiency, but do not replace a holistic assessment and treatment that includes integrated dietary advice.

• Calcium requirements are easy to meet if the athlete's eating patterns include at least three servings of dairy foods or a calcium-fortified soy equivalent each day (one serving is equal to a glass of milk or a carton of yoghurt). Low-fat and reduced-fat dairy products are available, as well as an increasing range of soy products.

• Calcium requirements are increased in young athletes undergoing a growth spurt, and in females who are pregnant or breastfeeding. These athletes should increase their intake of dairy products to four or five servings a day. Female athletes who have irregular menstrual periods also require extra calcium and should seek expert advice from a sports doctor.

• Fish eaten with its bones (e.g. tinned salmon, sardines) is a useful calcium source.

• Athletes who are vegetarian or are unable to eat dairy products and red meat in the recommended amounts should seek the advice of a sports dietitian. Creative ways can be found to include other foods or food uses to meet iron and calcium needs, or to use mineral supplements correctly.

Strategies for achieving safe and effective loss of body fat

• The athlete should seek expert advice to identify an "ideal" body fat/body weight target, which is consistent with long-term health and performance and allows them to eat well and enjoy food.

• If loss of body fat is required, a realistic rate of loss should be set (e.g. 0.5–1.0 kg per week), including both short-term and long-term goals. The best time for weight loss is during the off season or early preseason, so that energy restriction does not interfere with competition or adaptation to key training periods.

• The athlete and coach should assess energy expenditure from training and lifestyle. Although athletes are usually perceived to have high energy needs, this is not necessarily the case. Many athletes in skill-based sports spend long hours at training that has a low energy cost. Other athletes are virtually inactive outside their training program. Changes to training patterns or supplementary training may be necessary to increase energy expenditure so that it can contribute to the fat loss program. Lifestyle changes such as walking and taking the stairs rather than driving the car and using the elevator may also play a role in increasing energy expenditure.

• It is important for the athlete to have an understanding of the eating patterns that have contributed to their current physique. This can be achieved by keeping a food record for a defined period (e.g. a week). Many athletes who feel that they "hardly eat anything" will be amazed at their unrecognized eating habits and food intake opportunities.

• A moderate energy restriction of 2–4 MJ·day^{-1} (500–1000 kcal·day^{-1}) is usually able to produce a reasonable loss of body fat but still ensure adequate food and nutrient intake. An athlete should not attempt severe energy restriction without expert advice or supervision. Generally, energy intake should remain above 5–6 MJ·day^{-1} (1200–1500 kcal·day^{-1}), regardless of circumstances, and above 6–8 MJ·day^{-1} (1500–2000 kcal·day^{-1}) during intensive training or competition.

• The meal plan for weight loss should not rely on skipping meals or enduring long periods without food intake. Rather, food intake should be spread over the day to allow for efficient refueling before and after training sessions and to avoid hunger (which generally precipitates overeating).

• Reducing intake of fat and oil is an effective way to reduce energy intake and decrease the energy density of meals. Strategies include choosing low-fat and lean versions of protein foods, minimizing added fats and oils in cooking and food preparation, and enjoying high-fat snack and sweet foods as occasional treats rather than everyday foods.

• Although low-fat eating is an aid to reducing energy intake, it is not a foolproof strategy. Low fat is not synonymous with low energy, and many athletes fail in their attempts to lose weight if they simply replace high-fat energy-dense foods with large amounts of sugar-rich or carbohydrate-rich energy-dense foods (e.g. jumbo-size low-fat muffins, economy-size bags of 97% fat-free pretzels, and giant bags of jelly-type confectionery).

• Portion control is an important strategy in achieving weight loss. Many athletes will benefit by reducing their typical serving sizes at meals, or by avoiding situations where they overeat. It may not be necessary to consume the portions that are typically served at meals.

• Meals and snacks can be made more "filling" by several strategies: Low glycemic index carbohydrate choices (oatmeal, legumes, *al dente* pasta, etc.) are considered to have a higher satiety value than high glycemic index choices (cornflakes, potatoes, etc.). Protein should be combined with carbohydrate-rich meals and snacks to produce greater satiety than carbohydrate-rich foods alone.

• Fruits, vegetables, and salads have a low energy density and are rich in fiber and micronutrients. Basing meals and recipes around fruits and vegetables is a great way to maintain or even increase the volume of food eaten while moderating energy intake.

• The athlete should be aware of the potential for excessive consumption of energy via the intake of energy-containing fluids (juices, sports drinks, soft drinks). Although there are occasions when it is useful to consume a compact energy source (e.g. during exercise), it is generally more satisfying to consume energy from solid foods.

• The athlete should also be prudent with alcohol and sugar intake; these energy sources are typically low in micronutrients. Since alcohol intake causes a relaxed feeling, it is often associated with unwise food choices. Sugar-rich foods and drinks are best consumed in situations related to exercise where a compact fuel source is needed.

• Nutrient-rich foods are valuable for the athlete who needs to meet nutrient requirements from a restricted energy intake. A broad-range low-dose vitamin/mineral supplement should also be considered if the energy intake is below 1200–1800 kcal·day^{-1} (5–7 MJ·day^{-1}) for prolonged periods.

• Many athletes do not appreciate that they may be engaging in inappropriate eating behavior—such as eating when bored or upset, or eating too quickly. Behavioral strategies should be considered to help adopt more appropriate eating habits and to redirect stress or boredom to alternative activities.

• The expertise of a sports dietitian is valuable for individualized and supervised weight loss programs. Expert advice is needed if the athlete is struggling with an eating disorder or disordered eating behavior.

Strategies for consuming a high energy intake, especially in situations of weight gain

• Athletes must be organized. They will need to apply the same dedication to their eating program as is applied to training in order to increase their intake of energy-dense foods. This additional food should supply carbohydrate to fuel the training sessions, and adequate protein and micronutrients for the development and support of new tissue.

• Many athletes with high energy demands do not eat as much—or, more importantly, as often—as they think. It is useful to examine the actual intake of athletes who fail to maintain their ideal weight yet report "constant eating". Commitments such as training, sleep, medical or physiotherapy appointments, work, or school often get in the way of eating opportunities. Lack of appetite before or after a hard training session is also likely to restrict intake. A food record will identify the hours and occasions of minimal food intake. This information should be used to reorganize the day or to find creative ways to make nutritious foods and drinks part of the activity.

• Overall, the athlete should increase the number of times that they eat rather than the size of meals, thus enabling greater intake of food with less risk of "overfilling" and gastrointestinal discomfort. This will require a supply of energy-dense and nutrient-rich snacks to be available between meals, particularly during and after exercise sessions.

• Ensuring a ready supply of palatable and easy-to-consume foods is an important way to help the athlete eat to their appetite level and beyond. Providing a constantly changing variety of food forms and flavors can help to overcome "eating fatigue".

• The energy content of carbohydrate-rich meals and snacks can be increased by adding sugars or lean protein choices. For example, thick jams and syrups can be added to toast or pancakes, sandwiches may have two- or three-layer fillings, and skimmed milk powder can be added to soups or drinks. This adds extra energy to a nutritious meal without adding greatly to the bulkiness of the food.

• The athlete can make their food intake more "compact" by avoiding excessive intake of high-fiber foods. It is often impractical to consume a diet that is solely based on wholegrain and high-fiber foods.

• High-energy fluids such as milkshakes, fruit smoothies, or commercial liquid meal supplements are useful. These drinks provide a compact and low-bulk source of energy and nutrients, and can be consumed with meals or as snacks—including before, during, or after a training session.

• Special sports foods such as sports bars, gels, high-carbohydrate powders, or liquid meal replacement powders also provide a compact carbohydrate and energy boost. They may be eaten as snacks, or in the case of powders, added to everyday foods to increase total intake.

• Recent research suggests that the stimulatory effects of resistance training on muscle protein uptake are enhanced by consuming a carbohydrate and protein snack immediately after, and even before, the session. Useful choices include fruit-flavored yoghurt or flavored milk drinks and fruit smoothies, sandwiches with meat or cheese fillings, breakfast cereal and milk, or special sports bars and liquid meal supplements.

• Athletes who undertake lengthy training or competition sessions each day should find ways to refuel during the workout. Food and drinks consumed during the session may be important for immediate performance as well as providing a substantial contribution to total daily energy intake. Suitable drinks and snacks will vary according to the sport, but may include sports drinks and bars, fruit, sandwiches, and confectionery. The athlete may need to organize a system of aid stations or "handlers" to make these supplies available throughout their event or practice.

Strategies for refueling and rehydrating during training and competition

• The athlete should begin all exercise sessions well hydrated, with particular focus on strategies to recover fluid losses from previous training sessions and to drink adequate amounts of fluid when living in hot conditions. Hyperhydration techniques (acute fluid overloading) may be useful for specific situations of high sweat rates and reduced opportunities to drink during the session, but these tactics should be well practiced in advance and are best undertaken under the supervision of appropriate medical and scientific support staff.

• During exercise, the athlete should develop a fluid intake plan to keep pace with sweat losses as much as is practicable and tolerated. It is difficult to gauge sweat losses during an exercise session, but monitoring changes in body mass before and after similar sessions can provide a guide to typical sweat

losses and the athlete's typical success in replacing these losses. A loss of 1 kg is approximately equal to 1 l of sweat loss. The athlete should undertake such fluid balance checks from time to time to get an estimate of expected sweat losses in different events and conditions.

• The athlete should examine their sport to identify opportunities to drink fluids during the session. Sometimes this can occur during formal breaks in play (time-outs, player substitutions, half-time), while in other sports, the athlete must learn to drink "on the move". A successful fluid intake plan will also mean ensuring supplies of suitable drinks are available—for example, at aid stations, carried by the athlete, or provided by trainers.

• The provision of cool, palatable drinks will encourage fluid intake. Sports drinks are ideal for providing fluids during events, as well as contributing to fuel needs. The replacement of electrolytes via sports drinks is probably valuable in very long events and contributes to the taste appeal of drinks. In prolonged events, it is useful to vary the flavors of drinks to continue to stimulate voluntary intake. Using insulated containers to keep drinks cool can also help.

• Carbohydrate intake can be achieved during longer exercise sessions using sports drinks, special sports products (e.g. gels, bars), and other everyday foods. A carbohydrate intake of 30–60 g·h^{-1} is generally associated with successful refueling during events of 60–90 min or longer. Each athlete should experiment to find a plan that works for their event and their comfort.

• Training sessions should also be targeted for fluid and fuel intake plans. Good hydration/fueling practices during training will mean better performance during that session, and a chance to practice the strategies intended for competition. There is considerable difference in individual (gastrointestinal) tolerance to drinking large volumes of fluid; however, there is some evidence that practice can increase the tolerance of even the most reluctant drinkers.

• After each training session or event, the athlete should enhance recovery by undertaking active rehydration and refueling strategies. Rehydration requires an intake of greater volumes of fluid than the postexercise fluid deficit. In general, the athlete will need to drink 150% of the postrace fluid deficit to ensure fluid balance is achieved—for example, if the postrace fluid deficit is 2 kg (2 l), the athlete should drink 3 l of fluid over the next hours to rehydrate. The replacement of sodium is important in restoring fluid balance, and can be achieved via the selection of sodium-containing fluids (sports drinks and oral rehydration solutions) and snacks (pretzels, bread, breakfast cereal), or by adding a little extra salt to meals.

Strategies for promoting recovery between workouts or competitions

• When time between intense workouts or competitions is brief (< 8–12 h), it makes sense for the athlete to optimize recovery between sessions. Rapid refueling requires a carbohydrate intake of at least 50–100 g (1 g CHO·kg body weight^{-1}) immediately after exercise until the normal meal plan can be resumed. For situations calling for maximal muscle glycogen storage, a total daily carbohydrate intake of 400–700 g (7–10 g·kg^{-1}) is required.

• When the athlete's appetite is suppressed or limited by stomach fullness, it is useful to focus on compact food forms—low fiber carbohydrate foods, sugar-rich foods, and special sports supplements such as sports bars and gels.

• Carbohydrate-containing fluids are also low in bulk and may be appealing to athletes who are fatigued and dehydrated. These include sports drinks, soft drinks, and fruit juices, commercial liquid meal supplements, milkshakes, and fruit smoothies.

• Studies show that low glycemic index (GI) carbohydrate foods such as lentils and legumes may be less suitable for speedy glycogen recovery and should not be the main carbohydrate source in recovery meals. This is generally not a problem for athletes following typical Western diets, as these are generally based on carbohydrate-rich foods of moderate and high glycemic index.

• Athletes should aim for small, frequent meals if they need to achieve high carbohydrate intakes without the discomfort of overeating. However, the athlete should organize a routine of meals and snacks to suit individual preferences, timetable, and appetite. As long as enough carbohydrate is consumed, it does not appear to matter how it is spaced over the day.

• When food intake is limited by gastric comfort or a restricted energy budget, the athlete should avoid large intakes of high-fat foods and excessive amounts of protein foods at the expense of fuel needs.

• Although carbohydrate is usually the nutrient most often considered in recovery meals and snacks, the athlete should be aware of growing evidence for the role of other nutrients, especially protein, in postexercise recovery and adaptation. Many recovery snacks and meal combinations are able to provide a range of nutrient goals simultaneously. As well as meeting the immediate needs of recovery, these foods will be important in the meeting everyday nutrient requirements.

• In situations where enhanced protein status is desirable—for example, to support the gain of muscle size and strength in combination with resistance training, it may be useful for the athlete to consume a snack providing carbohydrate and a source of high-quality protein (10–20 g) immediately before and/or after the workout.

• Examples of suitable recovery snacks are provided in Table 13.2.

Reading list

Burke, L.M. (1995) Practical issues in nutrition for athletes. *Journal of Sports Sciences* **13**, S83–S90.

Burke, L. (2002) Principles of eating for cycling. In: *High Performance Cycling* (ed. A. Jeukendrup), pp. 183–199. Human Kinetics, Champaign, IL.

Hawley, J.A. & Burke, L.M. (1998) *Peak Performance: Training and Nutrition Strategies for Sport*. Allen and Unwin, Sydney.

Chapter 14
Eating well while traveling

Introduction

The modern athlete is a global traveler. It is now commonplace for an athlete to travel interstate or to countries within the same region, often participating in a national or regional competition fixture. Athletes frequently travel to training camps at a location offering specialized training facilities or sports science support, or to a special environment such as altitude or hot weather. International competition is no longer limited to the Olympic Games every 4 years: between Olympiads there is a busy program of World Championships, World Cup or Grand Prix events, and various regional championships or competition tours. The ratio between travel and home stay can vary between sports and between athletes or teams. At one extreme, there are athletes who prepare for one or two important events each year that take them interstate or overseas. At the other end of the spectrum are tennis players, golfers and beach volleyball players who compete on an international circuit that is almost continuous. In this chapter, the various nutrition challenges faced by the traveling athlete will be explored.

Eating while in transit

While travel opportunities allow athletes to explore their country or the world in a day or so, this is ultimately achieved by placing the athlete in a restricted and sedentary environment. Sitting still for long periods is not a natural activity for most athletes. For many, it is a complete contrast to the high levels of energy expenditure normally achieved on a training day, and the forced inactivity often leads to boredom that is relieved by eating. Some athletes overeat while traveling on planes, trains, or automobiles, often buying high-energy high-fat snack foods or takeaway foods at outlets at stations and airports in addition to the menu already provided during the trip. For some athletes, therefore, travel can be a time of unwanted weight gain. On the other hand, some athletes with intrinsically high energy requirements find their energy or nutrient needs cannot be met by conventional catering on planes and trains. The 200-cm basketball player or rower may find themselves limited to child-size portions or without access to their usual frequent intake of snacks and high-energy drinks. These athletes can suffer from hunger as well as unwanted weight loss during trips.

The loss of fluid is often high and unnoticed during travel. Pressurized cabins on planes and, to a lesser extent, air-conditioned buses and trains, expose the athlete to a dry environment, which causes an insensible loss of fluid from the skin and lungs. Most athletes are not aware of the resulting levels of dehydration that occur on long trips. Although drinks are provided as part of the cabin service, the volumes are generally restricted to small cups and cans. Information often provided to travelers warns of the "dehydrating" effects of caffeine-containing beverages such as colas, tea, and coffee. People are often discouraged from having these drinks in the fear that the caffeine content will stimulate urine losses. Although caffeine may cause a small increase in urine production, these drinks still contribute to a positive fluid balance for the athlete. More importantly, if these drinks are part of the athlete's usual fluid intake patterns, the sudden avoidance of these choices may reduce the athlete's total fluid intake. The athlete should aim first for a high fluid intake before worrying about the choice of fluids that contribute to it. Alcohol-containing drinks are best avoided, especially during air travel, because of their intoxicating effects rather than their impact on fluid balance. In addition to the drink opportunities provided by the cabin service, the traveling athlete should take a drink bottle or bottled water in their hand luggage. Sports drinks are useful in providing a small amount of sodium to assist in promoting thirst and reducing urine losses. The athlete's own drink supplies can be further supplemented or topped up from the drinking fountains supplied near the lavatories, providing the added advantage of encouraging athletes to stretch their legs during long flights or trips.

In addition to looking after fluid needs, athletes should think ahead to consider the likely program of meals and snacks provided on their travel schedule. This should include the type and quantity of food as well as the time of eating. As will be discussed below, athletes might want to alter their meal times to help adjust their body clock. Many airlines offer a special menu of low-fat, vegetarian, or even sports meals, which may be suited to the needs of the traveling athlete. These need to be arranged at least 24 h prior to departure, with longer notice required in the case of a team. It may also be possible to ring airports or train stations to find out what catering options are available and their times of operation. Athletes should also be prepared to take along their own supply of meals or snacks to replace or supplement the official food provisions. It is useful to be independent and flexible; all travelers have tales of delayed schedules and hours spent in limbo.

There are many ideas for snacks that are portable and low in perishability. During train and bus travel, small coolers may be taken to store sandwiches, yoghurt, fruit, cereal, and cool drinks. Of course, quarantine laws may need to be taken into account when crossing borders: be careful, as attempts to import prohibited foods can lead to long delays and missed connections. Other snacks that require less storage or preparation facilities include cereal bars, sports bars, liquid meal supplements, dried fruit, and nut mixes. Self-catering for plane flights will depend on the length of the trip. When the urge to nibble exceeds the real need for food, the athlete should work on taking plenty of items to keep them occupied and relaxed (e.g. music, books, puzzles). Otherwise it is easy to succumb to food for entertainment rather than nutrition.

Coping with jetlag and time changes

International travel exposes the athlete to the modern condition known as jet lag: problems related to the rapid change in time zones encountered when traveling between countries across the world. The sudden shift from one time zone to another can lead to disturbance of the day/night cycle, sleeping difficulties, fatigue and mood changes, and gastrointestinal disturbances. The favored practice is to adapt to the new time as soon as possible, even adjusting lifestyle patterns before departure so that they coincide with the practices of the new location. At the least, athletes should set their watches to the time zone of their destination as they begin their journey, and set a timetable for sleep and eating on the trip which matches the activities of their new location. This often places the traveler at odds with the timetable of meals, movies, or designated sleep time that is occurring on board the plane. It can be useful for the athlete who is traveling on long-haul flights to take an eye-mask, pillow, and snacks of their own, to provide the independence to create their own routine. Eating and exposure to sunlight are factors that help trigger the body clock to adjust to a new wake/sleep cycle. Therefore it is helpful, on arrival, to establish a schedule of meals, time spent outside, and sessions of physical activity that immediately adopt the new time zone. Missing meals and napping during the day, or staying up late and snacking during the night, will be counterproductive to an early adjustment to the new location. Although adjustments vary between individuals, it may take a full day to adjust to the effects of each time zone that is crossed.

Nutritional challenges in a new country

It can be exciting to experience the tastes of an exotic new country. However, when athletes are in hard training or important competition, they are more interested in the familiarity and safety of their usual meal plan than the chance to try the unknown. Several nutritional challenges await the visitor to a new country.

Food safety and hygiene issues

The traveling athlete is at risk of becoming infected by unaccustomed organisms, especially those spread by insects or feco-oral contamination. Problems are common in "developing" countries, but even occur in "safe" destinations as the athlete is exposed to different varieties or amounts of the "bugs" with which we share our environments. Gastrointestinal problems are a common challenge to the nutrition of the athlete, causing the loss of fluid and nutrients from the body and interfering with the intake of the athlete's normal diet. Most travel-related diarrhea is caused by non-viral pathogens such as enterotox-igenic *Escherichia coli*, *Campylobacter*, *Salmonella*, *Shigella*, and *Giardia lamblia*. These pathogens are transmitted via contaminated food and water, and poor sanitation. This partly reflects the environment, but can be exacerbated by poor personal hygiene and food safety practices.

Obviously, the athlete's best plan is to prevent the infection from occurring. Prior to departing for a new country, the athlete should consult with a sports doctor for specific advice on hygiene issues related to the safety of food and water in the new environment. Table 14.1 summarizes the precautions that are advised to combat pathogens that are found in water and raw foods. Some athletes practice many of these tactics even in well-developed countries—for example, always sticking to bottled water when they are away from their home country. It is impossible to overemphasize the importance of personal hygiene practices. Many athletes forget or forego their usual behavior when they are away from the safety of home. It can be a nuisance, when out, to find a bathroom for washing hands before eating. Athletes who share food, or cups, bottles and utensils are at risk of spreading diseases—from gastrointestinal bugs to upper respiratory tract complaints. If the athlete's immune system is compromised by the phase of their training or taper, the risk of cross-infection is increased. Many athletes use a prophylactic course of antibiotics during their travel to "high-risk" countries to reduce the chance of succumbing to gastrointestinal problems.

Table 14.1 Strategies for minimizing the risk of succumbing to gastrointestinal bugs in countries with hygiene challenges.

- Athletes should wash their hands with soap thoroughly before eating, and dry with a clean towel or air-dryer. It is useful to carry antibacterial towel wipes so that it is possible to clean hands before each occasion of eating.
- If the local water supply is unsafe, athletes should only drink water that has been boiled or that comes from sealed bottles. If using bottled or canned drinks such as fruit juice or soft drinks to provide daily fluid needs, the energy content of these drinks will need to be taken into account.
- Athletes should take care not to swallow water while showering, and should use bottled water to clean their teeth.
- Salad and raw vegetables should be avoided unless athletes can be confident that these foods have been washed in bottled or boiled water.
- Fruit intake should be limited to types that can be peeled (e.g. oranges, bananas, pineapples, apples).
- Unpasteurized dairy products should be avoided.
- Fish and shellfish are considered risky—especially types that are served raw (e.g. oysters, sushi).
- It is preferable to order à la carte from restaurants so that the food is cooked to order, rather than having been precooked and left to simmer. If buffet food is consumed, athletes should only choose items that are well cooked and served at very hot or very chilled temperatures.
- Athletes should avoid buying foods from hawker stalls and open air cooking outlets.

Coping with gastrointestinal upsets

Vomiting and diarrheal illnesses must first be treated by the replacement of lost fluids and electrolytes. The use of oral rehydration solutions is recommended, but of course a safe water supply must be sought. A bland diet such as dry toast, biscuits, rice, and bananas can then be introduced, and alcohol, fat-rich and dairy foods should be avoided until the diarrhea settles. Antidiarrheal drugs are appropriate if there is no blood or mucus in the stools, but may prolong the duration of illness by reducing the rate at which the pathogens are flushed out of the system. Medical advice should be sought if the diarrhea is associated with fever, blood, or mucus, and antibiotics may be required. If low-grade diarrhea persists for more than 3 days, *Giardia lamblia* may be the underlying organism and a specific course of antibiotics is required. Many organisms cause symptoms that do not present until the athlete returns to the country of origin, and all athletes should be advised to seek medical advice in any case of post-travel illness.

Coping with a new food supply

Being in a foreign country with a different food supply and different eating customs is a challenge to the traveling athlete. It may be difficult for the athlete to obtain the types of food that they like and know will meet their dietary goals. For example, the endurance athlete who typically consumes a high-carbohydrate breakfast of breakfast cereal and toast may be confronted with problems in countries where cold meat and cheese are the usual morning meal. The local food customs may not assist with their nutritional needs for sport, and it can be hard even to find out the composition of foods and dishes (especially if the athlete can't speak the local language). Many an athlete with a fussy palate has lost weight because they don't find the local fare to their liking. Athletes from Western countries are often unprepared for the lack of variety, or access to fresh produce, in less developed regions. On the other hand, athletes have been known to gain significant amounts of body fat when tempted with a new array of food delights.

Before undertaking any travel, athletes should investigate the food patterns in their new location. The internet can provide many sources of information about different countries, as can embassies and trade departments. If the athlete is traveling to a well-known competition, the organizers can often provide information about their local surroundings. Athletes who have traveled there or undertaken the same competition in previous years are also a good source of stories about common problems and ways to cope. It is important to find out local food customs, typical meals served in local restaurants and the restaurant of the athlete's hotel, and the availability of foods that play a key role in the athlete's present diet. If these staple foods do not form part of the everyday eating patterns in a new country, it is likely that they will be more expensive that usual, even if they are available. The athlete should consider which local foods might be used to replace staples, and what consequences might occur. For example, if bread and breakfast cereal are not readily available in an Asian country, will the athlete feel happy to consume a bowl of rice as part of their breakfast? Can croissants be a suitable replacement when the athlete is in France? And even if the carbohydrate is successfully replaced by this food swap, will the change from high fiber content of wholegrain cereals to white rice or croissants have an effect on satiety or the athlete's usual bowel habits? Will the high fat content of croissants interfere with weight control goals for this athlete?

Cooking styles may also need to be explored to find out about added fats and oils (for weight control), or food hygiene issues (see Table 14.1). In many cases, a knowledge of the local fare can help the athlete to choose the food items most suited to their nutritional goals, or to ask for modifications to suit these needs. It may also alert the athlete to take a supply of their own foods from home (see below).

Eating away from home

At home the athlete is used to a routine, and to a certain level of access to food. Travel can destroy both the routine and the availability of food. Athletes are often organized to stay in hotels where

Table 14.2 Strategies for organizing team eating in a restaurant (from *Survival from the Fittest* 2001).

Feeding a team can be a logistical nightmare, especially when events finish late at night. It can be hard for restaurants to handle large numbers and individual meal requests quickly.
• Book a restaurant ahead of time and negotiate a menu. It also helps to ring ahead to fine-tune your arrival time so that food will be ready as you walk in the door.
• Buffet eating is recommended—it's quick for hungry athletes, cost-saving when negotiating prices with the restaurant, and offers flexibility so that each athlete can choose the type and amount of food that they need.
• Plan a menu based on carbohydrate-rich dishes and offer sufficient choice to meet the preferences of the majority of your athletes. Note that too much choice encourages overeating, because people try a little bit of everything. If you are away for more than a week, put effort into increasing the variety from day to day, rather than within the same meal.
• Make separate arrangements for athletes with special needs (i.e. vegetarians or those with food intolerances). It is hard to accommodate all needs within one menu, so be prepared to arrange special needs as required.
• Remember that snacks as part of the dietary plan are often neglected when catering arrangements provide for three meals a day. Provide items at meals that can be taken away for eating later—for example fruit, cartons of yoghurt, muffins, and breakfast bars. Alternatively, organize a communal room with a fridge so you have somewhere to put these snack-type items, and other choices such as breakfast cereal.

---

catering has been arranged to provide three meals a day, rather than the regular supply of snacks that are needed to meet energy requirements or post-training recovery goals. Being completely reliant on restaurants (or fast food outlets) for food needs is limiting, expensive, and often a challenge to busy timetables. Sometimes, training and competition hours clash with normal restaurant operating schedules. Other times, athletes who just want to arrive, eat, and get home to rest within the shortest time possible, are left to compete with other restaurant patrons who are there for an evening of entertainment. Large groups are particularly unwieldy to handle.

Even when athletes are organized to self-cater in apartments, they find their cooking skills limited by an inadequate budget, poor access to food shops, or a poor imagination for quick and easy recipes. It is easier to cook at home with a wide array of utensils, sauces, spices, and handy baking items. What do you do when these are missing, and it is wasteful to buy a whole box or bottle of something for a few teaspoons, especially when you move on to a new destination in a couple of days and start again in a new apartment?

The answer to these challenges lies, again, in pre-trip preparation. The destination should be explored with detailed information about food supplies and meal schedules. Many athletes and teams work with dietitians who can organize special menus or special food requests to be sent in advance to hotels and restaurants (see Table 14.2). When self-catering is chosen, it can be useful to take along a supply of herbs and spices in small containers (e.g. film canisters) or a few indispensable utensils (e.g. a sharp knife or a can-opener that works). Many cookbooks for athletes are now written with special menus that dovetail ingredients for a 4-day or 7-day stay.

Supplies for the traveling athlete

There are many foods that athletes can take on their travels to supplement the available food supply, provide favorite tastes from home, or supply important nutrients. Important characteristics include good storage and perishability features, and minimal preparation needs. This will be important when the athlete lacks any access to a fridge or kitchen. The weight of luggage is often an issue when the athlete is traveling on planes. In this situation, powdered or concentrated versions of foods are preferable (e.g. skimmed milk powder rather than UHT cartons of milk, concentrated fruit juice rather than tetrapack cartons of juice). Although some athletes travel with their food supply, other teams or individuals may send a package of food supplies ahead of time, making use of cheaper travel options rather than paying for excess baggage. Of course, all food supplies are subject to customs and quarantine laws, and the athlete should seek official advice before taking foods and supplements across borders and into new countries. Table 14.3 provides

Table 14.3 Foods and products suitable for the traveling athlete.

Breakfast cereal and skimmed milk powder
"Canned" fruit in plastic snack packs or cans with ring-pull lids
Baked beans or spaghetti in cans with ring-pull lids
Quick-cook rice and noodles (low-fat varieties)
Pasta sauces in plastic pouches
Dried fruit: sultanas, raisins, dried apricots, dried apple, trail mix (nuts and dried fruit)
Processed cheese sticks
Crackers, rice cakes, and jam, honey, and peanut butter (especially in individual packets)
Cereal bars, muesli bars, and breakfast bars (low fat)
Jelly confectionery
Powdered sports drinks
Powdered liquid meal supplements
Sports bars
Broad-range multivitamin/mineral supplement

---

suggestions of food supplies that may be useful to the traveling athlete.

Keeping a record

It is valuable for the athlete to keep a log of their food intake and dietary experiences on their trip. This can help to keep the athlete focused while away, by keeping track of food intake in a confusing and changing environment. Such a diary can pinpoint problem areas, or missing foods and nutrients. Alternatively it can provide a confidence boost to the athlete that they are meeting their nutritional needs well, despite being away from all that is familiar. Once the trip is over, the athlete or team should undertake a debriefing, summarizing the successes, challenges, and failures of their travel experiences. This information is important for planning new trips for the same athlete, or for assisting other athletes and teams who will travel to this same destination in the future.

Summary

Travel provides both challenges and lessons. Athletes should prepare well before their trip, in anticipation of the difficulties of eating while in transit and at the new destination. Meals can be organized in advance, and food supplies can be taken to supplement or replace meals and snacks in the new location. Hygiene issues—both personal and related to food and water supplies—are important to consider, since illness can have a profound effect on the athlete's nutrition and performance. Athletes should record a log of all their experiences to prepare for future trips, or to assist other athletes who will follow in their footsteps.

Reading list

Grandjean, A.C. & Ruud, J.S. (2000) The travelling athlete. In: *Nutrition in Sport* (ed. R.J. Maughan), pp. 484–491. Blackwell Science, Oxford.

Survival for the Fittest. The Australian Institute of Sport official cookbook for athletes. (1999) Murdoch Magazine, Sydney, Australia.

Survival from the Fittest. A companion cookbook to *Survival for the Fittest* from the AIS. (2001) Murdoch Magazine, Sydney, Australia.

Young, M. & Fricker, P. (2000) Medical and nutritional issues for the travelling athlete. In: *Clinical Sports Nutrition* (eds L. Burke & V. Deakin), pp. 702–709. McGraw-Hill, Sydney, Australia.

Young, M., Fricker, P., Maughan, R. & MacAuley, D. (1998) The traveling athlete: issues relating to the Commonwealth Games, Malaysia, 1998. *Clinical Journal of Sports Medicine* 8, 130–135.

CASE STUDY 1 Eating for recovery on the road. Melinda M. Manore

Team

The coaches of the collegiate male basketball team were working hard to educate their athletes about good nutrition, optimal body weight for performance, and what to eat for competition. All away tournaments involved plane travel, eating at hotels, and on many occasions a competition schedule of two games in a 24-h period.

Reason for consultancy

The coach wanted to know what to feed the athletes after an evening game that ended at 10.30 at night, when the athletes had to be ready for another game at 11.00 AM the next morning. Typically after an evening game, the coach allowed the athletes to eat what they wanted. During tournaments, he found that his athletes did not want to eat breakfast before the game after eating so much the previous evening and getting to bed so late. Instead they preferred to sleep in as late as possible, then rush to the game.

Current dietary patterns

Prior to the consultation with a nutritionist, the athletes ate whatever and whenever they wanted at tournaments, regardless of the game schedule. During games, water and sports drinks were made available. A typical day's diet from a tournament day is outlined below.

Professional assessment

Without a proper eating plan for tournaments, these athletes were judged to be at risk of failing to recover optimally from each game and prepare for the next. The typical eating practices were found to be inadequate in carbohydrate and fluid, and high in fat. They needed an organized approach to postgame eating that could be achieved on the road and manipulated according to the game schedule.

Intervention

In order to achieve a plan for postgame recovery, the following suggestions were made. These suggestions focused on replacing carbohydrate and fluid for the athletes in a team environment, with a series of strategies that could be achieved away from home.

1 Immediately after the game, the trainers should provide each athlete with a "ready to drink" liquid meal supplement. This supplement would provide a practical supply of carbohydrate, protein, and micronutrients to achieve optimal refueling and repair. The athletes should also be encouraged to drink sports beverages to rehydrate.

2 The hotel should be provided with a request to serve a postgame meal for the team, minutes after the athletes arrive back at the hotel. A series of menus could be generated for the team to be rotated throughout the tournament or season. Choices are high in carbohydrate (fruit, vegetables, grains), with lean meats and moderate amounts of fat. If this recovery meal is eaten late at night, menu choices may be lighter in style—for example, sandwiches and toasted sandwiches, healthy pizza slices, fruit platters. Athletes are encouraged to quickly refuel, without overfilling and feeling uncomfortable. Athletes are encouraged not to consume caffeinated beverages at this postgame meal if this interferes with sleep patterns.

3 A team breakfast is served the next morning to provide a high-carbohydrate pre-event meal. A menu of juice, cereal, milk, toast, and pancakes is provided. High-carbohydrate beverages, sports bars, and liquid meal supplements are always available.

4 During the game sports drinks are provided and athletes are encouraged to drink at every opportunity.

Outcome

The athletes reported that routine and team-based events provided a positive preparation for each game. The organization of postgame sports drinks and liquid meal supplements, followed by a light meal, allowed them to refuel and rehydrate quickly after the game. They found that they were able to get to bed earlier, and get better-quality sleep, compared to their previous routines. Although they were still tired in the morning, they were able to enjoy the team breakfast and start focusing on the next game. They arrived at the courts feeling more alert and energetic.

Breakfast	Lunch	Dinner	After game meal
Egg McMuffin Orange juice	Burger King double burger, fries and coke at the airport or hotel	Steak Baked potato with sour cream and butter Garlic bread Salad with ranch dressing Milk	Pepperoni pizza Coke Ice cream

Chapter 15
Strategies for special populations

Introduction

Athletes are concerned with the special nutritional needs of sport, but an optimal eating plan achieves these needs while also meeting the basic requirements for health and long-term well-being. Sometimes, however, there are additional considerations that need to be taken into account. The population involved in sport and physical exercise includes subpopulations with special nutritional needs; these can arise from age, gender, medical conditions, or dietary restrictions. In this chapter, we will discuss nutritional considerations and dietary strategies for special subgroups of the population who participate in exercise and sporting activities.

Special nutritional needs of female athletes

The last few decades have seen an increase in the rate and level of participation of women in sport. Women have participated in the fitness boom that has seen the growth of many new recreational sports and exercise activities. At the elite level of competitive sport, the professionalism and preparation of the female athlete now rivals that of her male counterpart. Consequently, in many sports the gender differences in exercise performance have considerably narrowed.

It is important to note that the overwhelming majority of studies related to sports nutrition have been conducted on male subjects. Therefore, while this book and, indeed, all other sources of sports nutrition information provide guidelines on dietary practices for optimal performance that are not gender specific, it has not been clearly established that females respond in an identical manner to males in all situations. We generally accept that such guidelines provide the most up-to-date information on sports nutrition available, and a sensible starting point for female athletes, but it is interesting to consider the ways in which special differences might occur.

Differences related to energy intake

A primary difference between female athletes and their male counterparts is that females are generally smaller in body size and have less muscle mass, and consequently have lower energy requirements. In addition, the push to achieve the light and lean body type that is considered ideal for performance in many sports seems to present particular challenges for the female athlete. After all, the post-adolescent female naturally carries a higher level of body fat than a male, and in addition to the general dissatisfaction of females in the community with their body shape, the female athlete appears to struggle to achieve her desired level of leanness even in the face of a substantial training load. Cross-sectional surveys of the attitudes and self-reported practices of various groups of female athletes report that many are concerned about their weight and fatness and are dieting to reduce body fat levels. As discussed in Chapter 1, dietary surveys of groups of athletes often show that the energy intakes reported by female athletes are lower than expected, on the basis of predicted energy requirements or in comparison to a group of males undertaking a similar exercise program. In addition to low-energy and fad diets, female athletes may resort to pathogenic weight loss techniques such as fasting, dehydration strategies, purging, and the use of diuretics and laxatives. Many studies report a higher prevalence of eating disorders or disordered eating behaviors and body perceptions among female athletes in sports where body mass or body fat content is an issue than would be expected in the general community or than that observed in control groups. It is difficult to determine the true prevalence of eating disorders among athletes; reports vary from less than 1% to 50% of athletic populations according to the type of athletes involved and the method used to assess dietary habits and to define eating disorders. It is not certain whether an involvement in sport, or in certain types of sport that promote leanness, presents a risk factor *per se* for disordered eating. After all, it is likely that the psychological characteristics that are associated with successful sports performance (e.g. obsessiveness, perfectionism, ability to tolerate discomfort) are also those that present a risk for disordered eating.

Notwithstanding the potential errors involved with dietary survey techniques, it appears that female athletes must generally meet their nutrient requirements from a smaller energy budget, and sports nutrition guidelines must be formulated accordingly. If the macronutrient requirements associated with heavy training are assumed to be similar for males and females (based on $g \cdot kg^{-1}$ targets), the practical outcome is that the female athlete will find it more difficult to meet protein and carbohydrate (CHO) needs than her male counterpart. In fact, many females in heavy training do not report eating sufficient energy to provide the notional daily targets for protein ($1.2–1.6$ $g \cdot kg^{-1}$) and CHO (up to $7–10$ $g \cdot kg^{-1}$). In fact, many female athletes appear to put their goals for achieving an ideal physique above that of providing adequate

fuel for training, and often report intakes of CHO that fall well below the targets for optimal performance and recovery as a side-product of severe energy restriction. Some females also avoid consuming sports drinks or other forms of CHO during prolonged exercise, in fear of consuming additional energy.

Dietary counseling may help the female athlete to permit herself an increased intake of CHO and total energy, or to adopt the well-supported practices of refuelling during lengthy workouts (see Case Study 4). The result is often a substantial improvement in training performance and competition outcome, despite the failure to achieve the "ideal" body shape and even in spite of an increase in body mass. Even so, it is often not feasible for the female athlete to meet the notional targets for protein and CHO within their training energy budget. Many female athletes alternate their eating patterns according to the priority of their nutrition goals; during competition or key workouts, greater priority is given to achieving CHO intake goals to promote optimal performance and recovery. Meanwhile the bulk of the training program is undertaken with a more restricted energy intake, designed to achieve or maintain lower body fat levels. Strategies that help to achieve loss of body fat while meeting fuel needs are discussed in Chapter 13.

In addition to meeting macronutrient needs, female athletes must achieve their requirements for vitamins and minerals from a lower energy intake than is consumed by most males. Ironically, the absolute requirement for some micronutrients— e.g. iron and perhaps calcium—may be greater for females. Female athletes, at least those who have a regular menstrual cycle, have greater iron requirements than males to cover the blood losses of menstruation. Restriction of energy intake and lack of dietary variety are key risk factors for an inadequate intake of well-absorbed iron. Although it is tempting to consider that iron supplementation should be routine for female athletes, the management of suspected cases of iron deficiency is best undertaken on an individual basis by a sports medicine specialist, and preferably by a team including the physician and dietitian. After all, this offers the possibility of improving eating patterns and overall nutritional status, as well as excluding the presence of pathogenic causes of iron loss (see Chapter 4). Dietary strategies that promote intake of bioavailable iron are outlined in Chapter 13, and include ideas that are consistent with a restricted energy intake.

Calcium intake plays an important role in achieving healthy bone status throughout life. However, because of the complex relationship between female sex hormones and bone health, female athletes who suffer from disturbances to regular menstrual function are often found to have suboptimal bone density (see Chapter 4). Many of these athletes may also have restricted energy intakes or irregular eating patterns, so it is likely that the situation of hormonal irregularity is compounded by low intakes of calcium. A desire to restrict fat intake may lead to avoidance of dairy products, the major source of dietary for calcium for most of the population. An increase in calcium intake, even to levels above the recommended daily intake for an adult female, may assist in the treatment or prevention of suboptimal bone density, but the cornerstone of treatment is to correct the hormonal imbalance (see Chapter 4). Nevertheless, the female athlete should be aware of strategies for high-calcium eating, especially ideas that can be achieved in combination with energy intake goals.

Possible gender differences in metabolism

A different perspective on sports nutrition for female athletes is to consider the possibility of gender-related differences in metabolism. This could range from differences in substrate utilization during exercise, which underpins many of the nutritional strategies of eating before, during, and after exercise, to differences in response to ergogenic aids and pharmacological agents such as caffeine. Female sex hormones can have a substantial influence on substrate utilization during exercise, meaning not only a difference in fuel usage patterns between males and females, but alterations over the course of the menstrual cycle as levels of estrogen and progesterone fluctuate. There is some evidence that female athletes derive more energy from the oxidation of fat during submaximal exercise, with sparing of muscle glycogen and protein, compared to males and that this can vary with the different phases of the menstrual cycle.

Based on these reports, it has been hypothesized that females are better suited to endurance and ultraendurance sports where fat is a more important fuel source, and that increases in protein requirements in response to heavy training are smaller in females than in males. It could also mean that female athletes have less need for, or are less responsive to, dietary strategies that promote CHO availability. There is evidence from some studies that female athletes are less likely than males to benefit from CHO loading strategies, and that they store glycogen less effectively than males. However, data from studies that are better designed refute these findings. Further doubt is cast upon these speculations by the data from existing world records, which suggest that the female athlete does not become relatively better than her male counterpart as the reliance on fat as a fuel increases (see Table 15.1).

While the scarcity of data on female athletes and the apparent contradictions in findings are far from ideal, they are understandable in view of the difficulty of undertaking such research. It is more

Table 15.1 World record or world best performances for men and women at various distances (July 2002). The relative performances of the best women and the best men remain remarkably constant across this wide range and these data certainly do not support the suggestion that women are better suited than men to endurance activities.

Distance	Male record	Female record	% Difference
100 m	9.79 s	10.49 s	5.1
1000 m	2 min 11.96 s	2 min 28.98 s	12.9
10 km	26 min 22.75 s	29 min 31.78 s	11.9
100 km	6 h 10 min 20 s	7 h 23 min 28 s	19.7
1000 km	5 days 16 h 17 min 00 s	8 days 00 h 27 min 06 s	41.2

complicated to undertake an intervention study using female athletes compared to male subjects. For example, researchers often find it difficult to recruit enough females of sufficient or similar training status to provide the sample sizes needed for statistical power. It appears to be important to control for a certain phase of the menstrual cycle, but such a design adds considerably to the logistical demands of the study. Studies directly comparing the response of males and females are even more problematic, because there is no ideal way to match subjects. Subjects might be matched for absolute or relative aerobic capacity, training status, percentage body fat, or yet other characteristics, but none of these approaches is entirely satisfactory. Clearly, further research is to be encouraged, and we await with interest the results of studies that will finally determine whether female athletes should follow the sports nutrition guidelines directed at male athletes. In the meantime, in spite of interesting hypotheses, there is little persuasive evidence that females will not benefit from the present range of nutrition strategies promoted for optimal performance, particularly the ideas for promoting CHO availability before, during, and after exercise.

Special nutritional needs of children who exercise

The public health strategies of most industrialized countries include attention to the importance of participation in regular sport or exercise activities for children. At the other end of the spectrum are sports such as swimming, tennis, and gymnastics, in which elite achievement is only possible after many years of training, and children as young as 11–14 years of age may undertake 10 or more hours a week of specialized training. In some of these sports, athletes with precocious talent are able to reach world-class level at less than 18 years of age. Despite their presence in the "adult" world of sport, these children are not simply young adults. Special attention must be paid to the nutritional requirements of growth and adolescence, as well as the social issues of eating. There are also some special issues related to the thermoregulatory physiology of children and adolescents that have implications for fluid intake during exercise.

Special needs for growth

During periods of growth there are additional needs for energy and the nutrients involved with the manufacture of new body tissues (e.g. protein, calcium, and iron). The recommended nutrient intakes for children and adolescents reflect these needs. Adolescent males undergo a greater growth spurt during puberty than females. In fact, many active males can find it difficult to meet the high energy requirements arising from growth as well as the energy cost of their training program. It is not uncommon to see young players in team sports such as football, basketball, and volleyball struggle to consume the energy needed to fuel their regular workouts, as well as support the fast increases in their height and desired increases in muscle mass and strength. The strategies identified in Chapter 13 can assist such athletes to increase their energy intakes within the constraints imposed by a busy day and by gastrointestinal comfort.

For females, puberty is associated with an increase in height and weight, and with a substantial increase in body fat levels. These changes to body shape and image are not always well accepted by the young athlete and by those around her, especially in sports where a small and lean body type is associated with top performances. Many young females become preoccupied with restricting energy intake to reduce or minimize the increase in body fat levels. There is some concern in sports such as gymnastics that a heavy training program and energy restriction can cause a deliberate or coincidental retardation of the child's growth and sexual maturation. Studies of female gymnasts show that they are smaller than age-matched girls, and have a delayed menarche (onset of menstrual cycle). However, the natural selection process, by which girls who are genetically predisposed to be small and lean gravitate to sports like gymnastics at which they will be successful, could also explain these characteristics. This explanation is supported by other data showing that most gymnasts, even those competing at the highest level, do ultimately reach their genetically programmed adult height. Nevertheless, it is important that young females are helped to develop a healthy attitude to their body shape and eating patterns as they pass through adolescence.

Eating habits of children and adolescents

Most children are highly dependent on their parents and carers for their eating patterns and nutritional requirements. Adolescence marks the development of independence in many aspects of life, including dietary habits. Among non-athletic groups, adolescent eating patterns are distinguished by irregular meal times and food choices, snacking, increased use of takeaway foods, and exploration of alternative food beliefs and eating styles. Females frequently begin "dieting" to lose weight or body fat, and may experiment with vegetarian eating, fad diets, or other forms of restrictive eating. Males are often interested in increasing their size and strength and may turn to supplements or "muscle building" diets. These characteristics are shared and perhaps even exaggerated in populations of young athletes. It is important that dietary advice offered to young athletes is targeted to their concerns and interests.

Thermoregulatory issues in children

Hyperthermia and dehydration have a detrimental effect on health and performance (see Chapters 5 & 8), and children are particularly at risk. The sweating response is less effective in children than in adults. Children have a lower sweat rate than adults (~ 2.5 times less), due to a lower rate of sweat production by each sweat gland. In addition, the sweating threshold (the core temperature when sweating starts) appears to be higher in children than adults, gradually approaching adult levels early in adolescence. Although it sounds as if children are less likely to develop a large fluid deficit, the problem is that the risk of heat injuries is greater at lower levels of dehydration in children. For every degree of fluid deficit that is incurred

during exercise, there will be a faster increase in core temperature in children compared with adults. The smaller the child, the greater is the excess in body heat content. Small size also means a greater surface area to body volume ratio, and a faster rate of heat gain when environmental temperature exceeds skin temperature.

Children and adolescents exercising in the heat should be monitored closely for signs of heat stress. Those with high levels of body fat and heavy builds are more susceptible to heat stress because they are less able to dissipate body heat. Sunscreens, lightweight clothing, and hats should be worn when possible, and supervisors should take a conservative approach to the duration and intensity of exercise that is undertaken in the heat. Children should learn the importance of drinking during exercise. Good fluid intake practices will assist the physically active child to reduce their risk of thermal injuries and fatigue, and to achieve the satisfaction of doing their best. This principle applies equally well to the elite junior athlete and to the child playing in a recreational sporting activity or a school sports competition. An important goal of children's sport and physical activities is to ensure that participation remains a safe and rewarding experience that will be continued throughout adulthood. Therefore, children should be introduced at an early stage to the practices that promote good performance and enjoyment of sport.

Special nutritional issues for vegetarians

Vegetarian eating should be considered a mainstream dietary practice, being followed by many millions of people worldwide. In some cases it is the predominant eating practice of a country or culture, while in most industrialized countries it represents a move away from the normal diet. "Vegetarian" is used to describe a wide range of eating behaviors that, in turn, are underpinned by a variety of beliefs or factors (see Expert Comment 1).

Vegetarian dietary practices appear to have a protective effect against many of the lifestyle diseases seen in affluent countries. A well-chosen vegetarian diet is likely to be rich in carbohydrate, fiber, and phytochemicals, and low in total and saturated fats. Vegetarian populations typically show lower mortality rates from coronary artery disease and certain forms of cancer, and lower risks of obesity and diabetes. Of course, lifestyle factors other than diet may partially account for the observed health differences seen between vegetarians and non-vegetarians. According to expert nutrition bodies such as the American Dietetic Association, a vegetarian eating style appears to be suitable for sports performance. In fact, many endurance athletes choose such an eating style to achieve their daily targets for CHO intake or to assist with weight control via a reduction in dietary intake of fat. Many athletes include vegetarian-style meals within an omnivorous diet to achieve these same goals.

The nutrient that is of most obvious concern in a vegetarian diet is protein. Lacto-ovo vegetarians who consume dairy products and eggs receive high-quality complete proteins and are unlikely to be challenged by inadequate protein intakes. Vegetarians who consume only plant proteins could become protein deficient unless a balance of amino acids is consumed by complementing protein sources over the day's menu. Examples of complementary mixtures of plant-derived foods are provided in Chapter 3.

The risk of inadequate intake of vitamins and minerals in a vegetarian diet depends on which of the traditional food sources are avoided and on the food sources that replace these. Iron and zinc are provided in well-absorbed forms in meat, and the vegetarian athlete must incorporate into their diet plant foods that are medium or good sources of these minerals. In the case of iron, clever combinations of foods at meals can match these iron-containing foods with factors that enhance the absorption of this non-heme iron form. Vitamin C-containing foods should be eaten with wholegrain and fortified cereals, legumes, and green leafy vegetables (e.g. a glass of orange juice with an iron-fortified breakfast cereal). Dairy products are the major sources of calcium in the Western diet, which means that vegans who avoid these foods must find a calcium-fortified soy alternative. Dairy products

are also a major source of riboflavin, but this vitamin can also be found in wholegrain cereals and yeast extracts. Finally, vitamin B_{12}, which is found in foods of animal origin, will be missing from the diets of strict vegans and fruitarians who avoid all such foods. Although it appears to take years to develop a deficiency, these subgroups of vegetarian eaters should find fortified food products that they are happy to consume on a regular basis.

Special nutritional issues for athletes with diabetes

Suffering from a medical condition or metabolic abnormality does not preclude participation in sport for most people. In fact, in many cases, exercise will have a positive effect on health and disease outcomes. Diabetes mellitus is a disease of abnormal regulation of glucose metabolism, which is classified into two distinct types:

1 insulin-dependent diabetes mellitus (IDDM) or type I diabetes, predominantly developing early in life, which requires insulin replacement because of an almost total lack of insulin secretion; and

2 non-insulin-dependent diabetes mellitus (NIDDM) or type II diabetes, predominantly developing later in life, which is characterized by insulin resistance.

Exercise is considered a cornerstone of the management of NIDDM because of its positive effect on insulin sensitivity and glucose tolerance and its potential role in treating some of the associated issues such as obesity. On the other hand, exercise is a challenge for people with type I diabetes, because of their need to externally manipulate blood glucose concentrations via insulin therapy and CHO intake. Of course this need not be a deterrent even to top-level performers; at the 2000 Olympics in Sydney, two of the athletes who won gold medals in sports demanding extremely high metabolic turnover are known to be insulin-dependent diabetics.

It appears that people with IDDM respond to exercise training in the same manner as non-diabetics. Therefore, the goal is to learn to manage insulin therapy and food intake to maintain blood glucose concentrations as close as possible to the normal range. Modern treatment programs utilize multiple injections each day using a mixture of insulin types with variable activity periods (rapid acting, long acting, etc.). It is critical to monitor blood glucose concentrations, using portable blood glucose analysers, at frequent intervals over the day and at critical times before, after, and even during exercise. With careful monitoring and supervised adjustment of insulin therapy and food intake, an athlete with IDDM can learn how to perform optimally during exercise. IDDM need not prevent an athlete from achieving their sporting goals. Individual attention to CHO intake in the days and hours before an event and during the event will be critical to avoiding the problems of hypoglycemia or hyperglycemia or the failure to meet general goals of sports nutrition. Adjustments may also need to be made in the postexercise period to account for glycogen repletion in the depleted muscles. Since this information is specialized and unique to each individual athlete, professional attention from an endocrinologist and sports nutrition expert is needed.

Reading list

Bass, S. & Inge, K. (2000) Nutrition for special populations: children and young athletes. In: *Clinical Sports Nutrition* (eds L. Burke & V. Deakin), pp. 554–601. McGraw-Hill, Sydney, Australia.

Berning, J.R. (2000) The vegetarian athlete. In: *Nutrition in Sport* (ed. R. J. Maughan), pp. 442–456. Blackwell Science, Oxford.

Brown, L. & Wilson, D. (2000) Special needs: the athlete with diabetes. In: *Clinical Sports Nutrition* (eds L. Burke & V. Deakin), pp. 640–655. McGraw-Hill, Sydney, Australia.

Cox, G. (2000) Special needs: the vegetarian athlete. In: *Clinical Sports Nutrition* (eds L. Burke & V. Deakin), pp. 656–671. McGraw-Hill, Sydney, Australia.

Gabel, K.A. (2000) The female athlete. In: *Nutrition in Sport* (ed. R. J. Maughan), pp. 415–428. Blackwell Science, Oxford.

Jensen, J. & Leighton, B. (2000) The diabetic athlete. In: *Nutrition in Sport* (ed. R. J. Maughan), pp. 457–466. Blackwell Science, Oxford.

Reaburn, P. (2000) Nutrition and the ageing athlete. In: *Clinical Sports Nutrition* (eds L. Burke & V. Deakin), pp. 602–639. McGraw-Hill, Sydney, Australia.

Unnithan, V.B. & Baxter-Jones, A.D.G. (2000) The young athlete. In: *Clinical Sports Nutrition* (eds L. Burke & V. Deakin), pp. 419–441. McGraw-Hill, Sydney, Australia.

EXPERT COMMENT 1 What does it mean to be a vegetarian athlete? Gregory R. Cox

For athletes, the decision to follow a vegetarian diet may differ from the reasons typically explaining vegetarian eating in non-athlete populations. Typically, cultural and religious prescriptions, beliefs concerning animal rights and environmental issues, and the purported health benefits are central to the decision to choose a vegetarian lifestyle. However, athletes may choose a vegetarian or near-vegetarian diet in the belief it will directly or indirectly optimize their sporting performance.

The term "vegetarian" has been used broadly to describe diets that exclude or partially exclude animal flesh foods. Because "vegetarian" has been used to describe such a vast array of eating patterns, it is difficult to ascertain the merits and disadvantages of vegetarian eating amongst the athletic community. Many "vegetarians", for example, regularly consume fish. To date, most research investigating the adequacy of a vegetarian diet has failed to differentiate between a "true vegetarian" diet (exclusion of animal flesh foods) and a "near-vegetarian" diet (typically, exclusion of red meat only). In fact, some people describe a series of types of vegetarian eating patterns, as summarized below.

To further complicate matters, some athletes describe their dietary intake as vegetarian, simply to hide restrictive eating patterns and/or mask a disordered eating behavior. Describing themselves as vegetarian provides a socially accepted avenue for athletes who want to restrict the quantity or range of foods consumed, particularly when eating in public. Many of these athletes simply delete meats (and often dairy foods) from their menus without making any attempt to replace these foods with alternatives; this places them at risk of consuming an inadequate energy and nutrient intake. In fact, this often is just the tip of the iceberg, as the athlete goes on to remove other key foods from their eating plan. This pattern of dietary restriction hiding behind vegetarianism is so prevalent in some sports or social circles, that practitioners involved with these subpopulations regard a self-proclaimed vegetarian eater as being at risk of disordered eating until otherwise proven. Such poor eating patterns do justice neither to the athlete's nutritional needs nor to the real features of vegetarianism.

Rather than simply describing a vegetarian eater by the foods that they *omit* from their diets, it is important for practitioners and researchers to consider the range of foods they *include* in their eating patterns, especially the foods that are chosen to provide a replacement source of energy and nutrients for those typically supplied by foods of animal origin. It is also useful to understand the individual's rationale for choosing a vegetarian lifestyle, since this often highlights a lack of nutrition knowledge or a disordered attitude to food and eating. For example, an athlete who simply omits meat or other animal foods from their diet in order to focus all their attention on carbohydrate-rich foods, or as a reaction to the belief that meat is high in fat or cholesterol, may fail to implement suitable dietary changes to meet daily energy and nutrient needs. Intervention and education for this athlete would differ considerably from that for an athlete who follows a true vegetarian diet for cultural or social reasons.

A vegetarian diet offers certain advantages and disadvantages to athletes striving to meet their daily energy and nutrient requirements. Typically, a vegetarian diet is higher in carbohydrate, but still adequate in protein, compared to non-vegetarian diets. This offers a potential advantage to athletes striving to meet high carbohydrate requirements, within a modest energy intake. As many endurance athletes strive to maximize their intake of carbohydrate while maintaining a low body weight and body fat level, it is not surprising that near-vegetarian eating patterns are common amongst these athletes.

Vegetarian diets are typically high in fiber, which raises concern about the ability of vegetarian athletes or near-vegetarian athletes to meet high daily energy requirements during periods of strenuous activity. Athletes who replace energy-dense animal flesh foods with low-fat, high-bulk fruits and vegetables will struggle to meet daily energy demands when energy requirements are high. Athletes with high energy requirements should be educated to incorporate compact, energy-dense vegetarian meat alternatives such as nuts, seeds, tofu, tempeh, textured vegetable protein, and commercially prepared meat alternatives, to ensure their daily energy requirements are met.

A well-planned vegetarian diet will meet the nutrient requirements of most athletes. However, a near-vegetarian diet excluding suitable vegetarian meat alternatives may provide an inadequate dietary intake to meet daily energy and nutrient requirements of an athlete. As vegetarian diets contain iron in its non-heme (low bioavailability) form, the iron status of all vegetarian athletes should be assessed, particularly when iron requirements are high.

Fruitarian	Diet consists of raw or dried fruits, nuts, seeds, honey, and vegetable oil.
Macrobiotic	Excludes all animal foods, dairy products, and eggs; uses only unprocessed, unrefined, "natural" and "organic" cereals, grains and condiments such as miso and seaweed.
Vegan	Excludes all animal foods, dairy products, and eggs. In the purest sense, excludes all animal products including honey, gelatine, and animal-derived food additives.
Lacto vegetarian	Excludes all animal foods and eggs. Does, however, include milk and milk products.
Lacto-ovo vegetarian	Excludes all animal foods, but includes milk, milk products, and eggs.

Athlete

Annie was a 17-year-old elite-level female gymnast. Her height was 150 cm, and her body mass (weight) was 44 kg. She trained 6 days a week for 4–5 h a day, and was in an important period of her preparation, 1 month away from national competitions.

Reason for consultancy

Annie was experiencing fatigue and failure to fully recover after workouts. At times she found herself becoming light-headed between rotations, forgetting skills she had practiced numerous times. She was frustrated by her poor performance, and anxious to find a way to get out of her training slump.

Existing dietary patterns

Annie consumed a strict vegan diet, based mainly on low-fat grain-based foods, garbanzo beans, fruits, and vegetables. She didn't eat before morning practice (lasting 2 h) and ate only a banana and a low-fat granola bar for breakfast afterwards. Although she always ate lunch and usually had a snack before afternoon practice, she admitted to being too tired after practice to eat much. This meant that she often resorted to eating a low-fat granola bar in place of dinner, before going to bed. Annie drank one glass of calcium-fortified soy milk each day but did not take any other vitamin or mineral supplements. She drank water before and usually after practice, but felt there was no time during practice to grab a drink. A typical day of food intake during training is outlined below.

Professional assessment

Mean daily intake from this self-reported eating plan was assessed to be ~ 5860 kJ (1400 kcal); 208 g carbohydrate (4.7 g·kg body mass^{-1}); 44 g protein (1.0 g·kg body mass^{-1}); 43 g fat (28% of total energy). This diet was lower in energy than the requirements estimated for her activity level, ~ 8800 kJ (2100 kcal), although some of the energy mismatch might be explained by under-reporting. Annie's apparently low energy consumption resulted in intakes that failed to meet the dietary reference intakes (DRI) for calcium (532 mg vs. DRI 1300 mg), riboflavin (0.7 mg vs. DRI 1.0 mg), niacin (7.2 mg vs. DRI 14 mg), and vitamin D (1 μg vs. DRI 5 μg). She also appeared to consume less than the recommended levels for intake of iron (13 mg vs. 15 mg) and zinc (8 mg vs. 9 mg). Annie was hesitant to increase her energy intake because she considered herself to be overweight, and believed that her excess weight was the source of her poor performance during practice.

Intervention

In order to increase Annie's energy and carbohydrate intake without making her feel she is eating too much food, as well as meeting DRIs for minerals and vitamins, the following recommendations were made.

1 Eat a low-fat granola bar and calcium-fortified orange juice before practice.

2 Replace low-fat granola bar at breakfast with iron-rich cream of wheat or iron-fortified cereal.

3 Add another half-cup of either garbanzo or another type of beans to salad at lunchtime and only have half the candy bar.

4 Eat a small wholegrain bagel with peanut butter for an afternoon snack.

5 Drink water and sports beverages during practice.

6 Add a glass of calcium-fortified soy milk with dinner.

7 Take a daily multivitamin plus mineral supplement in the morning, and a 500-mg elemental calcium supplement with vitamin D at bedtime.

Outcome

With some hesitation Annie implemented the recommended dietary modifications. Her daily energy intake increased to ~ 7500 kJ (1800 kcal) and carbohydrate intake increased to 296 g (6.5 g·kg body mass^{-1}). Through dietary change, and with the multivitamin and mineral and calcium supplement, Annie was able to achieve an intake meeting the DRIs for calcium, riboflavin, niacin, and vitamin D and meet the recommended intakes for iron and zinc. Despite increased energy intake, Annie only experienced a small (1-kg) weight gain over the next month. Although this could have been a threatening outcome for her, in fact, her fatigue improved and she improved her recovery for the next day's workout. Annie began to feel comfortable and stronger at her new weight, and at the national competition, she achieved personal bests in two events.

Breakfast	Lunch	Snack	Dinner

Banana
Low-fat granola bar
250 ml calcium-
fortified soy milk
	Garden salad (lettuce, carrots, tomatoes) with:
	    $^1\!/_2$ cup of garbanzo beans
	    1 tbspn sunflower seeds
	One carob candy bar
	360 ml diet ice tea
		Low-fat granola bar	Large wholewheat tortilla with hummus and cucumber slices
			Two peach halves canned in natural juices
			or
			Granola bar if too tired

CASE STUDY 2 Basketballer with diabetes. Helen O'Connor

Athlete

David was a 16-year-old basketball player. He had recently been selected to train with the elite squad at the state sports institute (two hour-long sessions each week) in addition to the two individual sessions he had with his own coach. He also undertook weight training two mornings a week and played as a guard in one or two games each weekend. David had developed insulin-dependent diabetes when he was around 8 years old. He used an insulin pen and took 4–5 units of Humalin NPH (long-acting insulin) in the morning and 16–18 units at night. He also took 4–8 units of short-acting Humalog (insulin) just before breakfast, lunch, and dinner. David used a glucometer to monitor his sugar levels morning and evening, and sometimes before and after training. Where necessary he adjusted his insulin dose.

Reason for consultancy

David had been struggling to manage both his energy intake and blood glucose levels since he started training with the elite institute squad. The training was more intense than his other sessions and he experienced problems with erratic blood glucose concentrations, including frequent overnight falls in glucose levels. His weight had dropped by 3 kg, and his current body mass of 62 kg was too low for his 181-cm frame. The weight training seemed to have little effect on helping him to "bulk up". Although David had previously maintained reasonably good diabetic control, his last blood glucose reading, a measure of overall control, showed an increase to 10% (optimal range around 7%). Despite experimenting with different carbohydrate and insulin strategies he did not seem able to find a routine to manage the elite squad training days. A sample daily intake is outlined below.

Professional assessment

Mean daily intake from this self-reported eating plan was assessed to be ~ 12 800 kJ (3100 kcal); 320 g carbohydrate (5.2 g·kg^{-1}); 165 g protein; 127 g fat (37% of energy). His intake was assessed to provide insufficient energy and carbohydrate to meet his new training requirements. David needed to reassess insulin requirements and prevent the overnight hypoglycemia.

Intervention

To normalize blood glucose levels, and increase energy and carbohydrate intake to facilitate weight gain and help David cope with the higher intensity training, the following suggestions were made.

1 Increase energy intake to approximately 15 500 kJ and carbohydrate to 455 g (7 g·kg^{-1} calculated for 65 kg) per day. Rather than simply increasing carbohydrate at his pretraining snack, David could experiment with use of a sports drink during the high-intensity sessions to help maintain blood glucose. This strategy could be "session specific" as David would be able to adjust his intake of sports drink according to the intensity of the session. He also tried this out in games at the weekend.

2 Follow-up more carefully after each training session with blood glucose monitoring to determine whether David needed to increase the size of his recovery snack. He was also advised to experiment with a bedtime snack involving low glycemic index carbohydrate-rich foods (e.g. a bowl of porridge and milk and a fruit smoothie). As well as increasing total carbohydrate intake, this snack would make use of a slow-release form of glucose to prevent hypoglycemia ("hypos") during the night.

3 Review insulin therapy with his endocrinologist. The endocrinologist recommended more intensive blood glucose monitoring to help restructure David's new insulin routine. To start with, a reduction in David's night time long-acting insulin after the intense training sessions was recommended to prevent the overnight hypos. An increase in morning long-acting insulin and short-acting dose before meals was also required as his intake of carbohydrate was to be significantly increased. To prevent overnight hypos, David should aim for a blood sugar level of at least 8 mmol·l^{-1} prior to bed.

Outcome

David found the modifications to his diet and insulin made a significant difference to his energy levels and greatly reduced the frequency of the overnight hypos. He began to regain the lost weight, and started to respond for the first time to the weight training, making some gains in strength and size. His blood glucose control also improved, although he realized he needed to stay in regular touch with his endocrinologist who could help him with insulin adjustment when his needs or training program changed. David gained more confidence with his basketball game, since he now knew his struggles had been caused by an inadequate diet and insulin routine, not because he "was not good enough". He went on later in the year to win an award for "most improved basketballer" in the elite state institute squad.

Breakfast	Lunch	Dinner	Snacks
Four slices of toast with butter 500 ml milk	Two lean meat or cheese sandwiches 250 ml fruit juice	Large serving lean meat, fish, or chicken Vegetables (includes 5–6 × 15-g carbohydrate exchanges as potato, rice, or pasta)	2–4 × 15-g carbohydrate exchanges between meals—fruit, sandwiches, fruit smoothies, crackers

CASE STUDY 3   Young athlete. Melinda M. Manore

Athlete

Jackie was a 12-year-old gymnast, training at an elite gymnastics program away from her home. She lived in a boarding home and attended the local high school. She was happy with her current weight (40 kg), but did not want to get any heavier. She trained 4 h each day during the week, and twice on Saturday. She had recently added weight training (1.5–2 h a week) to her program. Jackie had not received much nutrition education but was concerned about what she ate. She suspected that her eating patterns were not ideal since she often got very hungry and shaky during her afternoon practice. She was frustrated about her recent lack of improvement during practice or competition. Jackie had not grown in the past year and had not started menstruating.

Reason for consultancy

Jackie's mother was concerned about her lack of growth, and her restrictive eating patterns. She also considered that Jackie was too young for weight training.

Current dietary and activity patterns

In order to prevent weight gain, Jackie had decided to limit fat intake. She kept only fat-free snacks in her room and ate low-fat foods at meals. Her daily schedule was as follows: 7.30 AM school starts, 11.00 AM lunch, 1.30 PM school ends, 2.00 PM practice starts, 7.00 PM dinner. She studied and watched TV after dinner, usually going to bed around midnight. Jackie's typical diet is outlined below.

Professional assessment

Mean daily intake from this self-reported eating plan was assessed to be about 5900 kJ (1400 kcal), low in fat (~ 15% of energy), and adequate in protein (1.3 g·kg^{-1}). Jackie's intake of fruits and vegetables and dairy products was less than recommended daily intakes, and her cereal choices were highly processed (white bread, rice or pasta, sugar-rich breakfast cereals). Overall, her energy and fat intake was assessed to be too restrictive, and her intakes of many micronutrients and fiber were inadequate. The acute effect of inadequate intake of energy was the hunger and fatigue experienced during training, interfering with optimal performance. However, it was likely that chronic energy restriction failed to provide sufficient fuel for growth and the development of puberty.

Intervention

Jackie needed to increase her understanding of nutrition to appreciate some of the wider issues of health and performance. Her desire to keep her weight at 40 kg was unrealistic, since she needed to allow for growth. An initial plan to increase daily intake by 840–1680 kJ (200–400 kcal) was trialed. The importance of adequate intake of all nutrients, including fat, was explained to Jackie, and she learned which foods were good sources of key micronutrients and "good" fats. Jackie was also referred to a professional trainer to help plan a weight-training program appropriate for her age. The following dietary suggestions were made to Jackie and her mother.

1 Continue to base breakfast on juice, breakfast cereal, and low-fat milk each morning, but choose an iron-fortified wholewheat brand.

2 Increase lunch to a whole sandwich, with extra salad fillings, and have a low-fat milk drink instead of low-energy soft drink.

3 Eat an afternoon snack between classes (fruit, raisins, bagel, or a sports bar). During practice, use a sports drink and eat small pieces of an energy bar if feeling fatigued or shaky.

4 Choose evening meals based on lean meats, wholegrain cereals, and increased servings of vegetables. Add skimmed milk and a piece of fruit or a dairy-based dessert such as low-fat yoghurt or custard.

5 Snack on nutrient-rich choices including fruit, cheese, or low-fat fruit yoghurt rather than fat-free cookie and confectionery items.

6 Use a multivitamin/mineral supplement until diet improves in energy content and variety.

7 Review dietary plan and exercise goals with gymnastics coach. Get approval to use a sports drink and snack during practice, and add 1 day of rest per week.

Outcome

After 6 months, Jackie was able to report dietary changes and better performances. She grew taller and gained 1.5 kg, and her routines greatly improved. The snack before practice and larger lunches helped to fuel her workouts. Jackie now drank skimmed milk at each meal, ate more fruits and vegetables, and even liked wholegrain cereals. She still liked to nibble on fat-free "snack" foods between meals, but these snacks were smaller because her meals were more substantial and satisfying.

Breakfast	Lunch	Dinner	Snacks
Bowl sugar-coated cereal with skimmed milk	Slice of cheese pizza or half turkey sandwich (lettuce + mustard)	Half piece grilled chicken	Popcorn
Orange juice	Low-fat chips	Small salad with fat-free dressing	Fat-free chocolate cookies
Coffee with cream	Apple	Green beans	Pretzels
	Low-energy soft drink or water	White rice or pasta	Hard candy
		Water	Low-energy soft drink

CASE STUDY 4 Female athlete. Linda Houtkooper

Athlete

Jennifer was a 20-year-old collegiate cross-country and middle-distance runner for a nationally ranked Division I program. She was 170 cm in height and had maintained a stable weight of 55 kg for the past year. Her body fat, as estimated from anthropometry (skinfolds), was 11%. In preparation for the 1500 m, she undertook a 60-mile (100-km) training week, including 2 speed days, 1 hilly tempo distance day, a race on Saturday and a long run (20 km) on Sunday. She also completed two weight-training sessions each week.

Reason for consultancy

Jennifer had been experiencing light-headedness, fatigue, and failure to recover from workouts. She was unable to keep up with team-mates during training, causing substantial mental stress. On medical examination she was found to be both physically and mentally exhausted. A blood test revealed that Jennifer had iron deficiency anemia. Her menstrual status was reported to be normal over the previous 4 months, although she had suffered from amenorrhea for $1^1/2$ years prior to taking birth control pills.

Current dietary patterns

Jennifer typically ate three meals a day without snacks. She ate breakfast after her morning runs, went to class for 4 h, then had lunch and a multivitamin supplement. She ate dinner about 6 h later, typically 1–2 h after afternoon workouts. Lately she had been so tired on arriving home from afternoon workout, she had gone straight to bed without eating dinner. Jennifer carried a water bottle with her during the day but often forgot to drink from it or to refill it throughout the day. She drank water during and after workouts. Food intake over a typical training day is outlined below.

Professional assessment

Mean daily intake from this self-reported eating plan was assessed to be about 6700 kJ (1600 kcal); 264 g carbohydrate (4.8 g·kg body mass^{-1}); 52 g protein (0.9 g·kg body mass^{-1}); 33 g fat (19% of total energy intake). Jennifer's reported intake failed to meet her estimated energy requirements, and was about 4200 kJ (1000 kcal) below the recommended intake for her activity level. This suboptimal energy intake may have been partly explained by under-reporting, but there was some evidence of energy restriction to maintain body fat levels as low as she could manage. Her apparently low energy intake resulted in dietary intakes below recommended levels for carbohydrate and protein.

Due to low energy intake and restrictive food choices, Jennifer's dietary patterns also failed to meet the dietary reference intakes (DRIs) for calcium (660 mg vs. DRI 1000 mg), iron (12 mg vs. DRI 18 mg), and zinc (7 mg vs. DRI 8 mg).

Intervention

In order to increase Jennifer's energy, carbohydrate and protein intakes, replenish her iron and zinc stores, and meet the DRI for calcium, the following recommendations were made.

1 Add a small high-carbohydrate snack before morning runs (fruit, cereal bar, or fruit juice).

2 Increase quantity of food at breakfast time. Eat iron-fortified oatmeal and add raisins, a cup of 1% milk, and piece of vitamin C-rich fruit or fruit juice.

3 Add a small mid-morning snack (cereal bar and vitamin C-rich juice).

4 Add a vegetable to lunch (baby carrots or salad) and a handful of almonds.

5 Drink water throughout the day and sports beverages during long training sessions.

6 Within 15 min of finishing afternoon workout, eat a breakfast bar or sports bar and sports drink.

7 Add a lean protein source at dinner (chicken or other lean meat), a high-energy side dish (potato or bread), dressing to salad, and chocolate syrup to 1% milk.

8 Eat an evening snack before bed (oatmeal cookies, pudding, or low-fat fruit yogurt).

9 In addition to multivitamin, take an iron supplement providing 100 mg elemental iron daily, and a 200-mg elemental calcium supplement before bedtime.

10 After 3 months, repeat blood test to re-evaluate iron status and make adjustments in iron supplementation.

Outcome

Jennifer was very reluctant at first to increase her energy intake, but her desire and encouragement from team-mates helped her slowly increase her food intake over the season. Near the end of her competitive season, Jennifer's new dietary patterns were assessed to provide a carbohydrate intake of 7.1 g·kg body mass^{-1} and protein intake of 1.6 g·kg body mass^{-1}. Through diet and supplementation, Jennifer was able to meet the DRI for calcium and recommended intakes for iron and zinc, with her iron status reaching normal levels. She experienced about a 1-kg weight gain, which was of some initial concern, but her improved energy and performance during training sessions and competitions helped ease her fears.

Breakfast	Lunch	Dinner
1 cup oatmeal prepared with water	Peanut butter and jelly sandwich	$1^1/2$ cups pasta
	Banana	$^1/2$ cup plain tomato sauce
	Multivitamin	Vegetable salad
		1 cup of 1% milk
		Two pieces of corn bread

Chapter 16
Strategies for special environments: heat

Introduction

Many major sporting events are now held in unfavorable environmental conditions. Exercise at altitude or in heavily polluted large cities, as well as at extremes of heat and cold, provides an additional challenge for the athlete. Across the whole spectrum of sporting events, however, no threat to the health and performance of the athlete is greater than that posed by prolonged hard exercise in a hot, humid environment. Exercise performance is almost invariably impaired in these conditions, and at worst, there is a serious threat to health. The history of major championship marathon races held in hot weather provides many examples of serious and potentially fatal heat illness, including Dorando Pietri in the 1908 Olympic marathon in London, Jim Peters at the Empire Games marathon in Vancouver in 1954, and more recently, Garbriella Andersen-Schiess at the 1984 Los Angeles Olympic marathon. The common features in all these races were prolonged hard exercise and the high ambient temperature. Other events, including the World Track and Field Championships in Tokyo in 1991, in Athens in 1997, and in Seville in 1999, the 1994 Soccer World Cup in Florida, the 1996 Atlanta Olympic Games, and the 1998 Commonwealth Games in Kuala Lumpur are recent examples of major events held in conditions where competitors were exposed to heat stress. Sportsmen and women who are used to living, training, and competing in temperate climates are placed at a disadvantage when an event is scheduled for hot, humid conditions, and a strategy must be devised to minimize this disadvantage. Recent deaths of American football players from heat-related illness during preseason training are a reminder that problems can arise during hot-weather training as well as in competition.

Exercise in the heat

Most (about 75%) of the energy turnover during exercise appears as heat, causing body temperature to rise. In cool environments, heat can be lost by physical transfer from the body, but when the environmental temperature exceeds skin temperature, heat is gained by these avenues. At high ambient temperatures, the only effective means of heat loss is by evaporation of sweat secreted onto the skin surface. Heat loss by evaporation is effective in dissipating large amounts of heat and will limit the rise in core temperature to no more than 3–4°C in all but the most extreme conditions.

The response to exercise in the heat is determined in part by the intensity of the exercise and in part by the degree of heat stress. At the same power output, exercise in the heat results in a higher heart rate and a higher cardiac output, as well as higher core and skin temperatures, compared with exercise in a cooler environment. There are also some metabolic differences, with exercise in the heat usually being accompanied by a higher blood lactate concentration, and, according to some evidence, a faster rate of depletion of muscle glycogen. Although this suggests that it might be of greater importance to undertake strategies promoting carbohydrate (CHO) availability during exercise (e.g. CHO loading, consumption of CHO during an event), in fact, depletion of CHO does not seem to be the limiting factor to the performance of exercise in the heat. Cardiovascular and metabolic alterations during exercise in the heat are accompanied by a greater subjective sensation of effort, and combine to cause a reduction in exercise capacity.

Performance in all endurance events—which we can define as those lasting longer than a total time of about 20–30 min—is reduced under conditions of heat stress, and there seems to be no way of avoiding some impairment of performance. Laboratory work has shown that endurance time on a cycle ergometer at an exercise intensity that could be sustained for 94 min at a temperature of 10°C was reduced to 81 min when the temperature was increased to 20°C, and to 52 min when the temperature was increased to 30°C. In another study, an effort that the subjects could keep up for 95 min at an ambient temperature of 3°C could only be sustained for 75 min at 20°C, while at 40°C, these subjects were exhausted after only 33 min.

It is usually recommended that hard exercise should not be undertaken when temperature and humidity are high, but major sporting events are seldom or never cancelled even when conditions are extreme, so athletes must be prepared to compete in these conditions and take steps to minimize both the effects on performance and the health risks. If the athlete is dehydrated before exercise begins, the reductions in performance and the risk to health that occur in the heat are both greatly magnified. There is a very strong likelihood that many competitors in events of shorter duration will also suffer from the conditions, although rather more can be done here to reduce the impact of the climatic conditions by careful attention to acclimatization and fluid intake.

Competitors in indoor events might expect to suffer less, as these venues will generally be air conditioned. This should not, however, engender a feeling of security: any such feeling would be entirely false as competitors in the indoor events are also at risk from the heat and humidity. Both dehydration and exposure to heat even without exercise may result in a variety of symptoms, including headache, nausea, dizziness, and a sensation of fatigue. Some exposure to the local conditions is inevitable, and in the hours when competitors are exposed to the local climatic conditions they are likely to become dehydrated, with negative effects on performance, even in the relatively cool indoor conditions and even when the exercise duration is relatively short. In one laboratory study, where dehydration equivalent to 2.5% of body weight was induced prior to exercise by sauna exposure, a 30% reduction in power output occurred in a test (which was carried out in cool conditions) lasting about 7 min. Another carefully controlled experiment, carried out under race conditions, showed that 1500-m runners ran 3.7% slower when they were dehydrated by 2% of body weight prior to exercise: 3.7% represents 6 s at world-class 1500-m pace.

To minimize the adverse impact of hot, humid conditions, a number of issues need to be addressed. These include:
1 an acclimatization strategy;
2 lifestyle issues;
3 modified warm-up and precooling; and
4 nutrition support—particularly aggressive rehydration strategies.

Even if the majority of the issues involved with exercise in the heat appear to be related to physiology or lifestyle, it is important to realize that the success of many strategies is underpinned by sound dietary practice.

Acclimatization

Regular exposure to hot, humid conditions results in a number of adaptations that together reduce the negative effects of these conditions on exercise performance and reduce the risk of heat injury. The magnitude of the adaptation to heat that occurs is closely related to the degree of heat stress to which the individual is exposed. The two primary determining factors for adaptation to hot, humid conditions are:
1 the rise in body temperature that occurs; and
2 the sweating response that is induced.

Adaptation therefore depends largely on the intensity and duration of exercise and on the environmental conditions, and there is clearly an optimum set of conditions for the most effective acclimatization. Some adaptation is seen within the first few days of exposure to exercise in the heat, and even a few sessions of exercise in the heat are beneficial. Adaptation is more or less complete for most individuals within about 7–14 days and exposure involving exercise for relatively short periods (60–90 min) on a daily basis is as effective as longer exposures, so there may be no advantage of living for prolonged periods in a hot climate. It is equally clear that regular endurance training in temperate conditions confers some protection: trained subjects are already partially adapted and it has to be admitted that we do not know how complete this process is for highly trained athletes. There can be no doubt that a period of acclimatization is necessary for all athletes if they are to achieve optimum performance in hot, humid conditions. This probably becomes even more important when repeated rounds or events have to be completed. The idea of arriving shortly before competition in order to minimize the effects of living in these conditions prior to competition is to be strongly discouraged. Except for a few exceptional situations, such a practice will lead to a decrement in performance. The coach and athlete must decide together whether this risk is worth taking, and this judgement can only be made on the basis of individual experience.

Acclimatization strategies

There are two ways of acclimatizing for competitions in the heat, and various combinations of these two approaches are also possible. One is to live and train in a climate similar to that expected at the competition venue: the other approach is to live at home and adapt by training in an artificial climate. There are positive and negative aspects to both approaches. Because exercise capacity is reduced so much in the heat, training intensity and volume must be reduced for at least the first few days of the acclimatization process. This effect may be minimized if the athlete lives at home and is exposed to heat only during training, or during one out of two daily training sessions, allowing some quality training to be continued in the other session.

If two training sessions per day are carried out, whether at home or in a hot weather camp, it seems sensible for the quality session to be done first, with the longer heat acclimatization session coming later in the day. The quality training session should be outdoors if at home, or in the early morning while it is still cool if at a hot weather venue. The weather is notoriously unpredictable, and the acclimatization venue selected may not provide suitable conditions for optimum acclimatization, whereas these can easily be simulated at home. If the heat acclimatization training is one of two sessions per day, the athlete is generally happier to adopt a less drastic regimen: the heat training can be gradually phased in, beginning with short (perhaps 30–60-min) sessions at low intensity without compromising the total training quality.

It is not necessary to train every day in the heat, but no more than 2–3 days should elapse between exposures: it has been shown that exercising in the heat every third day for 30 days resulted in the same degree of acclimatization as exercising every day for 10 days. This is because it takes time to reverse the adaptations to heat; for subjects who are completely acclimatized, some of the improved responses are still present after as long as 21 days in a cool climate. Acclimatization at home means that the athlete can introduce the heat acclimatization sessions gradually while continuing with normal training, and is not trying to cope with the effects of heat and of jet lag or travel fatigue at the same time.

A disadvantage of training in a hot room may be that the exercise inevitably depends on the facilities available and probably consists of cycle ergometer exercise, treadmill running, skipping, or circuit training. From the point of view of acclimatization to the heat, the type of exercise is not important, but rather that a period of prolonged (60–100 min), moderately strenuous exercise is carried out in hot conditions. The intention is to raise body temperature and to stimulate sweating: these are the factors that promote adaptation. There is evidence that full acclimatization is most effectively achieved when the duration of exercise in the heat is about 100 min, and that there is no advantage in spending longer periods than this exposed to heat. After exercise in the heat, the athlete should aim to reduce body temperature rather quickly by seeking shade or an air-conditioned environment to cool down and hasten the recovery process. Intermittent exercise is likely to be as effective as continuous exercise: the total exposure time, including short breaks, should again be 100 min for the most effective adaptation. More recent evidence, however, suggests that exercise at higher intensities for shorter periods of time may be equally effective in bringing about beneficial adaptations, and that even 30 min per day at an intensity equal to about 75% of maximum oxygen uptake ($\dot{V}o_{2max}$) was as effective as 60 min at 50% of $\dot{V}o_{2max}$.

If acclimatization is carried out at a hot weather camp, information on local weather patterns is essential. The training program may have to be modified to take account of the prevailing conditions. The timescale should be sufficient to allow for a few (at least 3–4, but perhaps as many as 5–10) days of reduced training: both total training volume and the amount of training at high intensity should be reduced, the extent of the reduction depending on the individual response. Because of the heat and the effects of travel, training for the first few days should be reduced to light recreational levels if sufficient time is available, progressively increasing in volume and intensity as the athlete adapts. Normal training can then be re-established for a few days while the acclimatization process continues and before tapering for competition begins; the vital "quality training" should continue, with enhanced periods of rest and recovery, over the final week before competition. Recovery will be faster and more complete if it is possible to find a cool shady place for this. Again, it must be stressed that every individual is different, and the extent and duration of the period of reduced training will vary between individuals; the coach must be alert to warning signs in those having difficulty in coping with the conditions. The whole process needs at least 10–14 days on average, but a longer or shorter period may be appropriate for some athletes.

The ideal plan may be a combination of both approaches, with an increasing level of heat exposure at home during the last 1–2 weeks before travelling. This might be of particular benefit to those most at risk, i.e. those whose sport will result in the greatest exposure, and those who have been found by experience to have difficulty in coping with the heat. It is strongly recommended that every opportunity to experience hot, humid weather conditions be taken, so that individuals who encounter problems can be identified and an effective strategy devised. Where a team travels together, it is especially important to remember that everyone will adapt at different rates, and some individualization of training schedules will be necessary to take account of this.

The ideal temperature and humidity for the acclimatization process are not well established, and practicalities will have a large influence on the choice of venue. If the temperature is too hot, training will be reduced. A temperature of at least 30°C but not more than 35°C, with a relative humidity of at least 70%, may be proposed, but if the competition venue is hot and dry, a lower humidity will be better. Somewhere in the same time zone as the competition is to be preferred. Attempts to take short cuts by compressing the whole process should not be undertaken lightly. The acclimatization process requires the athlete to be exposed to sufficient heat stress for the necessary adaptations to take place, but there is a real danger that taking the process too far or too quickly can result in acute heat injury.

As well as the physiological adaptations that occur in response to living and training in the heat, athletes gain valuable experience that allows them to develop coping strategies. The need for attention to fluid intake and for wearing the most appropriate clothing, and how to monitor fluid balance are not learned easily other than by experience. The most effective acclimatization program for any individual can also be learned only by trial and error. At hot weather training camps, those individuals whose performance is most affected by heat can be identified, and a strategy to meet their needs developed. Some athletes find great difficulty in performing well in hot, humid conditions and there may be implications for team selection. These aspects may be almost as important as the physiological adaptations that result.

Lifestyle in the heat

Athletes from temperate climates should be aware that some changes to their normal routine will be essential when living in a hot climate. Training times may need to be changed to avoid the hottest part of the day. Several shorter sessions may usefully replace a single longer session to reduce the adverse effects of hyperthermia. During acclimatization, quality training should be done in the early part of the day, with a longer session at lower intensity later in the day.

At training camps, it is often tempting to spend time between training sessions by sitting in the sun or sunbathing, Some degree of tanning of the skin can be beneficial in reducing the risk of sunburn. However, even mild sunburn sufficient to cause redness of the skin will impair thermoregulatory capacity for up to 10 days. A high-factor sunscreen should be used when exposure is unavoidable, and time spent sunbathing should be severely restricted. Clothing should be chosen to protect the skin from direct sun but to promote evaporation of sweat. It is important to choose clothes that are comfortable even when wet.

Living accommodation, as well as most indoor areas, will be air conditioned at many, but by no means all, venues. It is not unusual for the temperature to be set at a low level, usually about 20°C, but sometimes as low as 12–15°C. Repeated changes from the heat outdoors to the cool indoor conditions seem to increase upper respiratory tract symptoms such as sore throat, cough, and runny nose which may interfere with training. Self-monitoring of the morning pulse rate can be a useful objective sign of impending problems: a rise of more than 8 beats per minute indicates that the athlete may not have fully recovered from the last training session. Continued hard training may lead to fatigue and underperformance. Athletes who are asthmatic or suffer from hay fever or rhinitis must make sure that they take appropriate medication and should consult a physician about increasing the dosage if the symptoms persist.

Bedroom temperatures should not be set too low, as the frequent changes from indoors to outdoors will increase upper respiratory problems. There are advantages in having a cool place where recovery from training can take place; this may be a common room or dining area rather than a bedroom. It is completely wrong to think that there is an advantage in terms of acclimatization in switching the air-conditioning system off. A bedroom temperature of between 16 and 23°C is recommended: this is a wide range, which gives scope for individual preference. It should be noted, however, that disturbances of sleep have been shown to increase as the temperature of the room increases.

Modified warm-up and precooling strategies

Contrary to popular belief, there is little, if any, evidence that warm-up prevents or reduces the risk of injury. Warming up before training or competition does, however, ensure adequate physiological and psychological preparation. In cool climates, the purpose of the warm-up is to elevate body temperature and increase blood flow to the muscles and associated soft tissues. In contrast, in hot climates, the body temperature should not be markedly increased during the warm-up due to the real possibility of reduced performance because of hyperthermia and dehydration.

In explosive events, an elevated muscle temperature may have some benefits, but where exercise continues for more than perhaps 2 or 3 min, body temperature should not be markedly increased before exercise begins. The coach, athlete, and physiotherapist need to look at modifications to the warm-up and ensure that this is achieved without compromising the physiological and psychological preparation. It is absolutely essential that this is practiced well in advance so that the athlete is comfortable with any changes made. Basic modifications must include warming up in the shade and drinking plenty of fluids, and the warm-up must be tailored to each individual's state of acclimatization and sweating response.

The modified warm-up will have to be practiced and adjusted while at warm weather training camps, and perhaps also in heat chambers at home, so that the athlete becomes comfortable with any changes made. Practicing the modified warm-up prior to training or competition while living in a cool climate may cause problems because of the need for an increased body temperature to produce the optimum physiological preparation.

While there is ample evidence that excessive body heating will reduce performance, cooling the athlete prior to the event can have the opposite effect. Athletes have tried a number of strategies to achieve rapid cooling; these include the use of cold showers, and wearing clothes or towels that have been cooled. Recently, special "cooling jackets" have been manufactured for the purpose, with pockets to hold icepacks contained within an insulating fabric such as neoprene; such jackets allow the athlete to place ice strategically on selected body sites. While they can be used to cool the athlete prior to an event, in some sports there is the opportunity to wear the jacket during the event—for example, during formal breaks in play or substitutions. While studies have shown that precooling or within-event cooling strategies can enhance the performance of exercise undertaken in the heat, the effects are likely to be specific to the event and the individual. The athlete should experiment with such strategies in training or in minor competition; they should definitely not be used for the first time at a major event.

Nutrition strategies for the heat

Fluid considerations

Daily water turnover for sedentary individuals living in a temperate environment is typically about 2–3 l. Sweat losses during training can add 0.5–3 l·h^{-1} depending on the training intensity, the clothing worn, the climatic conditions, and characteristics of the individual. For athletes training intensively in hot climates, fluid needs can reach 10–15 l·day^{-1}, representing about 25–30% of total body water. Failure to replace sweat losses will severely impair exercise capacity and will increase the risk of heat illness. Athletes who incur a fluid deficit will also lose the beneficial effects of acclimatization: heat-acclimatized individuals who are hypohydrated respond to a heat stress as though they are unacclimatized.

Although athletes may be tempted to believe that the need for fluid replacement will decrease as they become adjusted to the heat, heat acclimatization will actually increase the requirement for fluid replacement because of the enhanced sweating response. This means that athletes not only have to

drink more in the heat, but must increase their fluid intake even further as they become acclimatized and begin to sweat more. If dehydration is allowed to occur, the improved ability to tolerate heat that results from the acclimatization process will disappear completely. There is no way of adapting to dehydration: any attempt to do so is futile and dangerous.

Monitoring of body mass changes before and after training can give some indication of the extent of sweat loss in training: each kg of weight loss represents a loss of approximately 1 l of sweat. Athletes should aim to drink sufficient fluid after training or competition to replace about 1.5 times the amount of sweat lost. The kidney will dispose of any excess fluid. Daily measurements of body mass—made at the same time of day, wearing the same clothes, and under the same conditions—can give some indication of progressive sweat loss, but may be complicated by changes in training load, food intake, bowel habits, and other factors related to the new environment (see Expert Comment 1). Monitoring of urine parameters, including volume, color, conductivity, specific gravity, or osmolality may help identify individuals suffering from dehydration and can provide feedback that athletes find helpful in establishing their fluid requirements. Such measurements are only useful, however, if care is taken to standardize sample collection and analysis. The apparently "scientific" measures such as osmolality or specific gravity are no better than those such as color that athletes can assess for themselves.

Athletes must recognize the need to use all available opportunities for fluid intake when sweat losses are high. This means increasing fluid intake, especially at mealtimes, and perhaps spending more time over meals to achieve this. Carrying drinks bottles (preferably insulated to keep drinks cool) should become a habit, even if it is not a routine at home. A water bottle kept by the bed at night allows athletes to take drinks during the night with minimum inconvenience.

Fluids or food consumed after training must include sufficient electrolytes—especially sodium —to replace the losses in sweat. The electrolytes effectively act like a sponge, holding the ingested fluid in the body. If large volumes of plain water are consumed, urine production is stimulated because of the fall in the plasma osmolality and sodium concentration. As well as preventing a diuresis, the presence of salt in drinks maintains the body's thirst mechanism (see Chapters 5 & 9 for greater discussion).

Restoration of fluid balance is a vital part of the recovery process after training and should begin as soon as possible. In the recovery period, muscle glycogen synthesis is a priority, but synthesis of new proteins should perhaps be seen as being of equal or even greater importance. Hydration status may be of importance for both of those processes. It is increasingly recognized that cell volume is an important regulator of metabolic processes, and there may be opportunities to manipulate this to promote tissue synthesis. During and after exercise there may be large changes in cell volume, secondary to osmotic pressure changes caused by metabolic activity, hydrostatic pressure changes, or sweat loss, and these may in turn be affected by fluid intake. The full significance of these findings for the postexercise recovery process and the roles they play in adaptation to a training program remain to be established. Manipulation of fluid and electrolyte balance and the ingestion of a variety of osmotically active substances or their precursors offer potential for optimizing the effectiveness of a training regimen.

Carbohydrate needs

We might expect CHO needs to be of greater concern for exercise in the heat than in temperate conditions, due to the evidence that rates of muscle glycogen utilization are increased in a hot environment. Although acclimatization may reduce glycogen utilization rates during exercise, there is evidence that glycogen use is still higher after acclimatization than that observed in cooler conditions. Sports nutrition guidelines promote a variety of options for acutely increasing CHO availability for exercise, including consuming CHO before (Chapter 7) and during (Chapter 8) exercise, and in the recovery period between prolonged exercise bouts (Chapter 9). When these strategies enhance or maintain CHO status, they may delay the onset of fatigue, and enhance exercise capacity (i.e. endurance). Most studies of these interventions

have been carried out in moderate climatic conditions and there is little specific research to document how well the performance benefits translate to exercise undertaken in the heat where the dual issues of increased CHO utilization and an increased risk of thermoregulatory concerns coexist. Although thermoregulatory issues may limit performance in many events conducted in hot conditions, in situations of compensable heat stress, such as exercise at lower intensities, substrate availability may also become a limiting factor. There is some evidence that a CHO loading regimen may improve exercise capacity in the heat, even though the exercise time is much shorter than in cool conditions. In any case, as long as strategies to enhance CHO status do not compromise hydration and thermoregulation, they should be practiced by athletes undertaking exercise in hot weather.

Athletes should take note that the CHO cost of training sessions may be increased in hot weather. This message may need to be stressed to athletes whose competition demands are not normally challenged by substrate availability and who are not familiar with high CHO eating strategies. Athletes should choose eating patterns that provide daily CHO intakes of 7–10 g·kg body mass^{-1} to ensure restoration of muscle glycogen stores between workouts (see Chapter 9), and to experiment with CHO intake during sessions of more than 1 h duration (see section below). The benefits of refueling during exercise include better performance in that session, and most probably a faster recovery afterwards, as well as a contribution towards total daily CHO intake. Furthermore, experimentation may allow athletes to fine-tune their competition intake plans; strategies that are suitable for events conducted in cold weather may need to be manipulated to meet the new priorities of hot weather competition.

Specific practices for an event: are fluid needs of greater priority than fuel requirements?

Fluid intake during exercise can overcome or reduce many of the problems associated with sweat-induced hypohydration, and its importance as a nutritional strategy for sport is greater during exercise in hot conditions where sweat losses and fluid deficits are greater. Indeed it provides an additional benefit of reducing muscle glycogen utilization, probably by attenuating the rise in both circulating epinephrine concentrations and muscle temperature. Since fluid needs take priority over CHO availability in many exercise situations in the heat, it has been suggested that plain water might be suitable as an exercise drink. Whatever fluid is consumed, the athlete will need to devise a more aggressive plan of intake during and after their event than they are accustomed to in cool conditions. Some athletes also experiment with hyperhydration or "fluid overloading", aided by the use of glycerol, in the hours prior to an event, attempting to reduce the total fluid deficit incurred during the exercise session (see Chapter 7).

However, CHO ingestion may also be of benefit to the performance of many exercise events, and there is some evidence that the benefits of fluid replacement and CHO intake are independent and additive. For example, one study investigated the performance of a time trial undertaken at the end of 50 min of cycling undertaken at moderately high intensities in hot and humid conditions. Subjects undertook four separate trials involving replacement of fluid and/or CHO during the ~ 1-h cycling bout. The replacement of fluid resulted in a 6% improvement in performance, CHO intake also enhanced performance by 6%, and the combination of both strategies enhanced performance by 12%.

Although the inclusion of solutes in fluids was previously considered to reduce gastric emptying and impair fluid delivery during exercise, the present consensus is that the ingestion of commercially available sports drinks containing 4–8% CHO and electrolytes is not detrimental to hydration status. Indeed the palatable taste of these drinks has been shown to increase the voluntary intake of fluid during and after exercise, and may actually enhance total fluid balance. Therefore sports drinks can be recommended as suitable exercise fluids across a range of exercise activities undertaken in the heat, and may offer specific advantages as well as the stimulation of greater fluid intake. Some athletes use a strategy of graduating the CHO concentration of drinks consumed during prolonged events in the heat; dilute solutions are used in the first hour of the event (e.g. 2–3% CHO concentration) to promote maximal gastric emptying and fluid delivery, and as the event progresses, the CHO concentration of drinks is increased to 6–8% in recognition of the dwindling body CHO stores.

Other nutrients

There is preliminary evidence that exercise in the heat increases protein oxidation and cellular damage due to generation of free oxygen radicals. Insufficient research has been undertaken to determine whether this translates into additional requirements for protein, antioxidant vitamins, and minerals or other micronutrients. There may be some advantages to increasing protein intake and supplementing with antioxidant vitamins in the early days of exposure to a hot climate; however, these strategies have not been adequately tested.

Summary

Heat exposure and dehydration impair performance, and their negative effects are additive. Acclimatization will reduce the negative impact of heat on athletic performance, and is most effectively achieved by exercise in the heat; heat without exercise and exercise without heat are less effective. The major physiological adjustments to heat acclimatization take about 7–14 days, and training volume and intensity should be reduced on first exposure to the heat and then gradually increased. Some high-intensity training should be maintained throughout the acclimatization period. Monitoring responses of individual athletes is essential—individuals respond differently to physical activity in the heat. Since acclimatization strategies and actual competition in the heat increase the athlete's need for fluid to match the increase in sweat rate, there is a need for athletes to rethink and update their fluid intake practices during and after exercise. Since exercise in the heat may cause an increased utilization of CHO, there may be some need to consider strategies to increase CHO availability during training sessions and competition. However, fluid needs must take priority over intake of CHO.

Reading list

Below, P.R., Mora-Rodriguez, R., Gonzalez-Alonso, J. & Coyle, E.F. (1995) Fluid and carbohydrate ingestion independently improve performance during 1 h of intense exercise. *Medicine and Science in Sports and Exercise* **27**, 200–210.

Febbraio, M.A. (2000) Exercise at climatic extremes. In: *Nutrition in Sport* (ed. R.J. Maughan), pp. 497–509. Blackwell Science, Oxford.

Galloway, S.D.R. (1999) Dehydration, rehydration, and exercise in the heat: rehydration strategies for athletic competition. *Canadian Journal of Applied Physiology* **24**, 188–200.

Galloway, S.D.R. & Maughan, R.J. (1997) Effects of ambient temperature on the capacity to perform prolonged cycle exercise in man. *Medicine and Science in Sports and Exercise* **29**, 1240–1249.

Maughan, R.J. (1999) Exercise in the heat: limitations to performance and the impact of fluid replacement strategies. Introduction to the symposium. *Canadian Journal of Applied Physiology* **24**, 149–151.

Montain, S.J., Maughan, R.J. & Sawka, M.N. (1996) Heat acclimatization strategies for the 1996 Summer Olympics. *Athletic Therapy Today* **1**, 42–46.

Sawka, M.N. & Pandolf, K.B. (1990) Effects of body water loss on physiological function and exercise performance. In: *Perspectives in Exercise Science and Sports Medicine*, Vol. 3 (eds C.V. Gisolfi & D.R. Lamb), pp. 1–38. Benchmark Press, Indianapolis.

Wenger, C.B. (1998) Human heat acclimatization. In: *Human Performance Physiology and Environmental Medicine at Terrestrial Extremes* (eds K.B. Pandolf, M.N. Sawka & R.R. Gonzalez), pp. 153–197. Benchmark Press, Indianapolis.

EXPERT COMMENT 1 How should athletes monitor their responses to exercise in the heat? Ronald J. Maughan

Some degree of monitoring of individual responses to heat stress and of the rate and extent of adaptation is an essential part of preparing athletes for hot weather competition. Warm weather training camps should be used to collect information on individuals and on squads. Measurements made on individuals are a crucial part of the education process in demonstrating the negative effects of dehydration and hyperthermia and the ways in which these effects can be minimized.

When exposed to the heat, athletes may become dehydrated despite the availability of fluids. Regular monitoring of body weight can give useful information on the athlete's hydration status, provided some precautions are observed. These results, however, only have value if they can be compared with baseline measurements made in normal training conditions at home. Each athlete must know their own optimum body weight for training and competing, and must also know how much their body weight normally varies on a daily basis. Small variations (perhaps as much as 1–2 kg for some individuals) have no significance, but for others whose weight is normally very constant, this can be an early warning sign: it is therefore crucial that the individual athlete knows what the normal range is. Body weight measurements should always be made at the same time of day, under the same conditions. Ideally, this will be done first thing in the morning, before breakfast or training but after a visit to the toilet. If this is not possible, it may be done before training each day. Measurement of weight loss during training sessions should also be monitored, so these measurements can be combined and compared with the normal daily pattern: 1 kg of weight loss represents approximately 1 l of sweat loss. A progressive decrease in body weight may be an indication of dehydration which is not being compensated for by an increased fluid intake: alternatively, it may reflect a loss of appetite and decreased food intake, which is common in hot conditions. A decrease in weight may also be an early warning of overtraining. An increase in body weight is also possible, reflecting overeating resulting from the increased availability of high-quality free food and increased leisure time. If large volumes of CHO-containing drinks are consumed, these can contribute a large amount of energy to the athlete's diet: 10 l of cola would supply 4000 kcal (17 MJ). This is of particular concern to those athletes competing in weight category sports.

Athletes should also be encouraged to keep, in their training diary, a record of subjective symptoms associated with travel, training, and competition, to see what patterns emerge. This diary might record, as well as body weight, some information on urine output: the time of day urine is passed, an estimate of the volume (simply done with a measuring cylinder—and beaker, if necessary), and the color (by comparison with a color chart). This information gives an indication of hydration status, but the return of the normal pattern of urine output is also a good index of the recovery from jet lag and the re-establishment of normal body rhythms. Again, this only has real value if the information collected in hot conditions can be compared with the normal pattern established over a period of at least a few weeks at home in normal training conditions immediately prior to departure. It is appreciated that this is not acceptable to everyone, but it is nonetheless vital that some sort of monitoring is carried out before and during visits to hot weather venues.

Team coaches and support staff have a responsibility to ensure that athletes appreciate the need to collect this information by explaining its value in advance. They must also keep an eye on the individual records and pay particular attention to anyone who appears to be having difficulty coping with training. Each athlete should try to encourage team-mates to take extra fluids.

Index

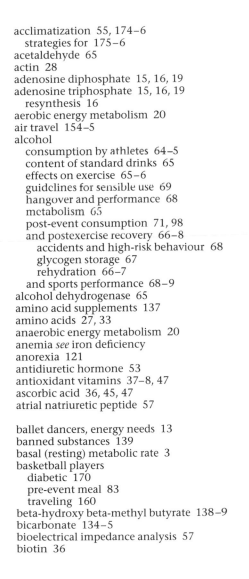